RA445 .B8573 2005

Building a better
delivery system : a new
c2005.

BUILDING A BETTER DELIVERY SYSTEM

D1296558

A New Engineering/Health Care Partnership

GEORGE BROWN COLLEGE
CASA LOMA LIBRARY LEARNING COMMONS

Proctor P. Reid, W. Dale Compton, Jerome H. Grossman,
and Gary Fanjiang, Editors

NATIONAL ACADEMY OF ENGINEERING *AND*
INSTITUTE OF MEDICINE
OF THE NATIONAL ACADEMIES

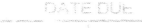DATE DUE

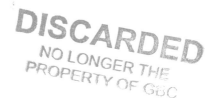

DISCARDED
NO LONGER THE
PROPERTY OF GBC

THE NATIONAL ACADEMIES PRESS
Washington, D.C.
www.nap.edu

THE NATIONAL ACADEMIES PRESS   500 Fifth Street, N.W.   Washington, DC 20001

NOTICE: The project that is the subject of this report was approved by the Governing Board of the National Research Council, whose members are drawn from the councils of the National Academy of Science, the National Academy of Engineering, and the Institute of Medicine. The members of the committee responsible for the report were chosen for their special competences and with regard for appropriate balance.

Support for this project was provided by the National Science Foundation (Award No. DMI-0222041), the Robert Wood Johnson Foundation (Grant No. 044640), and the National Institutes of Health (Contract No. N01-OD-4-2139, Task Order No. 111). Any opinions, findings, and conclusions or recommendations expressed in this report are those of the National Academy of Engineering/Institute of Medicine Committee on Engineering and the Health Care System and do not necessarily reflect the views of the funding organizations, nor does mention of trade names, commercial products, or organizations imply endorsement by the U.S. government.

International Standard Book Number 0-309-09643-X

Copies of this report are available from the National Academies Press, 500 Fifth Street, N.W., Lockbox 285, Washington, DC 20055; (888) 624-8373 or (202) 334-3313 (in the Washington metropolitan area); online at *http://www.nap.edu*.

Copyright 2005 by the National Academies. All rights reserved.

Printed in the United States of America

THE NATIONAL ACADEMIES
Advisers to the Nation on Science, Engineering, and Medicine

The **National Academy of Sciences** is a private, nonprofit, self-perpetuating society of distinguished scholars engaged in scientific and engineering research, dedicated to the furtherance of science and technology and to their use for the general welfare. Upon the authority of the charter granted to it by the Congress in 1863, the Academy has a mandate that requires it to advise the federal government on scientific and technical matters. Dr. Ralph J. Cicerone is president of the National Academy of Sciences.

The **National Academy of Engineering** was established in 1964, under the charter of the National Academy of Sciences, as a parallel organization of outstanding engineers. It is autonomous in its administration and in the selection of its members, sharing with the National Academy of Sciences the responsibility for advising the federal government. The National Academy of Engineering also sponsors engineering programs aimed at meeting national needs, encourages education and research, and recognizes the superior achievements of engineers. Dr. Wm. A. Wulf is president of the National Academy of Engineering.

The **Institute of Medicine** was established in 1970 by the National Academy of Sciences to secure the services of eminent members of appropriate professions in the examination of policy matters pertaining to the health of the public. The Institute acts under the responsibility given to the National Academy of Sciences by its congressional charter to be an adviser to the federal government and, upon its own initiative, to identify issues of medical care, research, and education. Dr. Harvey V. Fineberg is president of the Institute of Medicine.

The **National Research Council** was organized by the National Academy of Sciences in 1916 to associate the broad community of science and technology with the Academy's purposes of furthering knowledge and advising the federal government. Functioning in accordance with general policies determined by the Academy, the Council has become the principal operating agency of both the National Academy of Sciences and the National Academy of Engineering in providing services to the government, the public, and the scientific and engineering communities. The Council is administered jointly by both Academies and the Institute of Medicine. Dr. Ralph J. Cicerone and Dr. Wm. A. Wulf are chair and vice chair, respectively, of the National Research Council.

www.national-academies.org

COMMITTEE ON ENGINEERING AND THE HEALTH CARE SYSTEM

W. DALE COMPTON (NAE), *co-chair*, Purdue University, West Lafayette, Indiana
JEROME H. GROSSMAN (IOM), *co-chair*, John F. Kennedy School of Government,
    Harvard University, Cambridge, Massachusetts
REBECCA M. BERGMAN, Medtronic Inc., Minneapolis, Minnesota
JOHN R. BIRGE, University of Chicago, Chicago, Illinois
DENIS CORTESE, Mayo Clinic, Rochester, Minnesota
ROBERT S. DITTUS, Vanderbilt University and Veterans Administration Tennessee Valley
    Healthcare System, Nashville, Tennessee
G. SCOTT GAZELLE, MGH Institute for Technology Assessment, Boston, Massachusetts
CAROL HARADEN, Institute for Healthcare Improvement, Cambridge, Massachusetts
RICHARD MIGLIORI, United Resource Networks, Golden Valley, Minnesota
WOODROW MYERS (IOM), WellPoint, Thousand Oaks, California
WILLIAM P. PIERSKALLA, Anderson Graduate School of Management, University of
    California, Los Angeles
STEPHEN M. SHORTELL (IOM), School of Public Health and Haas School of Business,
    University of California, Berkeley
KENSALL D. WISE (NAE), University of Michigan, Ann Arbor
DAVID D. WOODS, Ohio State University, Columbus

Project Staff

PROCTOR P. REID, Study Director and Director, Program Office, National Academy of
    Engineering
JANET M. CORRIGAN, Senior Board Director for Health Services, Institute of Medicine
CAROL R. ARENBERG, Editor, National Academy of Engineering
PHILIP ASPDEN, Senior Program Officer, Board on Health Services, Institute of Medicine
GARY FANJIANG, Fellow, National Academy of Engineering
PENELOPE J. GIBBS, Program Associate, Program Office, National Academy of Engineering
JAMES PHIMISTER, J. Herbert Hollomon Fellow, National Academy of Engineering
AMANDA SARATA, Intern, National Academy of Engineering

Preface

In 2000 and 2001, the Institute of Medicine (IOM) issued two reports, *To Err Is Human* and *Crossing the Quality Chasm*, documenting a glaring divergence between the rush of progress in medical science and the deterioration of health care delivery. The first report included an estimate that systems failures in health care delivery (i.e., poorly designed or "broken" care processes) were responsible for at least 98,000 deaths each year. The second report revealed a wide "chasm" between the quality of care the health system should be capable of delivering today, given the astounding advances in medical science and technology in the past half-century, and the quality of care most Americans receive. Documenting deep crises related to the safety, efficacy, efficiency, and patient-centeredness of health care in America, *Crossing the Quality Chasm* set forth a vision for a transformed health care system and challenged system stakeholders to take bold actions to bring about that transformation.

In response to this challenge, the National Academy of Engineering (NAE) and IOM, with support from the National Science Foundation, Robert Wood Johnson Foundation, National Institutes of Health, and the NAE Fund, initiated a project in 2002 to (1) identify engineering applications that could contribute significantly to improvements in health care delivery in the short, medium, and long terms; (2) assess factors that would facilitate or impede the deployment of these applications; and (3) identify areas of research in engineering and other fields that could contribute to rapid improvements in performance. This report, *Building a Better Delivery System*, is the culmination of the joint NAE/IOM study.

The report builds on a growing realization within the health care community of the critical role information/communications technologies, systems engineering tools, and related organizational innovations must play in addressing the interrelated quality and productivity crises facing the health care system. The report provides a framework for change and an action plan for a systems approach to health care delivery based on a partnership between engineers, health care professionals, and health care managers. The goal of the plan is to transform the U.S. health care sector from an underperforming conglomerate of independent entities (individual practitioners, small group practices, clinics, hospitals, pharmacies, community health centers, etc.) into a high-performance "system" in which participating units recognize their interdependence and the implications and repercussions of their actions on the system as a whole. The report describes opportunities and challenges to using systems engineering, information technologies, and other tools to advance a twenty-first century system capable of delivering safe, effective, timely, patient-centered, efficient, equitable health care—a system that embodies the six "quality aims" envisioned in *Crossing the Quality Chasm*.

The committee co-chairs are grateful to the members of the committee, not only for their knowledge, expertise, and commitment to change, but also for their participation in wide-ranging discussions on various aspects of this complex topic. Their collegiality and openness to ideas from many directions enabled the committee as a whole to overcome some of the very communications and cultural barriers described in the report and reach consensus on key recommendations. We also thank the outside experts who contributed their time and efforts to the success of this project, and the NAE and IOM staff for their research, editorial, and administrative support.

W. Dale Compton, *co-chair*
Committee on Engineering and
the Health Care System

Jerome H. Grossman, *co-chair*
Committee on Engineering and
the Health Care System

Acknowledgment of Reviewers

This report has been reviewed in draft form by individuals chosen for their diverse perspectives and technical expertise in accordance with procedures approved by the National Research Council Report Review Committee. The purpose of this independent review is to provide candid and critical comments that will assist the institution in making the published report as sound as possible and to ensure that the report meets institutional standards for objectivity, evidence, and responsiveness to the study charge. The review comments and draft manuscript remain confidential to protect the integrity of the deliberative process. We wish to thank the following individuals for reviewing this report:

David E. Daniel, University of Texas
Paul Griner, Emeritus, University of Rochester School of Medicine and Dentistry
John D. Halamka, CareGroup Health System
Angela Barron McBride, Indiana University School of Nursing
James C. McGroddy, IBM Corporation (ret.)
John M. Mulvey, Princeton University
Robert M. Nerem, Georgia Institute of Technology
Don M. Nielsen, American Hospital Association
Vinod K. Sahney, Henry Ford Health System
Edward J. Sondik, National Center for Health Statistics
Paul C. Tang, Palo Alto Medical Foundation

Although the reviewers listed above provided many constructive comments and suggestions, they were not asked to endorse the conclusions or recommendations nor did they see the final draft of the report before its release. The review of this report was overseen by Don E. Detmer, American Medical Informatics Association, and Charles E. Phelps, University of Rochester, appointed by the National Research Council Report Review Committee, who was responsible for making certain that an independent examination of this report was carried out in accordance with institutional procedures and that all review comments were carefully considered. Responsibility for the final content of this report rests entirely with the authoring committee and the institution.

Contents

APPENDIXES

Executive Summary

American medicine defines the cutting edge in most fields of clinical research, training, and practice worldwide, and U.S.-based manufacturers of drugs, medical devices, and medical equipment are among the most innovative and competitive in the world. In large part, the United States has achieved primacy in these areas by focusing public and private resources on research in the life and physical sciences and on the engineering of devices, instruments, and equipment to serve individual patients.

At the same time, relatively little technical talent or material resources have been devoted to improving or optimizing the operations or measuring the quality and productivity of the overall U.S. health care system. The costs of this collective inattention and the failure to take advantage of the tools, knowledge, and infrastructure that have yielded quality and productivity revolutions in many other sectors of the American economy have been enormous. The $1.6 trillion health care sector is now mired in deep crises related to safety, quality, cost, and access that pose serious threats to the health and welfare of many Americans (IOM, 2000, 2001, 2004a,b,c).

One need only note that: (1) more than 98,000 Americans die and more than one million patients suffer injuries each year as a result of broken health care processes and system failures (IOM, 2000; Starfield, 2000); (2) little more than half of U.S. patients receive known "best practice" treatments for their illnesses and less than half of physician practices use recommended processes for care (Casalino et al., 2003; McGlynn et al., 2003); and (3) an estimated thirty to forty cents of every dollar spent on health care, or more than a half-trillion dollars per year, is spent on costs associated with "overuse, underuse, misuse, duplication, system failures, unnecessary repetition, poor communication, and inefficiency" (Lawrence, in this volume). Health care costs have been rising at double-digit rates since the late 1990s—roughly three times the rate of inflation—claiming a growing share of every American's income, inflicting economic

hardships on many, and decreasing access to care. At the same time, the number of uninsured has risen to more than 43 million, more than one-sixth of the U.S. population under the age of 65 (IOM, 2004a).

With support from the National Science Foundation, National Institutes of Health (NIH), and Robert Wood Johnson Foundation, the National Academy of Engineering (NAE) and Institute of Medicine (IOM) of the National Academies convened a committee of 14 engineers and health care professionals to identify engineering tools and technologies that could help the health system overcome these crises and deliver care that is safe, effective, timely, patient-centered, efficient, and equitable—the six quality aims envisioned in the landmark IOM report, *Crossing the Quality Chasm* (Box ES-1).

The committee began with the expectation that systems-engineering tools that have transformed the quality and productivity performance of other large-scale complex systems (e.g., telecommunications, transportation, and manufacturing systems) could also be used to improve health care delivery. The particular charge to the committee was to identify: (1) engineering applications with the potential to improve health care delivery in the short, medium, and long terms; (2) factors that would facilitate or inhibit the deployment of these applications; and (3) priorities for research and education in engineering, the health professions, and related areas that would contribute to rapid improvements in the performance of the health care delivery system. The committee held three intensive workshops with experts from the engineering, health, management, and social science communities. The presentations by these experts can be found in Part 2 of this volume.

ENGINEERING/HEALTH CARE PARTNERSHIP

This report provides a framework and action plan for a systems approach to health care delivery based on a partnership

> **BOX ES-1**
> **Six Quality Aims for the 21st Century Health Care System**
>
> The committee proposes six aims for improvement to address key dimensions in which today's health care system functions at far lower levels than it can and should. Health care should be:
>
> - Safe—avoiding injuries to patients from the care that is intended to help them.
> - Effective—providing services based on scientific knowledge to all who could benefit and refraining from providing services to those not likely to benefit (avoiding underuse and overuse, respectively).
> - Patient-centered—providing care that is respectful of and responsive to individual patient preferences, needs, and values and ensuring that patient values guide all clinical decisions.
> - Timely—reducing waits and sometimes harmful delays for both those who receive and those who give care.
> - Efficient—avoiding waste, including waste of equipment, supplies, ideas, and energy.
> - Equitable—providing care that does not vary in quality because of personal characteristics such as gender, ethnicity, geographic location, and socioeconomic status.
>
> Source: IOM, 2001, pp. 5–6.

between engineers and health care professionals. The goal of this partnership is to transform the U.S. health care sector from an underperforming conglomerate of independent entities (individual practitioners, small group practices, clinics, hospitals, pharmacies, community health centers, et al.) into a high-performance "system" in which every participating unit recognizes its dependence and influence on every other unit. The report describes the opportunities and challenges to harnessing the power of systems-engineering tools, information technologies, and complementary knowledge in social sciences, cognitive sciences, and business/management to advance the six IOM quality aims for a twenty-first century health care system.

This NAE/IOM study attempts to bridge the knowledge/awareness divide separating health care professionals from their potential partners in systems engineering and related disciplines. After examining the interconnected crises facing the health care system and their proximate causes (Chapter 1), the report presents an overview of the core elements of a systems approach and puts forward a four-level model—patients, care teams, provider organizations, and the broader political-economic environment—of the structure and dynamics of the health care system that suggests the division of labor and interdependencies and identifies levers for change (Chapter 2).

In Chapters 3 and 4, systems-engineering tools and information/communications technologies and their applications to health care delivery are discussed. These complementary tools and technologies have the potential of improving radically the quality and productivity of American health care. A discussion of structural, economic, organizational, cultural, and educational barriers to using systems tools and

information/communications technologies follows; recommendations are offered for overcoming these barriers. In Chapter 5, the committee proposes a strategy for building a vigorous partnership between engineering and health care through cross-disciplinary research, education, and outreach.

SYSTEMS-ENGINEERING TOOLS FOR HEALTH CARE DELIVERY

Systems-engineering tools have been used in a wide variety of applications to achieve major improvements in the quality, efficiency, safety, and/or customer-centeredness of processes, products, and services in a wide range of manufacturing and services industries. The health care sector as a whole has been very slow to embrace them, however, even though they have been shown to yield valuable returns to the small but growing number of health care organizations and clinicians that have applied them (Feistritzer and Keck, 2000; Fone et al., 2003; Leatherman et al., 2003; Murray and Berwick, 2003). Statistical process controls, queuing theory, quality function deployment, failure-mode effects analysis, modeling and simulation, and human-factors engineering have been adapted to applications in health care delivery and used tactically by clinicians, care teams, and administrators in large health care organizations to improve the performance of discrete care processes, units, and departments.

However, the strategic use of these and more information-technology-intensive tools from the fields of enterprise and supply-chain management, financial engineering and risk analysis, and knowledge discovery in databases has been limited. With some adaptations, these tools could be used to measure, characterize, and optimize performance at higher levels of the health care system (e.g., individual health care organizations, regional care systems, the public health system, the health research enterprise, etc.). The most promising systems-engineering tools and areas of associated research identified by the committee are listed in Table ES-1.

Although data and associated information technology needs do not present significant technical or cost barriers to the tactical application of systems-engineering tools, there are significant structural, technical, and cost-related barriers at the organizational, multi-organizational, and environmental levels to the strategic implementation of systems tools. The current organization, management, and regulation of health care delivery provide few incentives for the use or development of systems-engineering tools. Current reimbursement practices, regulatory frameworks, and the lack of support for research have all discouraged the development, adaptation, and use of systems-engineering tools. Cultural, organizational, and policy-related factors (e.g., regulation, licensing, etc.) have contributed to a rigid division of labor in many areas of health care that has also impeded the widespread use of system tools.

In fact, relatively few health care professionals or administrators are equipped to think analytically about health care delivery as a system or to appreciate the relevance of systems-engineering tools. Even fewer are equipped to work with engineers to apply these tools. The widespread use of systems-engineering tools will require determined efforts on the part of health care providers, the engineering community, state and federal governments, private insurers, large employers, and other stakeholders.

Chapter 3 Recommendations

Recommendation 3-1. Private insurers, large employers, and public payers, including the Federal Center for Medicare and Medicaid Services and state Medicaid programs, should provide more incentives for health care providers to use systems tools to improve the quality of care and the efficiency of care delivery. Reimbursement systems, both private and public, should expand the scope of reimbursement for care episodes or use other bundling techniques (e.g., disease-related groups, severity-adjusted capitation for

TABLE ES-1 Systems Engineering Tools and Research for Health Care Delivery

Tool/Research Area	System Levels of Application			
	Patient	Team	Organization	Environment
SYSTEMS-DESIGN TOOLS				
Concurrent engineering and quality function deployment		X	X	
Human-factors tools	X	X	X	X
Tools for failure analysis		X	X	
SYSTEMS-ANALYSIS TOOLS				
Modeling and Simulation				
Queuing methods		X	X	
Discrete-event simulation		X	X	X
Enterprise-Management Tools				
Supply-chain management		X	X	X
Game theory and contracts		X	X	X
Systems-dynamics models		X	X	X
Productivity measuring and monitoring		X	X	X
Financial Engineering and Risk Analysis Tools				
Stochastic analysis			X	X
Value-at-risk			X	X
Optimization tools for individual decision making		X	X	X
Distributed decision making: market models and agency theory			X	X
Knowledge Discovery in Databases				
Data mining			X	X
Predictive modeling		X	X	X
Neural networks		X	X	X
SYSTEMS-CONTROL TOOLS				
Statistical process control	X	X	X	
Scheduling		X	X	

NOTE: Italics indicate areas with significant research opportunities.

Medicare Advantage, fixed payment for transplantation, etc.) to encourage the use of systems-engineering tools. Regulatory barriers should also be removed. As a first step, regulatory waivers could be granted for demonstration projects to validate and publicize the utility of systems tools.

Recommendation 3-2. Outreach and dissemination efforts by public- and private-sector organizations that have used or promoted systems-engineering tools in health care delivery (e.g., Veterans Health Administration, Joint Commission on Accreditation of Healthcare Organizations, Agency for Healthcare Research and Quality, Institute for Healthcare Improvement, Leapfrog Group, U.S. Department of Commerce Baldrige National Quality Program, and others) should be expanded, integrated into existing regulatory and accreditation frameworks, and reviewed to determine whether, and if so how, better coordination might make their collective impact stronger.

Recommendation 3-3. The use and diffusion of systems-engineering tools in health care delivery should be promoted by a National Institutes of Health Library of Medicine website that provides patients and clinicians with information about, and access to, systems-engineering tools for health care (a systems-engineering counterpart to the Library of Medicine web-based "clearinghouse" on the status and treatment of diseases and the Agency for Healthcare Research and Quality National Guideline Clearinghouse for evidence-based clinical practice). In addition, federal agencies and private funders should support the development of new curricula, textbooks, instructional software, and other tools to train individual patients and care providers in the use of systems-engineering tools.

Recommendation 3-4. The use of any single systems tool or approach should not be put "on hold" until other tools become available. Some systems tools already have extensive tactical or local applications in health care settings. Information-technology-intensive systems tools, however, are just beginning to be used at higher levels of the health care delivery system. Changes must be approached from many directions, with systems engineering tools that are available now and with new tools developed through research. Successes in other industries clearly show that small steps can yield significant results, even while longer term efforts are being pursued.

Recommendation 3-5. Federal research and mission agencies should significantly increase their support for research to advance the application and utility of systems engineering in health care delivery, including research on new systems tools and the adaptation, implementation, and improvement of existing tools for all levels of health care delivery. Promising areas for research include human-factors engineering,

modeling and simulation, enterprise management, knowledge discovery in databases, and financial engineering and risk analysis. Research on the organizational, economic, and policy-related barriers to implementation of these and other systems tools should be an integral part of the larger research agenda.

INFORMATION AND COMMUNICATION TECHNOLOGIES FOR HEALTH CARE DELIVERY

Although information collection, processing, communication, and management are at the heart of health care delivery, and considerable evidence links the use of clinical information/communications technologies to improvements in the quality, safety, and patient-centeredness of care, the health care sector remains woefully underinvested in these technologies (Casalino et al., 2003; DOC, 1999; IOM, 2004c; Littlejohns et al., 2003; Pestotnik et al., 1996; Walker et al., 2005; Wang et al., 2003). Factors contributing to this longstanding information/communications technologies deficit include: the atomistic structure of the industry; current payment/reimbursement regimes; the lack of transparency in the market for health care services; weaknesses in health care's managerial culture; the hierarchical structure and rigid division of labor in health professions; and (until very recently) the immaturity of available commercial clinical information/communications systems.

In the past decade, efforts to close the information/communications technologies gap have focused on the need for a comprehensive National Health Information Infrastructure (NHII), that is, the "set of technologies, standards, applications, systems, values, and laws that support all facets of individual health, health care, and public health" (National Committee on Vital and Health Statistics, 2001). Recent progress toward this goal, including the creation of the Office of the National Coordinator for Health Information Technology, in the U.S. Department of Health and Human Services, and the release of a 10-year plan to build the NHII, is encouraging (Thompson and Brailer, 2004).

A fully implemented NHII could support applications of information/communications technologies that empower individual patients to assume a much more active, controlling role in their own health care; improve access to timely, effective, and convenient care; improve patient compliance with clinician guidance; enable continuous monitoring of patient conditions by care professionals/care teams; and enable care providers to integrate critical information streams to improve patient-centered care, as well as to analyze, control, and optimize the performance of care teams. The NHII could enable health care organizations to integrate their clinical, administrative, and financial information systems internally, as well as link their systems with those of insurers, vendors, regulatory bodies, and other elements of the extended health care delivery enterprise. The

NHII could allow provider organizations to make more extensive use of data/information-intensive systems-engineering tools and facilitate the aggregation and exchange of data among health care organizations, public and private payer organizations, regulatory bodies, and the research community. This data pool could support better regulation and oversight of the health care delivery system, population health surveillance, and the continuing development of the clinical knowledge base.

The NHII could also support another family of emerging technologies based on wireless communications and micro-electronic systems with the potential to radically change the structure of the health care delivery system and advance patient-centeredness and quality performance. Wireless integrated microsystems could have an enormous beneficial impact on the quality and cost of health care, especially home health care in the coming decade. Microsystems implemented as wearable and implantable devices connected to clinical information systems through wireless communications could provide diagnostic data and deliver therapeutic agents for the treatment of a variety of chronic conditions, thereby improving the quality of life for senior citizens and chronically ill patients.

Much of the information/communications technology necessary for the realization of NHII exists today and will certainly improve in the decade ahead; however, there will be many challenges to putting it in place. Interoperability and other data standards and serious privacy and reliability concerns must be addressed, as well as training issues at all levels of the health care system. These and many of the same structural, financial, policy-related (reimbursement schemes, regulation), organizational, and cultural barriers that have impeded the use of systems tools will have to be surmounted to close health care's wide information/communications technologies gap.

Chapter 4 Recommendations

Recommendation 4-1. The committee endorses the recommendations made by the Institute of Medicine Committee on Data Standards for Patient Safety, which called for continued development of health care data standards and a significant increase in the technical and material support provided by the federal government for public-private partnerships in this area.

Recommendation 4-2. The committee endorses the recommendations of the President's Information Technology Advisory Council that call for: (1) application of lessons learned from advances in other fields (e.g., computer infrastructure, privacy issues, and security issues); and (2) increased coordination of federally supported research and development in these areas through the Networking and Information Technology Research and Development Program.

Recommendation 4-3. Research and development in the following areas should be supported:

- human-information/communications technology system interfaces
- voice-recognition systems
- software that improves interoperability and connectivity among systems from different vendors
- systems that spread costs among multiple users
- software dependability in systems critical to health care delivery
- secure, dispersed, multiagent databases that meet the needs of both providers and patients
- measurement of the impact of information/communications systems on the quality and productivity of health care

Recommendation 4-4. The committee applauds the U.S. Department of Health and Human Services 10-year plan for the creation of the National Health Information Infrastructure and the high priority given to the creation of standards for the complex network necessary for communications among highly dispersed providers and patients. To ensure that the emerging National Health Information Infrastructure can support current and next-generation clinical information/communications systems and the application of systems tools, research should focus immediately on advanced interface standards and protocols and standards-related issues concerning access, security, and the integration of large-scale wireless communications. Special attention should be given to issues related to large-scale integration. Funding for research in all of these areas will be critical to moving forward.

Recommendation 4-5. The committee recommends that public- and private-sector initiatives to reduce or offset current regulatory, accreditation, and reimbursement-related barriers to more extensive use of information/communications technologies in health care be expanded. These initiatives include efforts to reimburse providers for care episodes or use other bundling techniques (e.g., severity-adjusted capitation; disease-related groups, etc.), public and private support of community-based health information network demonstration projects, the Leapfrog Group's purchaser-mediated rewards to providers that use information/communications technologies, and others.

Recommendation 4-6. Public- and private-sector support for research on the development of very small, low-power, biocompatible devices will be essential for improving health care delivery

Recommendation 4-7. Engineering research should be focused on defining an architecture capable of incorporating data from microsystems into the wider health care network and developing interface standards and protocols to implement this larger network. Microsystems research should be focused on the following areas:

- integration, packaging, and miniaturization (to sizes consistent with implantation in the body)
- tissue interfaces and biocompatibility for long-term implantation
- interfaces and approaches to noninvasive (wearable) devices for measuring a broad range of physiological parameters
- low-power, embedded computing systems and wireless interfaces consistent with *in vivo* use
- systems that can transform data reliably and accurately into information and information into knowledge as a basis for treatment decisions

A STRATEGY TO ACCELERATE CHANGE

The committee believes that the actions recommended in this report will accelerate the development, adaptation, implementation, and diffusion of systems-engineering tools and information/communications technologies for health care delivery. However, building the partnership between engineering and health care that will accelerate and sustain progress toward the high-performance, patient-centered health care system envisioned by IOM will require bold, intentional, far-reaching changes in the education, research priorities, and practices of health care, engineering, and management. Building on the experiences of recent large-scale, multidisciplinary, research/education/technology-transfer initiatives in engineering and the biological sciences, the committee proposes a strategy for building bridges between the fields of engineering, health care, and management to address the major challenges facing the health care delivery system. An environment in which professionals from all three fields could engage in basic and applied research and translate the results of their research and advances both into the practice arena and the classroom, where students from the three disciplines could interact, would be a powerful catalyst for cultural change.

Chapter 5 Recommendations

Recommendation 5-1a. The federal government, in partnership with the private sector, universities, federal laboratories, and state governments, should establish multidisciplinary centers at institutions of higher learning throughout the country capable of bringing together researchers, practitioners, educators, and students from appropriate fields of engineering, health sciences, management, social and behavioral sciences, and other disciplines to address the quality and productivity challenges facing the nation's health care delivery system. To ensure that the centers have a nationwide impact, they should be geographically distributed. The committee

estimates that 30 to 50 centers would be necessary to achieve these goals.

Recommendation 5-1b. These multidisciplinary research centers should have a three-fold mission: (1) to conduct basic and applied research on the systems challenges to health care delivery and on the development and use of systems-engineering tools, information/communications technologies, and complementary knowledge from other fields to address them; (2) to demonstrate and diffuse the use of these tools, technologies, and knowledge throughout the health care delivery system (technology transfer); and (3) to educate and train a large cadre of current and future health care, engineering, and management professionals and researchers in the science, practices, and challenges of systems engineering for health care delivery.

Recommendation 5-2. Because funding for the multidisciplinary centers will come from a variety of federal agencies, a lead agency should be identified to bring together representatives of public- and private-sector stakeholders to ensure that funding for the centers is stable and adequate and to develop a strategy for overcoming regulatory, reimbursement-related, and other barriers to the widespread application of systems engineering and information/communications technologies in health care delivery.

Accelerating Cultural Change through Formal and Continuing Education

Making systems-engineering tools, information technologies, and complementary knowledge in business/management, social sciences, and cognitive sciences available and training individuals to use them will require the commitment and cooperation of engineers, clinicians, and health care managers, as well as changes in their respective professional cultures. The committee believes that these long-term cultural changes must begin in the formative years of professional education. Individuals in all of these professions should have opportunities to participate in learning and research environments in which they can contribute to a new approach to health care delivery. The training and development of health care, engineering, and management professionals who understand the systems challenges facing health care delivery and the value of using systems tools and technologies to address them should be accelerated and intensified.

Recommendation 5-3. Health care providers and educators should ensure that current and future health care professionals have a basic understanding of how systems-engineering tools and information/communications technologies work and their potential benefits. Educators of health professionals should develop curricular materials and programs to train graduate students and practicing professionals in systems approaches to health care delivery and the use of systems tools and information/communications technologies. Accrediting organizations, such as the Liaison Committee on Medical Education and Accreditation Council for Graduate Medical Education, could also require that medical schools and teaching hospitals provide training in the use of systems tools and information/communications technologies. Specialty boards could include training as a requirement for recertification.

Recommendation 5-4. Introducing health care issues into the engineering curriculum will require the cooperation of a broad spectrum of engineering educators. Deans of engineering schools and professional societies should take steps to ensure that the relevance of, and opportunities for, engineering to improve health care are integrated into engineering education at the undergraduate, graduate, and continuing education levels. Engineering educators should involve representatives of the health care delivery sector in the development of cases studies and other instructional materials and career tracks for engineers in the health care sector.

Recommendation 5-5. The typical MBA curriculum requires that students have fundamental skills in the principal functions of an organization—accounting, finance, economics, marketing, operations, information systems, organizational behavior, and strategy. Examples from health care should be used to illustrate fundamentals in each of these areas. Researchers in operations are encouraged to explore applications of systems tools for health care delivery. Quantitative techniques, such as financial engineering, data mining, and game theory, could significantly improve the financial, marketing, and strategic functions of health care organizations, and incorporating examples from health care into the core MBA curriculum would increase the visibility of health care as a career opportunity. Business and related schools should also be encouraged to develop elective courses and executive education courses focused on various aspects of health care delivery. Finally, students should be provided with information about careers in the health care industry.

Recommendation 5-6. Federal mission agencies and private-sector foundations should support the establishment of fellowship programs to educate and train present and future leaders and scholars in health care, engineering, and management in health systems engineering and management. New fellowship programs should build on existing programs, such as the Veterans Administration National Quality Scholars Program (which supports the development of physician/scholars in health care quality improvement), and the Robert Wood Johnson Foundation Health Policy Research and Clinical Scholars Programs (which targets newly minted M.D.s and social science Ph.D.s, to ensure their involvement in health policy research). The new programs should include all relevant fields of engineering and the full spectrum of health professionals.

CALL TO ACTION

As important as good analytical tools and information/communications systems are, they will ultimately fail to transform the system unless all members of the health care provider community participate and actively support their use. Although individuals "on the ground" (i.e., those doing the work) often know best how to improve things, empowering them to participate in changing the system will require that they understand the overall goals and objectives of the system and subsystem in which they work. Based on this understanding, they can contribute substantively to continuous improvements, as well as to radical advances in processes. The communication of the overall system and subsystem goals to individuals and groups at all levels is a crucial task for the management of the organization, and encouraging and recognizing individuals for their contributions to continuous improvements in operations at every level must be a principal operating goal for management.

Overhauling the health care delivery system will not come quickly or easily. Achieving the long-term goal of improving the health care system will require the ingenuity and commitment of leaders in the health care community, including practitioners in all clinical areas, and leaders in engineering. The committee recognizes the immensity of the task ahead and offers a word of encouragement to all members of the engineering and health care communities. If we take up the challenge to help transform the system now, crises can be abated, costs can be reduced, the number of uninsured can be reduced, and all Americans will have access to the quality care they deserve and that we are capable of delivering.

REFERENCES

Casalino, L., R.R. Gillies, S.M. Shortell, J.A.Schmittdiel, T. Bodenheimer, J.C. Robinson, T. Rundall, N. Oswald, H. Schauffler, and M.C. Wang. 2003. External incentives, information technology, and organized processes to improve health care quality for patients with chronic diseases. Journal of the American Medical Association 289(4): 434–441.

DOC (U.S. Department of Commerce). 1999. The Emerging Digital Economy II: Appendices. Washington, D.C.: DOC.

Feistritzer, N.R., and B.R. Keck. 2000. Perioperative supply chain management. Seminars for Nurse Managers 8(3): 151–157.

Fone, D., S. Hollinghurst, M. Temple, A. Round, N. Lester, A. Weightman, R. Roberts, E. Coyle, G. Bevan, and S. Palmer. 2003. Systematic review of the use and value of computer simulation modelling in population health and health care delivery. Journal of Public Health Medicine 25(4): 325–335.

IOM (Institute of Medicine). 2000. To Err Is Human: Building a Safer Health System, edited by L.T. Kohn, J.M. Corrigan, and M.S. Donaldson. Washington, D.C.: National Academy Press.

IOM. 2001. Crossing the Quality Chasm: A New Health System for the 21st Century. Washington, D.C.: National Academy Press.

IOM. 2004a. Insuring America's Health: Principles and Recommendations. Washington, D.C.: National Academies Press.

IOM. 2004b. Keeping Patients Safe: Transforming the Work Environment of Nurses. Washington, D.C.: National Academies Press.

IOM. 2004c. Patient Safety: Achieving a New Standard of Care. Washington, D.C.: National Academies Press.

Leatherman, S., D. Berwick, D. Iles, L.S. Lewin, F. Davidoff, T. Nolan, and M. Bisognano. 2003. The business case for quality: case studies and an analysis. Health Affairs 22(2): 17–30.

Littlejohns, P., J.C. Wyatt, and L. Garvican. 2003. Evaluating computerized health information systems: hard lessons to be learnt. British Medical Journal 326(7394): 860–863.

McGlynn, E.A., S.M. Asch, J. Adams, J. Keesey, J. Hicks, A. DeCristofaro, and E.A. Kerr. 2003. The quality of health care delivered to adults in the United States. New England Journal of Medicine 348(26): 2635–2645.

Murray, M., and D.M. Berwick. 2003. Advanced access: reducing waiting and delays in primary care. Journal of the American Medical Association 289(8): 1035–1040.

National Committee on Vital and Health Statistics. 2001. Information for Health: A Strategy for Building the National Health Information Infrastructure. Available online at: *http://ncvhs.hhs.gov/nhiilayo.pdf.*

Pestotnik, S.L., D.C. Classen, R.S.Evans, and J.P. Burke. 1996. Implementing antibiotic practice guidelines through computer-assisted decision support: clinical and financial outcomes. Annals of Internal Medicine 124(10): 884–890.

Starfield, B. 2000. Is U.S. health really the best in the world? Journal of the American Medical Association 284(4): 483–485.

Thompson, T.G., and D.J. Brailer. 2004. The Decade of Health Information Technology: Delivering Consumer-centric and Information-Rich Health Care: Framework for Strategic Action. Washington, D.C.: U.S. Department of Health and Human Services.

Walker, J., E. Pan, D. Johnston, J. Adler-Milstein, D.W. Bates, and B. Middleton. 2005. The value of health care information exchange and interoperability. Health Affairs Web Exclusive (Jan. 19): W5-10–W5-18.

Wang, S.J., B. Middleton, L.A. Prosser, C.G. Bardon, C.D. Spurr, P.J. Carchidi, A.F. Kittler, R.C. Goldszer, D.G. Fairchild, A.J. Sussman, G.J. Kuperman, and D.W. Bates. 2003. A cost-benefit analysis of electronic medical records in primary care. American Journal of Medicine 114(5): 397–403.

PART I

CONSENSUS REPORT

1

A New Partnership between Systems Engineering and Health Care

THE PARADOX OF AMERICAN HEALTH CARE

The United States leads the world in medical science and technology, defining the cutting edge in most fields of clinical research, training, and practice. U.S.-based manufacturers of drugs and medical devices and equipment are considered the most innovative and competitive in the world (AdvaMed, 2004; NSB, 2004). U.S. leadership has been achieved largely by focusing public and private resources on research in the life sciences and physical sciences and on the engineering of devices, instruments, and equipment for treating individual patients. The U.S. market for health care services has supported this focus by rewarding innovation in medical procedures and interventions and the drugs, devices, and equipment linked to them with relatively little regard for cost. Thus, the U.S. health care system provides high quality, highly specialized care for some individuals, but at a very high cost.

At the same time, the U.S. health care enterprise has devoted relatively little technical talent, material resources, or intellectual effort to improving or optimizing the operations of health care systems (especially higher level systems, such as hospitals, health systems, health networks, etc.) or to measuring performance in terms of quality and productivity. The costs to the American economy and the health of Americans of this collective inattention have been enormous. The $1.6 trillion U.S. health care enterprise now faces crises in safety, quality, cost, and access that seriously threaten the health and welfare of many Americans (IOM, 2000, 2001, 2004a,b,c).

To plan a response to these challenges and missed opportunities, the National Institutes of Health, National Science Foundation, and Robert Wood Johnson Foundation asked the National Academy of Engineering and Institute of Medicine (IOM) of the National Academies to conduct a study to identify: (1) engineering applications and tools with the potential to improve health care delivery in the short,

medium, and long terms; (2) factors that would facilitate, or inhibit, the deployment of these applications and tools; and (3) priorities for research in engineering and other areas that would contribute to expeditious improvements in the health care delivery system. The sponsors further directed that the study "evaluate current needs and opportunities in the . . . areas [of]: existing engineering applications that have been proven to improve health care delivery but are not widely deployed; emerging technologies and tools that would help overcome barriers to the delivery of high-quality care; [and] envisioned engineering applications and technologies that could be used to redesign care processes at various levels of the delivery system."

This report presents a case for a vigorous new partnership between engineering and health care to redress system imbalances. The report outlines a strategy for using information/communications technology and systems-engineering tools to address the crises in health care and improve the quality and productivity of the health care system. In this chapter, the historical origins and structural underpinnings of the interconnected health care crises are described. This is followed by an outline of IOM's vision of a twenty-first century health care system that meets six quality performance goals: safety, effectiveness, timeliness, patient-centeredness, efficiency, and equity (IOM, 2001). The chapter concludes with a framework for a new partnership between engineering and health care based on systems engineering and advances in information/communications technology with the potential to improve health care and realize IOM's vision of a truly patient-centered health care delivery system.

INTERCONNECTED CRISES IN U.S. HEALTH CARE

Today, "broken" health care processes and system failures result in the deaths of more than 98,000 Americans and injuries to more than 1 million patients every year (IOM, 2000;

Starfield, 2000). The gap between the rapidly advancing medical knowledge base and its application to patient care can best be described as a chasm. Little more than half of the patients in the United States receive known "best practice" treatment for their illnesses, and less than half of large physician practices provide recommended care processes (e.g., as recommended in disease registries and guidelines) for patients with chronic diseases (Casalino et al., 2003; McGlynn et al., 2003). Many patients are aware that the quality of care they receive is not what it could, or should, be. According to one survey, 75 percent of patients describe the health care system as fragmented and fractured; a "nightmare" to navigate; and plagued by duplications of effort, lack of communication, conflicting advice regarding treatment, and tenuous links to the evolving medical evidence base (Picker Institute, 2000).

The poor quality of care has enormous costs. Health care costs have been rising at double-digit rates since the late 1990s—roughly three times the rate of inflation—claiming a growing share of individual incomes, inflicting economic hardships on many, and making access to care increasingly difficult. Lawrence (see paper in this volume) estimates that $.30 to $.40 of every dollar spent on health care, more than half a trillion dollars per year, is spent on costs associated with "overuse, underuse, misuse, duplication, system failures, unnecessary repetition, poor communication, and inefficiency."

In addition, the number of people without health insurance has risen to more than 43 million, more than one-sixth of the U.S. population under the age of 65 (IOM, 2004a). Because the uninsured receive little preventive care, they tend to require a disproportionate share of costly chronic and acute care. In addition, the growing number of uninsured increases the disease burden on the uninsured population and imposes a heavy cost burden on providers and payers.

In response to the escalating cost of health care, government and industry—the third-party payers for most people—have shifted a growing share of the cost burden back to care providers and patients by reducing health care benefits, requiring that providers and patients pay a greater share of rising health insurance premiums, increasing co-payments, increasing deductibles, and, in some cases, dropping employee health coverage altogether (Regopoulos and Trude, 2004).

Hospitals and ambulatory care facilities are being forced to do more work with fewer people to keep revenues ahead of rising costs. Unable or unwilling to invest in tools and the complementary capabilities that might increase their productivity, many care-provider organizations have instead cut support staff and increased the workload on existing professional staff. This has undermined morale, causing many nurses to cut back to part-time employment or leave the profession altogether. In addition, these policies have seriously undermined the recruitment of new people to the field. The shortage of nurses alone has been shown to have adverse consequences for safety, quality, and access to health care (IOM, 2004b).

Many physicians have responded by seeing more patients per hour and focusing on activities with high rates of reimbursement and paying less attention to activities related to prevention. Some have even dropped out of the main payment system altogether and demanded retainers from patients who can afford personalized care—a practice known as boutique or concierge medicine.

PROXIMATE CAUSES OF HEALTH CARE CRISES

There are multiple, complex causes of the interrelated crises in health care delivery, but most of them can be traced to the confluence of six factors:

- rapid advances in medical science and technology and the increasing complexity of health care during the past half century
- the "cottage-industry" structure and acute-care orientation of the health care delivery system
- a patient population that predominantly needs chronic care, rather than acute care
- the structure of the U.S. market for health care services, which has encouraged and supported innovation in medical procedures, drugs, devices, and equipment, but has been indifferent to, if not discouraged, innovation directed at improving the quality and productivity of care delivery
- persistent underinvestment by the health care delivery sector in information/communications technology
- the inability or unwillingness of the health care delivery sector to take advantage of engineering-based systems-design, -analysis, and -management tools that have transformed other sectors of the American economy

Science, Technology, Specialization, and Complexity

Advances in medical science and technology since World War II have been a major reason for the growing complexity of American health care, the growing number and increased specialization of people involved in health care delivery, rising expectations about what can be done to treat illnesses, and the enormous increase in scientific and technological information health care providers must manage. To appreciate the impact of advances in medical science, consider the following changes. In the last 30 years, the number of randomized control trials (RCTs) published annually in the U.S. medical literature increased 100-fold, from 100 RCTs per year in the late 1960s to nearly 10,000 RCTs per year by the late 1990s (Chassin, 1998). In the last half-century, the number of categories of health care professionals in the United States increased from 10 to more than 220, roughly a 20-fold increase. Over the same period of time, the number of specialties in medicine increased from fewer than 10 to more than 100 (see paper by Lawrence in this volume).

Cottage-Industry Structure

The increase in specialization in medicine has reinforced the cottage-industry structure of U.S. health care, helping to create a delivery system characterized by disconnected silos of function and specialization. Of the approximately 700,000 clinicians in the United States, who represent more than 100 clinical specialties, more than 80 percent practice medicine in groups of 10 or fewer (see paper by Lawrence in this volume). Less than 24 percent of all physicians directly involved in patient care have practices based in one or more of the 5,800 public or privately owned hospitals, and fewer than 40 percent of hospital-based physicians (roughly 9 percent of all clinicians nationwide) are employed as full-time staff by hospitals (AHA, 2004; Pasko and Smart, 2004). In other words, the vast majority of hospitals, which provide the infrastructure, management systems, and supporting human and material resources for the health care professionals who deliver care to patients, rely heavily on clinicians who function as "independent agents."

This highly fragmented, highly specialized, independent-practitioner-driven, hospital-centered system of health care delivery has not kept pace with rapid advances in medical knowledge or adapted well to the growing need for chronic care. For decades, McGlynn and many others have documented extensive variations among practitioners (locally, regionally, and nationally) in the treatment of patients with given conditions (McGlynn et al., 2003; Wennberg et al., 1989, 2002). Clearly, a strong attachment to the autonomy of individual clinicians and a deeply held belief that the ultimate responsibility of each clinician is to the individual patient—and that each patient is unique—have actually impeded the diffusion of standard care protocols based on the latest medical evidence (Reinersten, 1996).

Although many clinicians now acknowledge the value of "evidence-based medicine" (the notion that there is a fundamentally correct way to diagnose and treat patients with a given condition) and recognize that they cannot keep up with advances, let alone deliver evidence-based care on their own, the persistent "guild" structure of the health care profession and the hierarchical nature of interaction continue to interfere with the diffusion of evidence-based medicine and the team-oriented care it requires. Indeed, most health care professionals still have little or no training in, or timely access to, the tools and infrastructure necessary to the practice of evidence-based medicine.

The Chronic-Care Imperative

Overall, Americans are living longer, thanks to advances in sanitation and water-treatment systems, emergency care, antibiotics and other medications (e.g., insulin and anti-hypertensive drugs), and other factors. At the same time, chronic conditions in the United States, as in other developed countries, are widespread. About 50 percent of the U.S. population—125 million people—have at least one chronic condition, and about 60 million of these suffer from more than one (Partnership for Solutions, 2002). In addition, a disproportionate amount of health care dollars (more than 75 percent) is spent on patients with chronic conditions (Partnership for Solutions, 2002).

Chronic-care patients require integrated, longitudinal care, that is, coordinated, uninterrupted care, which depends on connectivity among distributed care providers (including family members, physicians, nurses, pharmacists, and others) and the coordination and integration of many functions and specialized areas of knowledge over time. In fact, despite this tremendous need, connectivity, integrated care, and coordination are inadequate at all stages of the treatment of illnesses, from preventive care to acute and chronic care to rehabilitation to long-term care to end-of-life care. Most physicians are not trained to work effectively as members of care-provider teams, and the health care sector as a whole has failed to invest its resources in information infrastructure, information and systems-management tools, and supporting educational, research, and organizational capital that could begin to offset the deep-seated structural and cultural obstacles to coordinated, integrated, continuous patient care.

Structure of the U.S. Market for Health Care Services

The peculiar structure of the U.S. market for health care services and products has also been a significant factor in the current crises. The true cost of health care services is borne not by the patient, or customer, but by third-party payers—employers, private insurers, and the federal government (through Medicare/Medicaid). Insulated from the cost of care, the insured majority of Americans has increasingly come to consider health care as an entitlement. At the same time, the extremely successful U.S. biomedical research establishment has contributed to rising public expectations about the power of medical science and technology to cure diseases and treat illnesses.

In this environment, public and private insurers have been under constant pressure to cover new devices and therapies as they become available, regardless of cost. In the absence of measures of the relative quality or productivity performance of different care providers, insurers have controlled costs by limiting the services they reimburse, offering no incentives for, and, in some cases, actively discouraging, innovation and the application of technologies that could improve the quality and increase the efficiency of care delivery processes and systems.

Information Technology Deficit

For decades, health care has made much less use of information technology than other sectors of the U.S. economy. As of the late 1990s, health services ranked thirty-eighth among 53 major non-farm industries tracked by the U.S.

Department of Commerce in terms of information technology investment per worker. The health services industry spent less than one-tenth the amount invested by banks and nine other manufacturing and services industries (DOC, 1999). Even today, health care has barely begun to take advantage of the information/communications technology systems that have radically reshaped and revolutionized the performance of most major manufacturing and services industries in the United States. In transportation, financial services, communications, and manufacturing industries, modern information/communications systems have enabled and hastened the development of new high-quality products and services and the management of increasingly dispersed and complex production systems. Along with rapid increases in productivity, many of those industries also operate more efficiently with geographically dispersed operations. Although the health care industry has begun to close the information/communications technology gap in the financial and administrative dimensions of its business, core clinical operations are still information technology starved.

Given that the fundamental currency of health care is information, the information/communications technology deficit is ironic. Health care can be thought of as a continual series of *information-processing* experiments. From the initial collection of data (the patient's history, physical exam, and diagnostic tests), a hypothesis (diagnosis) is formed and then validated by further data collection. Feedback (the success of the treatment) is a test of the efficacy of the earlier data collection and hypothesis procedures. Information technologies would greatly facilitate every step of these information-processing experiments.

The reasons for the clinical information technology deficit are difficult to untangle. One major contributor is the cottage-industry structure of American health care, which includes many thousands of small businesses (individual clinical practices and small clinics) that cannot rationalize substantial investments in information/communications systems. Moreover, the payment/reimbursement structure for health care services does not reward clinicians for using information/communication technologies in clinical operations.

Another contributor to the clinical information technology gap is limited understanding by clinicians of the potential uses, impacts, and benefits of advanced information/communications technologies for the delivery of care. Clinical information systems in health care delivery can create new relationships that facilitate the exchange of information among sources with different perspectives and develop patient-centered processes of integrated, coordinated care. Designing systems for patient-centered care will require not only investments in information technology hardware and software, but also corresponding investments in related fields, such as human/computer interactions, computer-supported cooperative work, and cognitive engineering (Cook et al., 1998; Woods, 2000). As information/

communications technology is used to expand patient-centered care, dependence on software intensive systems will also increase, which, in turn, will entail new investments in measures to ensure software reliability (NRC, 2004).

Limited Use of Systems Engineering

Given the complexity of health care delivery, which involves the coordination and management of large numbers of highly specialized, distributed personnel, multiple streams of information, and material and financial resources across multiple care settings, it is astounding that health care has not made better use of the design, analysis, and control tools of systems engineering. The experiences of other major manufacturing and services industries, which have relied heavily on systems-engineering concepts and tools to understand, control/manage, and optimize the performance of complex production/distribution systems to meet quality, cost, safety, and other objectives, can provide valuable lessons for health care.

General Motors, Wal-Mart, and Boeing, just to mention a few, could not operate their far-flung organizations in today's competitive environment without the benefit of comprehensive information/communications systems and the extensive use of engineering tools for the design, analysis, and control of complex production/distribution systems. Deliveries from suppliers are controlled automatically; complex design operations share data instantaneously, resulting in the flawless production of parts and products on different continents; and factory outputs are becoming increasingly responsive to customer demand. Analogous operations can be found throughout the health care system. Thus, it is reasonable to suggest that the use of information/communications technologies and systems tools could lead to higher productivity, better quality care, and improved patient satisfaction.

One must be careful, however, about oversimplifying the parallels between health care and manufacturing and other services industries. Because of the complexities of disease processes, variations in human physiology, and the difficulties in restoring health, simple cut-and-copy approaches to improving health care processes will not suffice. Meeting the challenges of providing health care will require innovative uses of systems-engineering principles and techniques.

THE ROLE OF ENGINEERING IN THE TRANSFORMATION OF HEALTH CARE

In 2001, IOM documented the connections among crises in American health care, set forth a compelling vision for a transformed, twenty-first century, *patient-centered* health care system, and appealed to engineering for help. IOM identified six interrelated dimensions of quality for the health care system that must be improved. A transformed system must be safe, effective, patient-centered, timely, efficient, and equitable (IOM, 2001):

- *Safe*—avoiding injuries to patients from the care that is intended to help them.
- *Effective*—providing services based on scientific knowledge to all who could benefit and refraining from providing services to those not likely to benefit (avoiding underuse and overuse, respectively).
- *Patient-centered*—providing care that is respectful of and responsive to individual patient preferences, needs, and values and ensuring that patient values guide all clinical decisions.
- *Timely*—reducing waiting times and sometimes harmful delays for those who receive and those who give care.
- *Efficient*—avoiding waste, including waste of equipment, supplies, ideas, and energy.
- *Equitable*—providing care that does not vary in quality because of personal characteristics, such as gender, ethnicity, geographic location, and socioeconomic status.

IOM identified "patient-centeredness" as the unifying and guiding principle for redesigning and improving the health care system to achieve these performance goals.

This patient-centered vision for the twenty-first century health care system not only provides a compelling case for increasing investment in information/communications technology and improving collaboration between medicine and engineering in health care delivery, but also offers a clear functional road map for transformation of the existing system. The IOM report underscores the importance of information/communications technology for meeting multidimensional performance challenges and identified proven, fundamental engineering concepts, such as designing for safety, mass customization, continuous flow, and production planning, that could be brought to bear immediately to redesign and improve care processes.

Currents of Progress in a Stagnant Sea

Since IOM's clarion call for action, there have been many isolated, localized examples of the selective use of information/communications technologies, systems-engineering tools, and organizational innovations to address one or more of the health care crises. (See, for example, Brandeau et al., 2004, and papers in this volume by Bohmer, Breslow, Coffey, Gustafson, Halamka, Hendrich, Lawrence, Sahney, Stead, Uzsoy, and Zachariah). Although a few institutions have made some progress toward meeting some of IOM's six quality aims, evidence indicates that the health care delivery system as a whole has not (IOM, 2004d).

Most health care providers continue to underinvest in the technologies, tools, people, and organizational changes necessary to manage and improve clinical care in any of the six dimensions of quality. Overall, crises of quality, cost, and access have become more intense, and scant progress

has been made in improving safety, bringing advances in medical science to bear more rapidly on care delivery (effectiveness and timeliness), addressing inequities, and increasing efficiency. Not surprisingly, then, little headway has been made toward patient-centeredness, as many patients can attest (Picker Institute, 2000; see also Safran in this volume).

Given these persistent problems and scattered, isolated attempts to address them, the committee believes it is time to take up the challenge presented in the IOM report to establish a vigorous new partnership between engineering and health care to help bring a systems perspective to health care and hasten the transition to a patient-centered, twenty-first century health care system.

THE ENGINEERING/HEALTH CARE PARTNERSHIP

Engineering and health care have had a long and productive history of collaboration in the development of medical technologies (devices, equipment, pharmaceuticals) and in support of medical research (instrumentation, computational tools, etc.) (IOM, 1995; NAE, 2003). The ongoing revolutions in bioengineering and genomics and the promise of quantum advances in diagnostic tools and therapies testify to the continued vitality of the partnership. Nevertheless, engineering has remained on the periphery of efforts to assess, manage, and redress the shortcomings of the health care delivery system. Information/communications technology, the product of engineering, has been widely used to improve the administrative and financial aspects of the health care industry, but has had relatively little impact on the core business of health care—clinical operations. In short, the principles, tools, and research from engineering disciplines associated with the analysis, design, and control of complex systems (systems engineering, industrial engineering, operations research, human-factors engineering, financial engineering/risk analysis, materials/microelectromechanical systems engineering, etc.)—disciplines that have helped improve, and sometimes transform, many manufacturing and other services industries—are largely unknown in the clinical operations of health care delivery.

The recent history of multiple, interrelated crises of quality, access, and cost in the health care system testifies to the inherent complexity of the health care system and a desperate need for systems-engineering tools and information/communications technology. This complexity reflects the tensions and trade-offs between IOM's six quality aims for the transformation of health care and the goals, priorities, and perspectives on quality of the many stakeholders in the system—patients, physicians, nurses, administrators, insurers, regulators, and others. Trade-offs among major objectives are not unique to health care. For example, a manufacturer (e.g., an automaker) must make trade-offs between product features that may reduce maintenance costs for the customer but increase manufacturing costs and thus the initial cost of the product. There are many,

many examples of trade-offs in other economic sectors and, in fact, in all complex systems and operations.

Because of the extensive experience of systems engineers in dealing with trade-offs in manufacturing and other technology-intensive service industries, they are adept with the tools, methods, and knowledge base to grasp the deep functions and dynamics of complex systems, provide insights into interactions between subsystems and processes, and understand and manage the tensions and trade-offs among competing system-performance goals and competing priorities of stakeholders in the health care system. Engineering tools and technologies can be used to measure and optimize system performance to meet performance goals, such as safety, effectiveness, patient-centeredness, and timeliness, and, at the same time, anticipate, measure, and manage the effects of these interventions on other performance goals, such as equity, efficiency, and productivity.

Although systems engineering seems a natural partner for addressing the challenges of the health care delivery system, practitioners of the two disciplines are still largely ignorant of each other's methods, metrics, values, and mind-sets. Most clinicians, as well as most health care administrators, have had little exposure to the research and problem-solving methodologies of engineering; thus, they do not readily grasp how their applications might lead to improvements. By the same token, few engineers are knowledgeable of the complex sociotechnical fabric of health care processes and systems. Thus, they cannot communicate with health care providers in terms and concepts that take account of their values and perceptions. They do not have a common vocabulary for defining problems.

STRUCTURE OF THE REPORT

In the following four chapters of this consensus report (Part 1), the committee attempts to bridge the knowledge/awareness divide separating health care professionals from their potential partners in the fields of systems engineering and related disciplines. Two overlapping sets of engineering applications are identified—systems-engineering tools and information/communications technologies—that could potentially transform the American health care system. The committee believes that by taking advantage of existing opportunities and pursuing longer range research, short-term and long-term improvements can be made.

In Chapter 2, the committee elaborates on a four-level model of the structure and dynamic of the health care system, the rough division of labor and interdependencies among major elements of the system, and the levers for change throughout the system. An outline of the core elements of a systems approach to the health care delivery system is provided to give both health care professionals and engineers a systems perspective on the major challenges and opportunities facing the health care system and its constituent parts.

In Chapters 3 and 4, two major, interrelated opportunities are described for transforming the system: (1) the use of systems-engineering tools; and (2) the application of information/communications technologies. In Chapter 3, the focus is on (1) the identification of tools that have been demonstrated to be useful in managing large, complex systems that could lead to short-term improvements; and (2) the identification of research opportunities for improving existing tools and making them more user-friendly to achieve long-term improvements and create new, more powerful tools. In Chapter 4, the committee describes opportunities for accelerating the development and widespread diffusion of modern information/communications systems for health care delivery that are integrated with core system tools and technologies and capable of improving connectivity, continuity of care, and responsiveness in the overall health care system. In Chapter 5, the committee proposes an institutional strategy for developing a vigorous partnership between the engineering, management, and health care fields that could lead to the realization of the IOM vision of a high-performance, patient-centered twenty-first century health care system.

Part 2 of the report includes 38 edited, individually authored papers that were presented at three fact-finding workshops. The papers, many of which are cited in Part 1, address various dimensions of the quality/productivity challenges at all levels of the health care system, describe specific applications of systems-engineering tools and information/communications technologies to advance the quality and patient-centeredness of health care delivery, and describe various barriers and incentives to change.

REFERENCES

AdvaMed. 2004. The Medical Technology Industry at a Glance 2004. Available online at: *http://www.advamed.org/newsroom/chartbook.pdf*.

AHA (American Hospital Association). 2004. Hospital Statistics 2004. Chicago, Ill.: AHA.

Brandeau, M.L., F. Sainfort, and W.P. Pierskalla, eds. 2004. Operations Research and Health Care: A Handbook of Methods and Applications. International Series in Operations Research and Management Science Vol. 70. Boston, Mass.: Kluwer Academic Publishers.

Casalino, L., R.R. Gillies, S.M. Shortell, J.A.Schmittdiel, T. Bodenheimer, J.C. Robinson, T. Rundall, N. Oswald, H. Schauffler, and M.C. Wang. 2003. External incentives, information technology, and organized processes to improve health care quality for patients with chronic diseases. Journal of the American Medical Association 289(4): 434–441.

Chassin, M.R. 1998. Is health care ready for six sigma quality? Milbank Quarterly 76(4): 575–591.

Cook, R.I., D.D. Woods, and C. Miller. 1998. A Tale of Two Stories: Contrasting Views on Patient Safety. Chicago, Ill.: National Patient Safety Foundation. Available online at: *http://www.npsf.org/exec/report.html*.

DOC (U.S. Department of Commerce). 1999. The Emerging Digital Economy II: Appendices. Washington, D.C.: DOC.

IOM (Institute of Medicine). 1995. Sources of Medical Technology: Universities and Industry, edited by N. Rosenberg, A.C. Gelijns, and H. Dawkins. Washington, D.C.: National Academy Press.

IOM. 2000. To Err Is Human: Building a Safer Health System, edited by L.T. Kohn, J.M. Corrigan, and M.S. Donaldson. Washington, D.C.: National Academy Press.

IOM. 2001. Crossing the Quality Chasm: A New Health System for the 21st Century. Washington, D.C.: National Academy Press.

IOM. 2004a. Insuring America's Health: Principles and Recommendations. Washington, D.C.: National Academies Press.

IOM. 2004b. Keeping Patients Safe: Transforming the Work Environment of Nurses. Washington, D.C.: National Academies Press.

IOM. 2004c. Patient Safety: Achieving a New Standard of Care. Washington, D.C.: National Academies Press.

IOM. 2004d. 1st Annual Crossing the Quality Chasm Summit: A Focus on Communities. Washington, D.C.: National Academies Press.

McGlynn, E.A., S.M. Asch, J. Adams, J. Keesey, J. Hicks, A. DeCristofaro, and E.A. Kerr. 2003. The quality of health care delivered to adults in the United States. New England Journal of Medicine 348(26): 2635–2645.

NAE (National Academy of Engineering). 2003. The Impact of Academic Research on Industrial Performance. Washington, D.C.: National Academies Press.

NRC (National Research Council). 2004. Summary of a Workshop on Software Certification and Dependability. Washington, D.C.: National Academies Press.

NSB (National Science Board). 2004. Science and Engineering Indicators 2004 (2 volumes). Arlington, Va.: National Science Foundation. Available online at: *http://www.nsf.gov/sbe/srs/seind04/start.htm*.

Partnership for Solutions. 2002. Chronic Conditions: Making the Case for Ongoing Care. Prepared for the Robert Wood Johnson Foundation. Baltimore, Md.: Johns Hopkins University Press.

Pasko, T., and D.R. Smart. 2004. Physician Characteristics and Distribution in the US., 2004 ed. Chicago, Ill.: American Medical Association.

Picker Institute. 2000. Eye on Patients. A Report by the Picker Institute for the American Hospital Association. Boston, Mass.: Picker Institute.

Regopoulos, L.E., and S. Trude. 2004. Employers Shift Rising Health Care Costs to Workers: No Long-term Solution in Sight. Issue Brief No. 83. May 2004. Washington, D.C.: Center for Studying Health System Change. Available online at: *http://www.hschange.org/CONTENT/677/* [accessed Sept. 9, 2004].

Reinersten, J.L. 1996. Health Care: Past, Present, and Future. 14th Annual Terry C. Shackelford, MD, Memorial Lecture. The Bulletin 40: 61–70.

Starfield, B. 2000. Is U.S. health really the best in the world? Journal of the American Medical Association 284(4): 483–485.

Wennberg, J.E., J.L. Freeman, and R.M. Shelton. 1989. Hospital use and mortality among Medicare beneficiaries in Boston and New Haven. New England Journal of Medicine 321(17): 1168–1173.

Wennberg, J.E., E.S. Fisher, and J.S. Skinner. 2002. Geography and the debate over Medicare reform. Health Affairs: W96–W114. Web Exclusive, February 13, 2002.

Woods, D.D. 2000. Behind Human Error: Human Factors Research to Improve Patient Safety. Washington, D.C.: American Psychological Association.

2

A Framework for a Systems Approach to Health Care Delivery

To consider how information/communications technologies and systems-engineering tools can be used to help realize the IOM vision of a patient-centered health care system, we must first understand the challenges facing the U.S. health care system (IOM, 2001). The committee has adapted a four-level model by Ferlie and Shortell (2001) to clarify the structure and dynamics of the health care system, the rough divisions of labor and interdependencies among major elements of the system, and the levers for change. A brief description of the model follows. The remainder of this chapter provides a "systems view" of health care and a brief description of the potential role of information/communications systems.

A FOUR-LEVEL MODEL OF THE HEALTH CARE SYSTEM

In this model, adapted from Ferlie and Shortell (2001), the health care system is divided into four "nested" levels: (1) the individual patient; (2) the care team, which includes professional care providers (e.g., clinicians, pharmacists, and others), the patient, and family members; (3) the organization (e.g., hospital, clinic, nursing home, etc.) that supports the development and work of care teams by providing infrastructure and complementary resources; and (4) the political and economic environment (e.g., regulatory, financial, payment regimes, and markets), the conditions under which organizations, care teams, individual patients, and individual care providers operate (see Figure 2-1).

The Individual Patient

We begin appropriately with the individual patient, whose needs and preferences should be the defining factors in a patient-centered health care system. Recent changes in health care policy reflect an emphasis on "consumer-driven" health care. The availability of information, the establishment of private health care spending accounts, and other measures reflect an increasing expectation that patients will drive changes in the system for improved quality, efficiency, and effectiveness. Overall, the role of the patient has changed from a passive recipient of care to a more active participant in care delivery.

At the same time, the fragmented delivery system, combined with the growing burden of chronic disease and the need for continuous care, have all but forced many patients to assume an active role in the design, coordination, "production," and implementation of their care, whether they want to or not. Unfortunately, most people do not have access to the information, tools, and other resources they need to play this new role effectively. Considering the roles, needs, and objectives of first-level actors—individual patients—and their interdependencies with actors at other levels of the system, opportunities abound for using information/communications technologies and systems-engineering tools to improve the overall performance of the health care system.

A starting point for increasing the "patient-centeredness" of health care delivery is changing the perspective of clinicians to consider patients and their families as "partners" and to incorporate their values and wishes into care processes. The level of responsibility patients and their families assume differs from patient to patient. Some prefer to delegate some, if not most, of the decision making to a trusted clinician/counselor in the care system; others want to be full partners in decision making. In either case, however, patients need a free exchange of information and communication with physician(s) and other members of the care team, as well as with the organizations that provide the supporting infrastructure for the care teams.

For patients to communicate "informed" needs and preferences, participate effectively in decision making, and coordinate, or at least monitor the coordination, of their care, they must have access to the same information streams—in "patient-accessible" form—as their physician(s) and care team. Information that supports evidence-based,

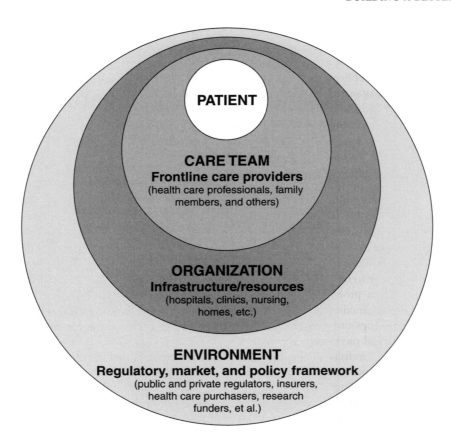

FIGURE 2-1 Conceptual drawing of a four-level health care system.

effective, efficient care encompasses the patient's medical record, including real-time physiological data; the most up-to-date medical evidence base; and orders in process concerning the patient's care. The patient and/or his or her clinician/counselor or family member must also have access to educational, decision-support, information-management, and communication tools that can help them integrate critical information from different sources.

From the patient's perspective, improving the timeliness, convenience, effectiveness, and efficiency of care will require that the patient be interconnected to the health care system. Synchronous communication between patient and physician could improve the quality of care in a number of ways. For example, continuous, real-time communication of a patient's physiological data to care providers could accelerate the pace of diagnosis and treatment, thereby reducing complications and injuries that might result from delays. Remote (e.g., in-the-home, on-the-go) monitoring, diagnosis, and treatment would make care much more convenient for patients, save them time, and conceivably improve compliance with care regimes (see paper by Budinger in this volume). Communication technologies also have the potential to change the nature of the relationship between patient

and provider, making it easier for patients to develop and maintain trusting relationships with their clinicians.

Asynchronous communication also has the potential to significantly improve quality of care. The easy accessibility of the Internet and the World Wide Web should enable all but continuous inquiries and feedback between patients and the rest of the health care system (IOM, 2001). The World Wide Web has already changed patients' ability to interact with the system and to self-manage aspects of their care. One of the fastest growing uses of the these communication technologies is as a source of medical information from third parties, which has made the consumer (i.e., the patient) both more informed, and, unfortunately, sometimes misinformed.

Some of the improvements just described are available today, some are under study, and some are as much as a decade away from realization. Thus, research is still an essential component in transforming the current system.

The Care Team

The care team, the second level of the health care system, consists of the individual physician and a group of care providers, including health professionals, patients' family members, and others, whose collective efforts result in the delivery of care to a patient or population of patients. The care team is the basic building block of a "clinical microsystem," defined as "the smallest replicable unit within an organization [or across multiple organizations] that is replicable in the sense that it contains within itself the necessary human, financial, and technological resources to do its work" (Quinn, 1992).

In addition to the care team, a clinical microsystem includes a defined patient population; an information environment that supports the work of professional and family caregivers and patients; and support staff, equipment, and facilities (Nelson et al., 1998). Ideally, the role of the microsystem is to "standardize care where possible, based on best current evidence; to stratify patients based on medical need and provide the best evidence-based care within each stratum; and to customize care to meet individual needs for patients with complex health problems" (Ferlie and Shortell, 2001). Most health and medical services today, however, are not delivered by groups or teams.

The role and needs of individual physicians have undergone changes parallel to those of individual patients. The exponential increase in medical knowledge, the proliferation of medical specialties, and the rising burden of providing chronic care have radically undercut the autonomy of individual physicians and required that they learn to work as part of care teams, either in a single institution/organization or across institutional settings. The slow adaptation of individual clinicians to team-based health care has been influenced by several factors, including a lack of formal training in teamwork techniques, a persistent culture of professional autonomy in medicine, and the absence of tools, infrastructure, and incentives to facilitate the change.

To participate in, let alone lead and orchestrate, the work of a care team and maintain the trust of the patient, the physician must have on-demand access to critical clinical and administrative information, as well as information-management, communication, decision-support, and educational tools to synthesize, analyze, and make the best use of that information. Moreover, to deliver patient-centered care (i.e., care based on the patient's needs and preferences), the physician must be equipped and educated to serve as trusted advisor, educator, and counselor, as well as medical expert, and must know how to encourage the patient's participation in the design and delivery of care.

At the present time, precious few care teams or clinical microsystems are the primary agents of patient-centered clinical care. Unwarranted variations in medical practice are common, even for conditions and patient populations for which there are standard, evidence-based, patient-stratified "best practice" protocols (McGlynn et al., 2003; Wennberg et al., 1989). Even though many clinicians now accept the value of "evidence-based medicine" and recognize that they cannot deliver evidence-based care on their own, they are many barriers to their changing accordingly: the guild

structure of the health care professions; the absence of training in teamwork; the strong focus on the needs of individual patients as opposed to the needs of patient populations; and the lack of supporting information tools and infrastructure. All of these can, and do, prevent systems thinking by clinicians, the diffusion of evidence-based medicine, and the clinical microsystems approach to care delivery. Thus, tailoring evidence-based care to meet the needs and preferences of individual patients with complex health problems remains an elusive goal.

For care teams to become truly patient-centered, the rules of engagement between care teams and patients must be changed. Like individual care providers, the care team must become more responsive to the needs and preferences of patients and involve them and their families (to the extent they desire) in the design and implementation of care. Care teams must provide patients with continuous, convenient, timely access to quality care. One member of the care team must be responsible for ensuring effective communication and coordination between the patient and other members of the care team.

The Organization

The third level of the health care system is the organization (e.g., hospital, clinic, nursing home) that provides infrastructure and other complementary resources to support the work and development of care teams and microsystems. The organization is a critical lever of change in the health care system because it can "provide an overall climate and culture for change through its various decision-making systems, operating systems, and human resource practices" (Ferlie and Shortell, 2001). The organization encompasses the decision-making systems, information systems, operating systems, and processes (financial, administrative, human-resource, and clinical) to coordinate the activities of multiple care teams and supporting units and manage the allocation and flow of human, material, and financial resources and information in support of care teams. The organization is the business level, the level at which most investments are made in information systems and infrastructure, process-management systems, and systems tools.

Health care organizations face many challenges. In response to the escalating cost of health care, government and industry—the third-party payers for most people—have shifted a growing share of the cost burden back to care providers and patients in recent years. As a result, hospitals and ambulatory care facilities are under great pressure to accomplish more work with fewer people to keep revenues ahead of rising costs.

In certain respects, management of health care organizations is not well positioned to respond to mounting cost and quality crises. Compared to other industries, health care has evolved with little shaping by the visible hands of management. Historically, most leaders of health care organizations were initially trained in medicine or public health. Moreover, except in the relatively few integrated, corporate provider organizations (e.g., Kaiser-Permanente, Mayo Clinic, et al.), the management of most hospitals faces the challenge of "managing" clinicians, the majority of whom function as "independent agents."

Less than 40 percent of all hospital-based physicians are employed as full-time staff by the hospitals where they practice, a reflection of the deeply ingrained culture of professional autonomy in medicine and the deeply held belief of care professionals that their ultimate responsibility is to individual patients. These circumstances have posed significant challenges to the authority of health care management in many organizations, often creating discord and mistrust between health care professionals and health care management. Other challenges to management include the hierarchical nature of the health professions and inherent resistance to team-based care, significant regulatory and administrative requirements (e.g., controlled substances, biohazardous waste disposal, patient privacy, safety, etc.), and health care payment/reimbursement regimes that provide little, if any, incentives for health care organizations to invest in non-revenue-generating assets, such as information/communications technologies and process-management tools.

To support patient-centered care delivery by well functioning clinical care teams or microsystems, health organizations must find ways to bridge the health care professional/delivery system management divide and invest in information/communications technologies, systems-engineering tools, and associated knowledge. Integrated, patient-centered, team-based care requires material, managerial, logistical, and technical support that can cross organizational/institutional boundaries—support that is very difficult to provide in a highly fragmented, distributed-care delivery system.

Financial investments in information/communications technologies and systems-engineering tools alone will not be enough, however. These investments must be accompanied by an organizational culture that encourages the development of care teams working with semiautonomous agents/physicians (see paper by Bohmer in this volume). "Developing a culture that emphasizes learning, teamwork, and customer focus may be a 'core property' that health care organizations . . . will need to adopt if significant progress in quality improvement is to be made" (Ferlie and Shortell, 2001). Finally, health care institutions must become "learning organizations" that are "skilled at creating, acquiring, and transferring knowledge, and at modifying [their] behavior to reflect new knowledge and insights" (Garvin, 1993).

The Political and Economic Environment

The fourth and final level of the health care system is the political, economic (or market) environment, which includes regulatory, financial, and payment regimes and entities that influence the structure and performance of health care organizations directly and, through them, all other levels of the system. Many actors influence the political and economic environment for health care. The federal government influences care through the reimbursement practices of Medicare/Medicaid, through regulation of private-payer and provider organizations, and through its support for the development and use of selected diagnostic and therapeutic interventions (e.g., drugs, devices, equipment, and procedures). State governments, which play a major role in the administration of Medicaid, also influence care systems. Private-sector purchasers of health care, particularly large corporations that contract directly with health care provider organizations and third-party payers (e.g., health plans and insurance companies), are also important environment-level actors, in some cases reimbursing providers for services not covered by the federal government.

Federal regulations influence the structure, level, and nature of competition among providers and insurers. They can also affect the transparency of the health care system by setting requirements related to patient safety and other aspects of the quality of care. By exercising its responsibility to monitor, protect, and improve public health, the federal government shapes the market environment for health care. Federal agencies, the primary sources of funding for biomedical research, influence the research and technological trajectories of health care, and, with them, the education of health care professionals and professionals in other areas invested in the health care enterprise.

At present, many factors and forces at the environmental level, including reimbursement schemes for health care services and some regulatory policies, do not support the goals and objectives of patient-centered, high-performance health care organizations or the health care delivery system as a whole. Although the federal government, the single largest purchaser of health care services, principal regulator, and major research patron, is, in many ways, best positioned to drive changes in the health care delivery system, some private-sector payer organizations and state governments are better positioned to experiment with new mechanisms and incentives for improving the quality of care and making health care more affordable (see papers by De Parle and Milstein in this volume).

A SYSTEMS VIEW OF HEALTH CARE

In Chapter 1, the health care delivery system was described as a "cottage industry." The main characteristic of a cottage industry is that it comprises many units operating independently, each focused on its own performance. Each unit has considerable freedom to set standards of performance and measure itself against metrics of its own choosing. In addition, cottage industries do not generally attempt to standardize or coordinate the processes or performance of Unit A with those of Units B, C, and so on.

Indeed, this is an apt characterization of the current health care delivery system. Even in many hospitals, individual departments operate more or less autonomously, creating so-called "silos." Many physicians practice independently or in small groups, and ambulatory clinics, pharmacies, laboratories, rehabilitation clinics, and other organizations—although part of the delivery system—often act as independent entities. We often call this arrangement a "health care system," even though it was not created as a system and has never performed as a system.

Moving from the current conglomeration of independent entities toward a "system" will require that every participating unit recognize its dependence and influence on all other units. Each unit must not only achieve high performance but must also recognize the imperative of joining with other units to optimize the performance of the system as a whole. Moreover, each individual care provider must recognize his or her dependence and influence on other care team members (e.g., specialists in different fields, pharmacists, nurses, social workers, psychologists, physical therapists, etc.) (IOM, 2003). These are the underlying attitudes that support a systems approach to solving problems.

Changing attitudes to embrace teamwork and systems "thinking" can be extremely difficult and may encounter resistance. Nevertheless, a concerted, visible commitment by management will be necessary to achieve this new way of thinking as a giant step toward the improvements identified in *Crossing the Quality Chasm* (IOM, 2001).

Optimization

It is easy to show mathematically that the optimization of individual units rarely, and only under highly improbable circumstances, results in optimization of the whole. Optimization is determined by a variety of metrics, including the productivity of a unit, the quality of service, the use of physical resources, or a combination of all of these. Optimization of the whole requires a clear understanding of the goal of the overall system, as well of interactions among the subsystems. The whole must be recognized as being greater than the sum of its parts (Box 2-1).

A handful of health care organizations have embraced the systems view (e.g., the Veterans Administration and Kaiser-Permanente Health Care). These significant exceptions to the general rule demonstrate that the systems view is applicable to health care and could be a model for other health care organizations. The goal of this report is to identify existing tools that can be used to address problems and to suggest areas for further exploration.

In any large system that has many subsystems, achieving high operating performance for each subsystem while taking into account the mutual influence of subsystems on each other and on the system as a whole can be a daunting task. A simple pictorial description of interacting elements in a system may be helpful for understanding how the system works. However, a deeper understanding invariably involves creating a mathematical description of subsystems, their performance, and their interactions. This, in turn, requires a model, that is, an abstract representation of how the system operates (a mathematical form that can be used to analyze the system) that includes parameters that determine the performance of each sub-element of the system, as well as descriptions of interactions. The model is a tool for simulating the performance of the actual system.

The principal objective of a simulation is to ask "what if" questions and assess the impact of alternative actions on the performance of the system to determine which ones might improve overall system performance. For example, if a change is planned in the layout of a facility, a model can be used to determine if it will improve the flow of people and equipment through the facility. A model might help

---

BOX 2-1
Optimizing System Performance

Optimization of the performance of a large system is often attempted through the optimization of each sub-element of the system. In industry, this is commonly accomplished by creating independent "profit/loss" centers whose performance can be measured independently of the performance of all other sub-elements. Unfortunately, this procedure rarely, if ever, results in optimization of the entire system. In fact, with a simple mathematical formula, it has been shown conclusively that optimization of the whole can only be achieved by optimizing the performance of each sub-element when the parameters that determine performance are independent of each other.

For example, assume that the productivity of a health care system is determined by: (1) the number of supporting staff (S); (2) the number of independent physicians (IP); (3) the level of capital investment in instrumentation (I); and (4) the level of investment in information/communications technologies infrastructure (IT). If, and only if, S, IP, I, and IT are totally independent, can the system by optimized by optimizing the four sub-elements. Even in this simple example, however, and certainly in practice, such independence does not exist. Therefore, to optimize overall system performance, regardless of whether one is attempting to optimize for safety, customer satisfaction, cost, or for all of these simultaneously, interactions among the parameters must be recognized and included.

determine how much inventory must be kept at Station A to ensure that it can respond to an emergency in less than five minutes. A model might also reveal if a different communication system might reduce the required inventory or the best way to assign a nursing staff when 10 percent of the nurses are not available. As Alan Pritsker, the author of many treatises on large-scale system modeling and simulation, writes, "The system approach is a methodology that seeks to ensure that changes in any part of the system will result in significant improvements in total system performance" (Pritsker, 1990).

Because the health care system involves a myriad of interacting elements, it is difficult, or even impossible, for any individual to have a complete picture of the system without using special tools to perform a systems analysis. A model of the health care system must include a description of "processes," including a wide variety of activities, from nurses administering medication on the hospital floor to examinations by a doctor to laboratory tests to the filling of prescriptions by a pharmacist to follow-on visits by a nurse. The model must include the role of each process in health care delivery and its interactions with other processes in the system. But clinical elements are not the only important elements in an analysis. The interaction between administrative elements (e.g., patient check-in and billing procedures) and other processes can also significantly influence the overall performance of the system from the patient and organization's point of view. All processes must be quantitatively described to be included in the model.

Any attempt to optimize the performance of a system must take into account objectives that are difficult to quantify and that may, in fact, conflict with each other. Quantifying the quality of care, for example, can be difficult, largely because the meaning of quality varies depending on whether the patient, the health care professional, or the clinic or hospital is assessing it. Improvements in productivity may mean an increase in the number of patients that can be accommodated or a decrease in waiting time for the average patient. IOM identified safety, effectiveness, patient-centeredness, timeliness, efficiency, and equity as proper quality objectives for the health care delivery system. Systems analyses can be used to improve the overall performance of systems with multiple objectives because they include possible trade-offs and/or synergies among these objectives. In addition, potentially conflicting goals—for example, cost containment and patient-centeredness—can also be analyzed.

THE ROLE OF INFORMATION AND COMMUNICATIONS TECHNOLOGY

Many industries have attempted to use information/communications systems in place of manual operations, such as record keeping. But information/communications systems can be used for much more than electronic record keeping. With incredible advances in computational speed and capacity and parallel advances in computer software, clinical information and communications systems can provide immediate access to information, including patient-based information (e.g., past laboratory values and current diagnoses and medications), institution-based information (e.g., drug-resistance patterns of various bacteria to different antibiotics), profession-based information (e.g., clinical-practice guidelines, including summaries of recommended best practices in various situations), real-time decision support (e.g., alerts about potential drug interactions or dosing patterns in a patient with a compromised drug-metabolism mechanism), practice-surveillance support (e.g., reminders about upcoming screening tests recommended for a patient), and population health data (e.g., for epidemiological research, disease and biohazard surveillance, notification of post-introduction adverse drug events).

Information/communications systems can also provide important information to the patient for self-treatment of diseases and enable ongoing asynchronous communication between patients and care providers. In the future, with the advent of remote monitoring devices and wireless communication systems, information/communications systems have the potential to support continuous monitoring of a patient's health status at home, rapid diagnosis by clinicians, and timely, effective therapeutic interventions in the home by the patient or a family member, with guidance by health professionals. Furthermore, by capturing process and system performance data for systems analysis, control and design, information/communications technologies can facilitate the use of systems-engineering tools by patient care teams, provider organizations, and environmental actors at all levels of the health care delivery system.

Chapter 3 provides descriptions of a large portfolio of systems-engineering tools and concepts with the potential to significantly improve the quality and cost performance of the health care system. These tools have been widely and effectively used to design, analyze, and control complex processes and systems in many major manufacturing and services industries. In Chapter 4 opportunities are described for accelerating the development and widespread diffusion of clinical information and communications systems for health care delivery that can support the use of systems tools and improve the connectivity, continuity of care, and responsiveness of the health care system as a whole.

REFERENCES

Ferlie, E.B., and S.M. Shortell. 2001. Improving the quality of health care in the United Kingdom and the United States: a framework for change. Milbank Quarterly 79(2): 281–315.

Garvin, D.A. 1993. Building a learning organization. Harvard Business Review 71(4): 78–91.

IOM (Institute of Medicine). 2001. Crossing the Quality Chasm: A New Health System for the 21st Century. Washington, D.C.: National Academy Press.

IOM. 2003. Health Professions Education: A Bridge to Quality. Washington, D.C.: National Academies Press.

McGlynn, E.A., S.M. Asch, J. Adams, J. Keesey, J. Hicks, A. DeCristofaro, and E.A. Kerr. 2003. The quality of health care delivered to adults in the United States. New England Journal of Medicine 348(26): 2635–2645.

Nelson, E.C., P.B. Batalden, J.J. Mohr, and S.K. Plume. 1998. Building a quality future. Frontiers of Health Services Management 15(1): 3–32.

Pritsker. 1990. Papers, Experiences, Perspectives. Chicago, Ill.: Donnelley and Sons.

Quinn, J.B. 1992. Intelligent Enterprise: A Knowledge and Service Based Paradigm for Industry. New York: Free Press.

Wennberg, J.E., J.L. Freeman, and R.M. Shelton. 1989. Hospital use and mortality among Medicare beneficiaries in Boston and New Haven. New England Journal of Medicine 321(17): 1168–1173.

3

The Tools of Systems Engineering

An understanding of the performance of large-scale systems must be based on an understanding of the performance of each element in the system and interactions among these elements. Thus, understanding a large, disaggregated system such as the health care delivery system with its multitude of individual parts, including patients with various medical conditions, physicians, clinics, hospitals, pharmacies, rehabilitation services, home nurses, and many more, can be daunting. To add to the complexity of improving this system, different stakeholders have different performance measures. Patients expect safe, effective treatment to be available as needed at an affordable cost. Health care provider organizations want the most efficient use of personnel and physical resources at the lowest cost. Health care providers want to serve patients effectively and minimize, or at least reduce, the time devoted to other tasks and obligations. Advancing all six of the IOM quality aims for the twenty-first century health care system—safety, effectiveness, timeliness, patient-centeredness, efficiency, and equity—will require understanding the needs and performance measures of all stakeholders and making necessary trade-offs among them (Hollnagel et al., 2005).

Understanding interactions and making trade-offs in such a complex system is difficult, sometimes even impossible, without mathematical tools, many of them based on operations research, a discipline that evolved during World War II when mathematicians, physicists, and statisticians were asked to solve complex operational problems. Since then, these tools have been used to create highly reliable, safe, efficient, customer-focused systems in transportation, manufacturing, telecommunications, and finance. Based on these and other experiences, the committee believes that they can also be used to improve the health care sector (McDonough et al., 2004). Indeed, improvements in health care quality and productivity have already been demonstrated on a limited scale in isolated elements at all four levels of the health care system (patient, care team, organization, and environment). These limited, but encouraging, first steps led the committee to conclude that the effective, widespread use of these tools could lead to significant improvements in the quality of care and increases in productivity throughout the health care system.

This chapter provides detailed descriptions of several families of systems-engineering tools and related research that have demonstrated significant potential for addressing systemic quality and cost challenges in U.S. health care. Although the descriptions do not include all of the tools or all of the challenges to the health care system, they illustrate potential contributions at all four levels of the health care system in all six characteristics identified by IOM.

The first part of this chapter is focused on three major functional areas of application for mathematical tools, namely the design, analysis, and control of large, complex systems; discussions include examples of current or potential uses in health care delivery. In the second part of the chapter, mathematical tools are considered from the perspective of the four levels of the health care system; the tools most relevant to the challenges and opportunities at each level are highlighted. Many of the tools described in this chapter are applicable to more than one level but generally address different questions or issues at each level. It will become obvious to the reader that each level of the system has different data requirements and a different reliance on information/communications technology systems.

The systems tools discussed below have been shown to provide valuable assistance in understanding the operation and management of complex systems. Some of these have been used sparingly, but successfully, in various circumstances in health care. Others will require further development and adaptation for use in the health care environment. To assist the reader in classifying these tools, they are divided into three sections: (1) tools for systems design; (2) tools for systems analysis; and (3) tools for systems control. Design tools are primarily used for creating new health care delivery systems or processes rather than improving existing systems or processes. Analysis tools can facilitate an understanding of how complex systems operate, how well they meet their overall goals (e.g., safety, efficiency, reliability, customer satisfaction), and how their performance can be improved with respect to these sometimes complementary, sometimes competing, goals. Controlling a complex system requires a clear understanding of performance expectations and the operating parameters for meeting those expectations; systems control tools, therefore, measure parameters and adjust them to achieve desired performance levels.

The reader will recognize that these categories are somewhat arbitrary—analysis is important to design, systems control is necessary for the effective operation of a system, and so on. Thus, the division is not prescriptive but is helpful for organizing the discussion.

THE NEED FOR GOOD DATA

Creating a mathematical representation that describes a feature of a system or a subsystem, although necessary, is seldom sufficient. A mathematical representation can only provide quantitative predictions of performance if it is based on good data. Therefore, sound data about the performance of the system or subsystem are also necessary.

The nature of these data depends on the problem being addressed, of course, but one important generalization can be made. In systems as complex as the health care system, processes are stochastic, that is, individual differences create significant variability over time. For example, the amount of time a physician spends with an individual patient varies greatly depending on the patient's medical condition. To analyze the system, therefore, it is necessary to know both the mean and variance for relevant process times, such as the time involved in the delivery of each process, the fraction of patients who require each process, the number and required capabilities of individual providers, and the incidence of patients who do not keep appointments. Statistical distributions of times and usage for processes and providers also vary, not only among processes, but also among facilities. No norms have been established, however, so they must be determined. These issues are addressed in the discussion on queuing theory.

The variables to be measured depend on the particular analysis and, because data collection is often time consuming,

determining which variables to measure is critical to the timely analysis of a system. However, understanding a complex system always entails time and effort to make measurements and observations.

The reader will note that the need for data is cited in many discussions of the applicability and uses of systems-engineering tools. Some of these needs can be met with a single sequence of measurements; others require massive databases. Good data are necessary to any systems analysis, but, because systems-engineering tools have not been routinely used in the health care delivery system, data for these analyses are often inadequate or missing altogether.

SYSTEMS-DESIGN TOOLS

Systems-design tools are primarily used to create systems that meet the needs/desires of stakeholders (Table 3-1). In the health care system, stakeholders include patients seeking care, health care providers, organizations that must operate efficiently and provide a satisfying environment for caregivers and patients, and participants in the regulatory/financial environment that must provide mass access to good care. The system must meet the needs of all of these stakeholders.

Concurrent Engineering

In the last 20 years, manufacturers in a variety of industries have used a procedure called concurrent engineering to design, engineer, and manufacture products that meet the needs and aspirations of customers, are defect free, and can be produced cost effectively. Concurrent engineering can be thought of as a disciplined approach to overcoming silos of function and responsibility, enabling different functional units to understand how their individual capabilities and efforts can be optimized as a system. Using concurrent engineering, a team of specialists from all affected areas (departments) in an organization is established; this team is then collectively responsible for the design of a product or process. The team considers "from the outset . . . all elements of the product life-cycle, from conception through disposal, including quality, cost, schedule, and user requirement" (Winner et al., 1988). The process begins with the initial concept and continues until a successful product or process is delivered to the customer.

Organizations that use the concurrent-engineering process have realized substantial benefits: fewer design changes are

TABLE 3-1 Systems-Design Tools

Tool/Research Area	Patient	Team	Organization	Environment
Concurrent engineering and quality function deployment		X	X	
Human-factors engineering	X	X	X	X
Tools for failure analysis		X	X	

required once the production or process has been introduced; the time from design to full production is significantly shortened; the number of defects in the product is greatly reduced; and the process (or production) costs less. In addition to these direct, readily measurable benefits, the concurrent engineering process can also yield indirect, or "spill over," benefits to an organization. These include improved cross-disciplinary/cross-unit learning, improved teamwork, improved quantitative and qualitative characterizations of processes and systems, and improved understanding and appreciation of the overall system (i.e., how the decisions and actions of individual units affect the performance of the organization as a whole.) Concurrent engineering has been used mostly in the manufacturing arena, but the idea can be applied to the health care delivery system to develop a process for delivering care rather than manufacturing a product.

Concurrent engineering teams have different compositions for different organizations (or "processes"). A concurrent engineering team for an operating room (OR), for example, would include surgeons, nurses, laboratory technicians, and others, depending on the goal. For other units of a hospital (e.g., an intensive care unit [ICU], a neonatal care unit, the business office, etc.), teams would include the individuals and members of groups relevant to that unit. For the hospital as a whole, teams would be established at many levels. Each unit team would provide input to a more comprehensive team with members from all parts of the hospital, including the admissions staff, laboratory technicians, nurses, pharmacists, physicians, physical therapists, representatives of the OR, ICU, and so on. Each unit team would receive feedback from the comprehensive team, which would provide a basis for modifying the original conclusions and moving closer to optimizing overall performance. For the extended enterprise, the team would include members of other caregiver groups (e.g., pharmacists, rehabilitation technicians, home nurses, etc.).

Simply defined, concurrent engineering is an attempt to break down silos in an enterprise through effective teamwork. Many tools have been developed to assist in this process for manufacturing operations, but for our purposes we will highlight only one—quality functional deployment (QFD).

Quality Functional Deployment[1]

QFD can be very useful for designing processes and procedures that meet the level of service a customer/patient wants. Although QFD is not a mathematical construct, it provides a structure to help the concurrent engineering team identify (1) factors that determine the quality of performance

and (2) actions that ensure the desired performance is achieved. The QFD procedure might be applicable to a team in an emergency room, the operation of an ambulatory clinic, or the operation of an entire hospital.

QFD is a *procedure* by which a stakeholder's wants/needs are spread throughout the elements of an organization to ensure that the final product/service satisfies those wants/needs. The concept of QFD, which was introduced in Japan by Katsukichi Ishihari in 1969, was later developed for U.S. manufacturers by L.P. Sullivan (1986) and Hauser and Clausing (1988). Sullivan describes QFD as "a system to assure that customer needs drive the product design and production process" by translating them into the technical requirements of the product and then into a process for delivering a product/service that meets those requirements.

QFD has been used to design a wide range of products and processes, including a new automobile (Sullivan, 1988) and wave-solder processes used in manufacturing integrated circuits (Shina, 1991). The QFD procedure is also applicable to the development of a service function, such as the design of a library system, the provision of fast food, the creation of a traffic-control system, or the delivery of health care (Chaplin et al., 1999).

The QFD process begins with the identification of team members who represent all activities involved in the creation of the final product/process/service. Team members are chosen for their expertise and not just to represent their organizational units, and the team strives to make the best decisions for the organization as a whole.

The QFD team begins by listing stakeholders' wants. The number of stakeholders can vary greatly, depending on the unit being studied. Stakeholders in the health care system could include inpatients, outpatients, ambulatory patients, physicians, nurses, payers, health care system managers, even communities, or they could include only a few of these. Once the stakeholders have been identified, the team compiles a list of their needs. Depending on who the stakeholders are, these might include ready access to physicians, low costs, absence of paperwork, prompt payment of claims, high-quality treatment, rewarding careers, keeping of appointments, financial system stability, and so forth. Obviously, some of these needs may conflict with each other. For example, physicians and nurses may not have compatible career objectives, and community expectations may differ from payers' expectations. In the initial identification step, no attempt is made to resolve these conflicts.

In step one, the team prepares a list of "what" is wanted. In step two, they prepare a list of "how" these wants can be satisfied. The second step involves translating needs (or wants) into requirements that must be met to satisfy them. An example of "whats" and "hows" for a component of an ambulatory clinic is provided in Table 3-2.

Of course, many more steps are involved in implementing QFD for a manufactured product, and similar steps are required for a QFD for the health care system. In complex

---

[1]For the purpose of illustration, the description of quality function deployment has been simplified to two steps. For complicated sub-elements of the system or for a much larger system, the process would be expanded.

TABLE 3-2 "Whats" and "Hows" for Stakeholders in an Element of an Ambulatory Care Clinic

Stakeholder Wants ("Whats")	System Attributes ("Hows")
Ready access to the physician of choice for the patient.	• Reduce caseload for physicians.
	• Better management of physician caseload.
No waiting for patients between steps during in-house procedures.	• Ensure seamless handoffs between departments.
	• Add staff and facilities.
	• Streamline processes.
Fewer repeat procedures during an examination.	• Create electronic health records (EHRs) with decision support.
Absence of errors in diagnosis.	• Use EHR system.
	• Practice evidence-based medicine.
Better understanding by the patient of his/her role in ensuring his/her health.	• Provide more counseling for patients.
	• Improve patient access to information and knowledge.
More time for nurses to spend with patients.	• Reduce paperwork.
More responsibility for nurses.	• Solicit agreement from physicians that nurses should have more responsibility.
More time for physicians to develop professional expertise.	• Reduce caseload for physicians.
More cooperation by physicians in independent practitioners' associations (IPAs) in eliminating errors.	• Provide incentives to encourage physicians in IPAs to participate.
Improved operating efficiency.	• Reduce costs.

systems in which several "hows" may be important to several "whats," the material is presented in matrices. In this simplified example, the material is presented in tabular form.

Once the "hows" have been identified, they must be translated into detailed instructions. In the QFD procedure, the right-hand column in Table 3-2 becomes the left-hand column in Table 3-3. The right-hand column in Table 3-3 then becomes the "hows" for satisfying the stakeholder needs that were identified initially. Note that even in this simple example, many of the "hows" in Table 3-3 will require a third step, and some may require more.

At this stage, some of the "whats" appear to conflict (e.g., the need for both more and less staff and facilities). In addition, the "hows" in both tables sometimes conflict. It is best

TABLE 3-3 The "Whats" and "Hows" for Meeting System Objectives

System Attributes ("Whats")	Actions ("Hows")
Smaller caseload for physicians.	• Redesign processes with input from physicians.
	• Add staff and facilities.
Creation of electronic health records (EHRs).	• Involve physicians and staff in planning the EHR system.
	• Identify responsibilities, available expertise, and consultants.
Use of the EHR system with decision support.	• Practice evidence-based medicine.
	• Ensure seamless handoffs between departments.
Less paperwork.	• Make full use of EHRs.
	• Use clinical physician order entry.
	• Write all prescriptions electronically.
Agreement by physicians that nurses take more responsibility.	• Establish multidisciplinary teams.
	• Implement training in teamwork.
	• Identify physician with responsibility.
More counseling for patients.	• Make follow-on contact by provider.
	• Use Internet.
	• Provide sources of medical information.
Incentives to encourage physicians in independent practitioners' associations to participate.	• Document improvements in quality of care.
	• Document improvements in safety.
	• Reduce wasted physician time.
	• Provide appropriate compensation for direct care and case management.
Additional staff and facilities.	• Increase number of counselors.
	• Increase number of staff capable of using engineering tools.
Lower cost.	• Make optimal use of facilities.
	• Improve scheduling of facilities.
	• Improve facility maintenance.
	• Decrease staff.

to allow conflicts to arise naturally and not to suppress them when they first occur but to resolve them in subsequent steps. Teams have a tendency to jump to conclusions in the second step instead of pursuing a careful examination of trade-offs and conflicts. Redesigning processes with input from physicians and nurses, providing training in teamwork, and documenting improvements in quality of care and safety will have immediate benefits, even though further efforts will be needed before the design of major organizational changes (the next major step) can be undertaken.

Throughout the QFD process, the team must work within certain constraints established by the organization, such as cost objectives for the final service and the time available to implement the QFD procedure. For example, the team might conclude that achieving zero errors in the writing of prescriptions by all physicians, including those associated with independent practitioners' associations, is not possible in the time frame for the project. If this is the case, the QFD steps must be repeated with modifications, which may result in changing some previously agreed upon decisions. It is essential that all members of the QFD team continue to participate in this sometimes painful process. In the unusual event that the objectives cannot be accomplished within the constraints, the team must meet with senior management and determine if the constraints can be relaxed or if the processes must be changed. These decisions must be made in conjunction with management.

The QFD process can be both time consuming and difficult, and success requires the availability of the resources of the organization. Accomplishing a QFD analysis for a complicated project requires considering a vast array of details, and QFD team members may find it necessary to consult with many people in their organizational areas and ask for detailed studies and analyses at various stages. Thus, team members will need the support of many people to accomplish their tasks, especially the support and encouragement of upper management.

Nevertheless, experience in other industries has shown that if QFD is done properly, that is, if all relevant stakeholders are involved and objectives and constraints have been well defined, the direct and indirect benefits generally far outweigh the costs and risks of the QFD process. The committee is confident that QFD applications to the design of health care delivery processes, particularly at the care-team and organization levels, will yield significant, measurable performance gains in quality and efficiency. In addition, QFD will have significant indirect or spill-over benefits in health care delivery, where disciplinary and functional silos of responsibility are deeply entrenched. Indirect benefits include improvements in the quantitative and qualitative characterization of processes and systems, improvements in cross-disciplinary/cross-unit learning, improvements in teamwork, and a better understanding and appreciation of how the actions/decisions of individual units affect the performance of the system as a whole.

Human-Factors Research

In general, complexity is the enemy of very high levels of human-systems performance. In nuclear power and aviation, this lesson was learned at great cost. Simplifying the operation of a system can greatly increase productivity and reliability by making it easier for the humans in the system to operate effectively. Adding complexity to an already complex system rarely helps and often makes things worse. In health care, however, simplicity of operation may be severely limited because health care delivery, by its very nature, includes, creates, or exacerbates many forms of complexity. Therefore, in the health care arena, success will depend on monitoring, managing, taming, and coping with changing complexities (Woods, 2000).

Human-factors engineering and related areas, such as cognitive-systems engineering, computer-supported cooperative work, and resilience engineering, focus on integrating the human element into systems analysis, modeling, and design. In health care, for example, the human-technology system of interest may be organizing an intensive care area to support cognitive and cooperative demands in various anticipated situations, such as weaning a patient off a respirator. Human-factors engineering could also provide a workload analysis to determine if a new computer interface would create bottlenecks for users, especially in situations that differ from the "textbook" scenario.

At the patient level, the focus might be on the provider-patient relationship, such as making sure instructions are meaningful to the patient or encouraging the patient's active participation in care processes (Klein and Isaacson, 2003; Klein and Meininger, 2004). At the team level, human-systems analysis might be used to assess the effectiveness of cross-checks among care groups (e.g., Patterson et al., 2004a). At the organizational level, the human-systems issue might be ensuring that new software-intensive systems promote continuity of care (e.g., avoid fragmentation and complexity). At the broadest level, human-systems engineering may focus on how accident investigations can promote learning and system improvements (Cook et al., 1989).

Patterns of human-systems interactions that have been analyzed in studies in aviation, industrial-process control, and space operations also appear in many health care settings. A single health care issue (e.g., mistakes in administering medications) is likely to involve many human-performance issues, depending on the context (e.g., Internet pharmacies, patient self-managed treatment, administration of medication through computerized infusion devices, computer-based communication in a computerized physician order entry system). For example, a human-factors analysis of the effects of nurses being interrupted while attempting to administer medication could lead to changes in work procedures. Once the processes in human performance that play out in the health care setting are understood, the human-factors knowledge base can be used to guide the development and testing of ways to improve human performance on all four levels of the health care system (Box 3-1).

Modeling, supporting, and predicting human performance in health care, as in any complex setting, requires language appropriate to different aspects of human performance. Patterns in human judgment, for example, are described in concepts such as bounded rationality, knowledge calibration, heuristics, and oversimplification fallacies (Feltovich et al., 1997). Patterns in communication and cooperative work include the concepts of supervisory control, common ground, and open versus closed work spaces (Clark and Brennan, 1991; Patterson et al., 2004b). Concepts relevant to patterns in human/computer cooperation include mental models, data overload, and mode error (Norman, 1988, 1993).

Generic patterns in human-systems performance are apparent in many health care settings, and identifying them can greatly accelerate the development of changes to improve health care. This will require integrating a medical or health care frame of reference and a human-systems frame of reference based on cognitive sciences and research on cooperative work and organizational safety. Numerous partnerships between human-factors engineers and the medical profession have already led to improvements in patient safety (Bogner, 1994; Cook et al., 1989; Hendee, 1999; Howard et

al., 1992, 1997; Johnson, 2002; Nemeth et al., 2004; Nyssen and De Keyser, 1998; Xiao and Mackenzie, 2004).

Thus, results already in the human-factors research base can provide a basis for rapid improvements in health care. A recent example is the improvement in handoffs and shift changes in health care based on a number of promising results in other industries that were directly applicable to this health care setting (Patterson et al., 2004b). Another example is in the cognitive processes involved in diagnosis. Faced with a difficult diagnosis, a provider may focus on a single point of view and exclude other possibilities (e.g., Gaba et al., 1987). Human-performance techniques (critical-incident studies and crisis simulation) have been used in other settings to study these kinds of situations and recommend ways that computer prompts and displays can be used to avoid this problem (Cook et al., 1989; Howard et al., 1992).

Another success story is the application of a human-systems perspective to improve medication-administration systems based on bar codes. The analysis of the problem involved identifying complexities and other side effects, such as workload bottlenecks and new error modes that arose when new computerized systems were introduced (e.g, Ash et al., 2004; Patterson et al., 2002). As advances in technology lead to improvements in telemedicine and the continuity

---

BOX 3-1
Improving Medical Instructions

Prescription medicines are generally accompanied by information sheets (e.g., take with food; do not use when certain other medications are being used; avoid alcohol; or store in an appropriate location). A study was undertaken to see if incorporating the principles of cognitive psychology could make medication information sheets more user friendly.

Human-factors/ergonomics (HF/E) research related to interface design, information processing, and perception suggest that the physical features (e.g., size and consistency of fonts, line spacing, etc.) of the information sheet and the language used in the text (e.g., simple, explicit, unambiguous phrases in brief sentences) can significantly affect the usability of the information. The organization of the material also influences understanding. For example, a list format is easier to understand than a prose format. These features can be especially important for patients with special limitations (e.g., elderly patients, people with short attention spans, patients under severe stress, etc.).

In the study, the readability and understandability of commercial information sheets and HF/E-modified sheets were evaluated by two groups. Sixty-two college-age students and 41 elderly subjects (ages 58 to 87) were asked to read and complete a multiple-choice test on a commercial or HF/E-modified sheet for two drugs. Subjects who read the commercial sheet for drug A were given the modified sheet for drug B. Subjects could take as much time as they needed to review each sheet and complete the test.

The review times and test times for the college-age group were 20 to 30 percent shorter than for the older group. This was statistically significant. Eighty-seven percent of the subjects overall expressed a preference for the HF/E-modified sheets. For older subjects, the reading time for the redesigned sheets was approximately 30 percent shorter than for the commercial sheets.

Even with improved physical features, simple, clear language, and clear organization, the participants in the study continued to make errors, showing that improvements were still necessary. The authors of the study concluded that "[a]dvances in medication self-management information will depend on knowledge of how users understand information and how they select a course of action. . . . Medications information sheets must accommodate the characteristics and limitations of users to be effective." Improving information sheets will require the participation of health care professionals, insurance providers, and users.

Source: Klein and Isaacson, 2003.

of care, similar applications will no doubt be useful in the future. Trade-offs will involve economic constraints and the development of new medical capabilities (e.g., Xiao et al., 2000).

As these and other examples show, human-factors research can contribute to the development of highly reliable processes, systems, and organizations in health care that would advance the goals of safety, effectiveness, efficiency, and patient-centeredness. Simplification and standardization can increase reliability in many complex systems, including complex health care systems. However, simplification and standardization alone will not be enough to manage many areas of changing complexity in health care delivery. Human-factors research and applications will also be useful for monitoring, managing, taming, and coping with these dynamic complexities.

Tools for Failure Analysis

The purpose of failure-mode effects analysis (FMEA) is to identify the ways a given procedure can fail to provide desired performance. The analysis may include disparate elements, such as the late arrival of information and laboratory errors because of a lack of information about the interactions of certain drugs. In FMEA, a mathematical model is usually created and used in the analysis.

Prior to releasing a new product design, manufacturers analyze how the product might fail under a variety of conditions. FMEA is a methodical approach to analyzing potential problems, errors, and failures and evaluating the robustness of a product design (McDonough et al., 2004). FMEA can be used to evaluate systems, product designs, processes, and services and is essential to finalizing the design of a product or identifying how a part, subsystem, or system might fail, as well as the impact of failure on safety and effectiveness. Thus, FMEA provides an opportunity to design a potential failure mode out of a product or process.

In the health care delivery system, FMEA can be helpful for designing systems (e.g., the seamless transfer of information, the implementation of electronic health records [EHRs], potential failures in the regional response to a public health emergency, etc.) on the level of health care provider teams and on the organizational level.

In addition to identifying potential design flaws, FMEA has several other benefits:

- identification of areas that require more testing or inspection to ensure high quality
- identification of areas where redundancies are justified
- prioritization of areas that require further design, testing, and analysis
- identification of areas where education could minimize the misuse or inappropriate use of a product
- foundation for reliability assessment and risk analysis
- effective communication and decision making

FMEA can be done using a bottom-up or a top-down approach, or both. A bottom-up analysis (called a failure mode, effects, and criticality analysis, or FMECA) starts at the component level, is carried through the subsystem level, and finally is used at the system level. Failure of an individual component is important, but it is equally important to understand possible failure modes when components are assembled into subsystems or systems. Wherever possible, the probability of failures and their criticality are quantified. A FMECA is redone every time a design is changed or new information from testing or preliminary field use becomes available. FMECA is used at each step until the final design meets design criteria and satisfies quality and reliability goals.

A top-down approach, called fault-tree analysis (FTA), is used to identify consequences or potential root causes of a failure event. With FTA, an undesirable event is identified and then linked to more basic events by identifying possible causes and using logic gates. FTA is an essential tool in reliability engineering for problem prevention and problem solving.

Root-cause analysis (RCA) is a qualitative, retrospective approach that is widely used to analyze major industrial accidents. An RCA can reveal latent or systems failures that underlie adverse events or near misses. In 1997, the Joint Commission on the Accreditation of Healthcare Organizations (JCAHO) mandated that RCAs be used to investigate sentinel events in its accredited hospitals. Key steps in an RCA include: (1) the creation of an interdisciplinary team; (2) data collection; (3) data analysis to determine how and why an event occurred; and (4) the identification of administrative and systems problems that should be redesigned. Although RCAs are retrospective, they identify corrections of systems problems that can prevent future errors or near misses. One caveat about RCAs is that they may be tainted by "hindsight bias," that is, after an accident, individuals tend to believe that the accident should have been considered highly likely, if not inevitable, by those who had observed the system prior to the accident (McDonough, et al., 2004).

In the past five years, the Veterans Health Administration (VHA) and JCAHO have taken several steps toward promoting the adaptation and application of FMEA, FMECA, FTA, and related tools of proactive hazard analysis and design to health care (McDonough, 2002) (see Box 3-2). In 2000, the VHA published a patient safety handbook that included instructions on FMEA and developed a health care failure-mode and effects analysis (HFMEA), "a systemic approach to identify and prevent product and process problems before they occur" (McDonough, 2002; Weeks and Bagian, 2000). In 2000, JCAHO encouraged the use of FMEA/HFMEA and related tools in its new standards that require all accredited hospitals to conduct at least one proactive risk assessment of a high-risk process every year. In 2002, JCAHO published a book specifically about FMEA for health care, which includes a step-by-step guide through the process and examples of FMEAs conducted by health care organizations (JCAHO, 2002).

BOX 3-2
Proactive Hazard Analysis

To address hazard and safety concerns in health care delivery, some have looked to other industries (e.g., aviation, manufacturing, food service, nuclear power plants, aircraft carriers) for models that can be applied to medical systems. From these sources, health professionals found frameworks for strategies and tools consistent with the needs of large clinical institutions. One prominent approach, called failure-mode and effects analysis (FMEA), which has been used in manufacturing for more than 30 years, was adapted for health care organizations. The health care failure-mode and effects analysis (HFMEA) is now being used by the Veterans Administration (VA) National Center for Patient Safety (NCPS).

In 2000, the Joint Commission on Accreditation of Healthcare Organizations (JCAHO) issued a new standard stipulating that all accredited hospitals must complete at least one "proactive risk assessment" of a high-risk process each year. JCAHO did not specify whether FMEA or HFMEA should be used, but its own approach to fulfilling this requirement is based on the terminology and structure of these two models. The first surveys were to be completed by July 1, 2002.

Hazard analysis and critical control points (HACCP), another form of proactive hazard analysis, also provides a useful framework for improving safety. HACCP, which is used in food production and food services worldwide, is now being used by medical-device manufacturers.

Although FMEA, HFMEA, and HACCP differ in significant ways, they also have striking similarities. The table below shows the basic steps in performing an HFMEA analysis and an HACCP. The five steps in the HFMEA are described in materials produced by the VA NCPS. The HACCP procedure has been slightly modified from a 14-step process to highlight the similarities with HFMEA. Both tools involve the selection of a process and/or product, the selection of a team, the creation of a process flow chart, the identification of hazards or failures, corrective or preventive action, ongoing monitoring and assessment, and process review. Both rely on decision making based on data, cross-functional teams, and, most important, a preventive approach to hazard/failure mode identification and elimination or reduction.

Because these analysis tools were developed for use in different sectors, they also have some differences in emphasis. In FMEA, the hazard is a failure mode in a process, and the principal goal is to redesign the process to reduce or eliminate the risk of the failure mode recurring. In HACCP, the hazard is unsafe food, and the primary goal is to control the process at critical points to eliminate or reduce the risk of the hazard. Thus the goal of FMEA/HFMEA is to reduce process failure. The goal of HACCP is to detect and control process failure to eliminate or reduce bad effects.

TABLE HFMEA and HACCP Steps

Step	HFMEA	HACCP
1.	Define the HFMEA topic.	Identify the hazard category.
2.	Assemble the team.	Assemble the team.
3.	Graphically describe the process: • Develop a flow diagram. • Number each process step. • Identify the key process step. • Identify sub-processes. • Create a flow diagram of the subprocesses.	Describe the product or process: • Identify the intended use. • Construct a flow diagram from point of entry to departure. • Confirm accuracy of flow diagram.
4.	Conduct a failure analysis: • List all potential failure modes. • Determine the severity and probability of each failure mode. • Use the HFMEA decision tree to determine if the failure mode requires further action. • Where the decision is to proceed, list all causes for each failure mode.	Conduct a hazard analysis: • Identify all relevant hazards and preventive measures. • Identify critical control points and apply a decision tree to determine if intervention is needed. • Establish target levels and critical limits for critical control points.
5.	Action and outcome measures: • Determine if you want to eliminate, control, or accept the failure mode cause. • Identify a description of action for each failure mode to be eliminated or controlled. • Identify outcome measures to test the redefined process. • Identify an individual to complete the recommended action. • Indicate whether top management concurs with recommended action.	Action and outcome measures: • Establish a monitoring system to ensure proper .implementation • Establish verification procedures. • Establish documentation and record keeping.
6.		Review HACCP plan: • Conduct reviews at predetermined intervals to determine whether working and still appropriate.

Source: McDonough, 2002.

SYSTEMS-ANALYSIS TOOLS

Engineers use system analysis to help themselves and others understand how complex systems operate, how well systems meet overall goals and objectives, and how they can be improved. On one level, a systems analysis may focus on the performance of a single unit in a large system (e.g., the flow of patients through a facility or the allocation of resources in an emergency room). The results of these studies can be used to evaluate how changes in procedures might improve performance (e.g., reduce patient delays, improve safety, eliminate nonessential steps). At a higher level, a systems analysis may consider interactions among elements in a large system, such as a hospital, a regional medical enterprise, or even the national health care delivery system. Obviously, the larger the system, the more complex and the more difficult the analysis. But a careful analysis of systems at all levels can reveal interactions and opportunities for improvement that might otherwise be missed. Table 3-4 shows the levels for which various systems-analysis tools are most useful.

Systems-analysis tools are generally used to analyze existing systems for improvement. Mathematical analyses of system operations include queuing theory, which could be used, for example, to understand the flow of patients through a system, the average time patients spend in the system, or bottlenecks in the system. Discrete-event simulation could be used for a more detailed examination of performance, such as an analysis of surges of patients on particular days or during emergencies or the scheduling of ambulances.

With enterprise-management tools, a system can be managed as a whole across the entire spectrum of elements, rather than at the level of individual patients. In spite of the fragmented nature of the health care system, interactions among all elements in the total chain can be clarified and managed. Supply-chain management tools, for example, are useful for determining the physical and informational resources necessary to the delivery of a product to a customer (e.g., reducing inventory, eliminating delays, reducing cost, etc.).

Economic and econometric models, based on historical data, are useful for bringing to light causal relationships among system variables. These tools include game theory, systems-dynamics modeling, data-envelopment analysis, and productivity modeling. Financial engineering, risk management, and market models, which are used to evaluate and manage risks, can be useful for examining financial risks to an organization, as well as for understanding the risks of certain actions for/by patients.

Knowledge discovery in databases is a method that can be used to examine large databases (e.g., a database of patient reactions to groups of drugs). It might be used, for example, to examine the history of particular drugs or treatments or to examine procedures for patients with particular life styles or health histories. With knowledge-discovery tools, one might search historical records for an effective procedure or identify outlier events, such as a small number of patients who share a condition and experience unexpected side effects from a medication.

Because system analyses must describe an existing system (or one that reasonably approximates an existing system), it is essential that data be available (or obtainable) for that system. The nature of the data depends on the problem being addressed. Analyzing a system to improve the efficiency of a surgical operation requires very different data from an analysis to assess the effectiveness of a disease-management program.

GEORGE BROWN COLLEGE
CASA LOMA LIBRARY LEARNING COMMONS

TABLE 3-4 Systems-Analysis Tools

Tool/Research Area	Patient	Team	Organization	Environment
Modeling and Simulation				
Queuing methods		X	X	
Discrete-event simulation		X	X	X
Enterprise-Management Tools				
Supply-chain management		X	X	X
Game theory and contracts		X	X	X
Systems-dynamics models		X	X	X
Productivity measuring and monitoring		X	X	X
Financial Engineering and Risk Analysis Tools				
Stochastic analysis and value-at-risk			X	X
Optimization tools for individual decision making	X		X	X
Distributed decision making (market models and agency theory)			X	X
Knowledge Discovery in Databases				
Data mining			X	X
Predictive modeling		X	X	X
Neural networks		X	X	X

0134109617552

Modeling and Simulation

Models and simulations are important tools for analyzing systems. Models are mathematical constructs that describe the performance of subsystems. Interactions among subsystems in a larger system, combined with the constraints within which the system operates, influence the performance of the total system and represent the overall system model. Using these models and simulations, it becomes possible to analyze the expected performance of a system if systemic changes are made. For example, would a change in inventory location and levels improve or reduce the effectiveness of the nursing staff? Would a change in scheduling of the emergency room increase or decrease the number of patients that must be diverted and at what cost?

Models have been developed for a variety of health care applications that do not directly involve physical facilities. For instance, multiple models have been developed to examine the effectiveness of screening and treatment protocols for many diseases, including colorectal cancer, lung cancer, tuberculosis, and HIV (Brandeau, 2004; Brewer et al., 2001; Eddy et al., 1987; Fone et al. 2003; Mahadevia et al., 2003; Neilson and Whynes, 1995; Ness et al., 2000; Phillips et al., 2001; Schaefer et al., 2004; Walensky et al., 2002). In addition, many models have implications for health care policy; for example, models might suggest that efforts to reduce tobacco use in adults would be most beneficial in the short term, whereas blocking the introduction of tobacco to young people is more likely to have long-term benefits (Levy et al., 2000; Teng et al., 2001). Hospitals and clinics have used simulations to improve staffing and scheduling (Dittus et al., 1996; Hashimoto and Bell, 1996), and models have been used to help clinicians distinguish injuries caused by falls down stairs from those resulting from child abuse (Bertocci et al., 2001). Virtual-reality patients have been used for training in psychiatry, the social sciences, surgery, and obstetrics (Letterie, 2002).

Queuing Theory

Queuing theory deals with problems that involve waiting (queuing), lines that form because resources are limited. The purpose of queuing theory is to balance customer service (i.e., shorter waiting times) and resource limitations (i.e., the number of servers). Queuing models have long been used in many industries, including banking, computers, and public transportation. In health care, they can be used, for example, to manage the flow of unscheduled patient arrivals in emergency departments, ORs, ICUs, blood laboratories, or x-ray departments. Queuing models can be used to address the following questions:

- How long will the average patient have to wait?
- How long will it take, on average, to complete a visit?
- What is the likelihood that a patient will have to wait for more than 20 minutes?

- How long are providers occupied with an average patient?
- How many personnel would be necessary for all patients to be seen within 10 minutes?
- Would flow be improved if certain patients were triaged differently?
- What resources would be necessary to improving performance to a given level or standard?
- What is the likelihood that a hospital will have to divert patients to another hospital?

Queuing is a descriptive modeling tool that "describes" steady-state functioning of the flow through systems. Although health care is rarely in a steady state, from a mathematical point of view, queuing models provide useful approximations that are surprisingly accurate.

Queuing models are generally based on three variables that define the system: arrival rate; service time; and the number of servers. The arrival rate, λ, describes the frequency of the arrival of patients. The most common type of unscheduled arrival pattern can be described with the Poisson distribution (Huang, 1995). Service time, T, is the average time spent serving a particular type of patient at a given station. In health care, the service time is most often random and is most commonly described by an exponential probability distribution. Number of servers, n, is the number of stations doing similar tasks for all patients who approach those stations.

For a station with a single server, average arrival rate of patients (λ) multiplied by the average time patients spend with a given server (T) must be less than or equal to unity (i.e., $\lambda T \leq 1$). Otherwise the queue would continue to build up without relief. If n servers are present, $\lambda T \leq n$. In the absence of variability, no queues would build up and the flow through the station would be regular. In the presence of variability, which always exists, queues will build up. The closer λT is to 1, the longer the queues for that station. The bottleneck station in the network can be identified by locating the station with the largest λT.

For a single station with the probability distributions described above, the response time for the station (the average time for a patient to pass through the station) is given by

$$Response\ Time = T/(1 - \lambda T).$$

As λT approaches unity, the response time becomes very long.

To manage flow well, service areas must measure critical indices derived from the model; these may include, but are not limited to, utilization (percentage of time servers are busy, waiting time, length of waiting lines), probability of diversion (rejection), abandonment rates, bottlenecks, and door-to-door time (time of actual arrival to time of actual departure).

It is critical that the full variability of the metrics be measured and displayed. Often the data mean or median is calculated and graphed, but this does not give a true picture of variability. If the measures were constant and could be predicted by the mean, the problem of managing flow would not exist!

Queuing theory can provide analytical expressions for a single station, but analytical expressions for a network of stations require computer programs that can approximate the performance of a network. Once the network description has been entered, the performance of the network can usually be analyzed quickly.

The law that applies to systems with queues, Little's law, enables one to determine either the number of patients being served in a facility, for example a clinic or a hospital, or the average time a patient spends in the facility. If L is the average number of entities (patients) in a system that contains a variety of locations at which procedures are performed, that is, servers, Little's law states that

$$L = \lambda W$$

where λ is the average arrival rate into the system and W is the average time each patient spends in the system (the sum of the average time patients spend waiting plus the average time they spend with caregivers). If either L or W is known, the other can be calculated easily.

One problem in health care today is that the number of facilities that have unscheduled patient flows is increasing, while the number of people available to treat them is decreasing. This situation requires new management approaches, methods of reducing waiting times and keeping emergency departments from turning away patients, such as building in segmentation, matching capacity to demand using queuing theory, and creating surge capacity and backup plans for exigencies. Because of variabilities in patient demand, fixed bed and staffing levels are almost always either too high or too low, which has ramifications for both the quality and cost of care. Queuing models allow for natural variabilities, which leads to greater predictability and control and, ultimately, more timely and safer patient care. Queuing theory has been used (although infrequently) to analyze a variety of clinical settings, including emergency departments, primary care practices, operating rooms, nursing homes, and radiology departments (Gorunescu et al., 2002; Huang, 1995; Lucas et al., 2001; Murray and Berwick, 2003; Reinus et al., 2000; Siddharthan et al., 1996).

Discrete-Event Simulation

In discrete-event simulation, the dependent variables are "actors" in, or are developed by, the system. In a health care system, these can include patients, caregivers, administrators, inventory, capital equipment, and others. The independent variable is time. In this type of simulation, it is expected that events take place at discrete points in time (e.g., the arrival of two patients at Station C, one at time t_1, the second at a later time, t_2).

A key aspect of a discrete-event simulation is the system-state description, which includes values for all of the variables in the system. If any variable changes, it changes the system state. In a simulation, the dynamic behavior of the system can be observed as entities (e.g., patients, staff, inventory) move through the nodes and activities (e.g., registration desk, nurse's preliminary examination, physician's examination, laboratory tests, etc.) identified in the model. The rules governing the motion of entities and the paths they follow are peculiar to the specific model and are specified by the modeler. Describing systems that involve human interactions requires the use of mathematics based on probability theory and statistics, which can describe the variabilities and discreteness of events. Computers are necessary to analyze the many states in complex systems.

In most cases, the initial system state must first be specified, that is, values must be supplied for the variables and their variances based on observations of an existing system or a system sufficiently similar. The model can then be tested to see if it describes the performance of the existing system. If it does not, it must be adjusted, perhaps by including different variables or by treating interactions among the variables in different ways. Once the model has been validated, it can be used to explore the consequences of different actions.

If each variable had only one possible value (e.g., the number of nurses available in the prenatal clinic at 10:05 a.m.), a single calculation would be sufficient to describe a system. But most system variables have a distribution of values, such as the differences in the number of nurses needed throughout the day in Surgical Ward 2 of the hospital. Thus, many computer runs must be made to explore combinations of values of the variables. Tools are readily available for determining how various computer outputs should be grouped and interpreted.

Discrete-event simulation has been used to analyze a number of health care settings, such as operating rooms, emergency rooms, and prenatal-care wards (Klein et al., 1993), and a variety of workforce planning problems. The overall objective has been to improve or optimize the safety, efficiency, and or effectiveness of processes and systems. Kutzler and Sevcovic (1980) developed a simulation model of a nurse-midwifery practice. Duraiswamy et al. (1981) simulated a 20-bed medical ICU that included patient census, patient acuity, and required staffing on a daily basis for one year. A simulation of obstetric anesthesia developed by Reisman et al. (1977) was used to determine the optimal configuration of an anesthesia team. Magazine (1977) describes a patient transportation service problem in a hospital; queuing analysis and simulation were used to determine the number of transporters necessary to ensure availability 95 percent of the time. Bonder (see paper in this volume), describes a simulation for a very large-scale, level-four analysis of a regional health care system in the Puget Sound area of Washington. Pritsker (1998) describes the development and use of a large-scale simulation model to improve the allocation policy for liver transplants (see Box 3-3).

Dittus et al. (1996) developed a simulation model of an academic county hospital to determine if alternative call schedules would address the problem of provider fatigue among the house staff. As a result, a new call schedule was implemented, and the model's predictions of work and sleep were validated against provider behavior under the new schedule. This prospective, empirical, hypothesis-driven validation demonstrated that a well constructed model can accurately characterize system behavior and predict future performance, even in a complex environment, such as the life of a medical resident in a busy county hospital.

These analyses have demonstrated that performance of complex units can be improved in terms of responsiveness and the allocation of resources. Discrete-event simulation can be used to simulate dynamic systems—systems in transition, new systems being developed, systems that have time irregularities, and others.

Enterprise-Management Tools

Enterprise-management tools are helpful for management on a system level and across component boundaries. For example, enterprise management has been used successfully for mass customization—a process by which every product is tailored to meet the specific needs and wants of an individual customer. In the portfolio of products offered by a manufacturer, many products have common components and common functions. For example, new cars may have a wide range of options, but the frame and many components of all new cars are the same. A mass customization production system offers customers a great deal of flexibility in specifying the final product.

An effective, efficient health care delivery system demands the same flexibility as "mass customization" of a manufactured product. The key to meeting individual customer or patient needs without sacrificing operating efficiency is maintaining a high level of flexibility (Champion et al., 1997). The mathematical tools described below can help health care managers maintain a system that balances the need for resources against the demand for those resources. In the health care setting, enterprise-management tools can be useful on the level of care teams, organizations, and the environment.

Early in the twentieth century, industrial pioneers could not have imagined that complex systems that include networks of suppliers, manufacturers, distributors, retailers, and service providers would be widespread in the manufacturing industry. These complex supply chains, which bring products made from raw materials to consumers around the globe, are some of the most efficient and complex socioeconomic systems in the world. Companies such as Dell Computer, Westin Hotels, Toyota, American Express, Procter & Gamble, and others have all benefited enormously from mass customization (Chandler, 1990; Gertz and Baptista, 1995; Reichheld, 1996).

Health care delivery, like other business enterprises, is a complex socioeconomic system in which multiple agents, often with very different agendas, interact. As in complex business enterprises, decisions taken by one party can significantly affect the costs incurred and the quality of service provided by other parties in the system. In addition, different entities in the system, so-called agents, often have different, sometimes conflicting, objectives. The history of enterprise-management systems has shown that a thorough understanding of how different agents in the system interact can yield significant benefits for the entire system.

Supply-Chain Management

Analyzing and optimizing systems with a great many participants and components is particularly difficult because no one can understand the entire system in detail. Supply-chain management is an engineering tool that recognizes and characterizes interactions among subsystems (see Ryan, in this volume). Supply-chain management tools can also be used to explore the consequences (expected and unexpected, and likelihood thereof) of reimbursement decisions, which may not become evident for years.

In an environment in which demands vary unpredictably, supply-chain management can help match resources with demands. In the health care delivery system, resources include human capital (e.g., nurses, therapists), physical capital (e.g., intensive care beds, ambulances, sponges), and intellectual capital (e.g., a patient medical record or an evidence-based medicine protocol). The stochastic nature of the demand for services and the inconsistent availability and effectiveness of resources always generate a great deal of variability in the health care system. Policy decisions in one part of the system, such as a decision by an insurer not to fund a preventive procedure, can have unexpected consequences for other parts of the system, which may only become apparent after a period of years.

Capacity and variability are at the heart of how components of supply chains operate (see Uzoy, in this volume). Whether we are considering two neighboring elements in a system or blocks of elements that interact with other elements, the input-output relationships are often nonlinear and must be treated that way in any mathematical representation of how variables interact in the presence of constraints on the system.

The coordination of geographically distributed operations owned by a single firm has been addressed for several decades by increasingly sophisticated optimization models, such as linear integer programs that optimize performance within a large number of constraints. Nonlinear programming has progressed to the point that models of significant scale and complexity can be developed. The primary disadvantage of these techniques is that, although they are

BOX 3-3
Allocation Policy for Organ Transplantations

The scarcity of livers for transplantation makes allocation extremely difficult. Approximately 4,000 donated livers were available in the United States in 1996 and 1997. In mid-1998, about 10,000 individuals were on the waiting list for liver transplants, and 8,000 were expected to be added in 1999. More than 1,100 patients awaiting transplants died in 1997. The allocation process is complicated by the geographical distribution of 63 organ procurement organizations and 106 transplant centers.

The purpose of the allocation policy is to set priorities for patients awaiting transplants. Measures for allocation procedures include: medical utility, such as the number of transplants and the number of deaths; patient utility, such as the probabilities of a patient receiving a transplant or dying while waiting; system utility, such as distance an organ had to be transported; medical equity, such as the total number of transplants; patient equity, such as differences in the probability of specific patients receiving a transplant; and system equity, such as geographic differences in the length of the waiting list.

A large-scale simulation model, ULAM for UNOS Liver Allocation Model, was developed to determine whether the allocation model used in the 1990s (SPF-Nat) could be improved. ULAM was based on modular techniques, wherein component models or submodels enabled new data to be inserted as they became available. The simulation was developed according to four guidelines: (1) the component models were based on historical data; (2) data and models for the policy analysis were kept up to date; (3) important operational procedures were embedded in the model; and (4) continual communication was maintained between policy makers and decision makers.

Historical data were available for 1950 to 1990, and the arrival streams of donors and patients were separately described by analytic expressions of their distributions over time. A characteristic for each donor was determined using a bootstrapping technique matching the donor with an individual in the 1990 to 1995 time frame according to age, weight, race, sex, and blood type. A similar approach was used for patients added to the waiting list.

ULAM included snapshots of patients on the waiting list at the beginning of the year; new patients were assigned characteristics and added to the list. The medical status of each patient was coded as 1, 2A, 2B, or 3, depending on medical condition using the Child-Turcotte-Pugh procedure. Status 1 is an acute patient who needs a liver immediately or a patient whose transplant has failed within seven days of transplant. Status 2A and 2B are less critical (2B is used for patients under 18). Status 3 is the least clinically ill. The probability of acceptance depended on the medical status of the patient, the transplant center, and the quality of the liver being offered. When a recovered liver was offered and accepted the patient was removed from the list. The probability that the graft might fail was then determined based on historical outcomes of patients with similar characteristics. If the graft then failed, the patient was relisted. Time-to-relist functions were developed for each medical status based on historical data from 1991 to 1995. If the patient was not relisted, mortality was determined by (1) the transplant center volume; (2) medical condition at the time of transplant; and (3) whether the patient had undergone a previous transplant. To model change in a patient's medical status while on the waiting list, a transition probability matrix (a Markov chain) was constructed to model day-to-day changes.

When ULAM was tested against historical data for verification and validation, the output of each component of the model, as well as the total output of the model, showed good agreement with actual results from 1992 to 1994. Once the model had been validated, a protocol was created (CP97). The table below shows expected outputs from CP97 and SPF-Nat for 1996 to 2003.

General Measures of Performance

	Policy	
	CP97	SPF-Nat
General measures		
Number of differential patients treated	25,023.5	23,515.3
Number of retransplants	2,998.9	4,508.6
Total	28,022.4	28,023.9
Number of survivors (> 36 mo.)	17,073.7	14,660.4
Number of pediatric patients (< 18 yrs)	2,765.9	3,173.1
Number of post-treatment deaths (< 12 mo.)	5,480.9	7,280.2
Percentage of survivals (> 12 mo.)	79.9	70.6
Percentage of survivals (> 36 mo.)	74.4	66.2

The CP97 showed an increase of 1,509 because CP97 patients were not as sick as SPF-Nat patients; thus, they had less chance of being relisted and requiring more than one transplant (retransplanted patients tend to be sicker, have a lower chance of survival, and require additional transplants). With the CP97 policy, 2,414 more patients would be expected to survive for more than 36 months, again because the patients were not always the sickest patients on the list.

As Alan Pritsker, senior consultant, Pritsker Corporation, noted, "The modeling process and the creation of the ULAM tool is an excellent example of how doctors, engineers, researchers and scientists have worked together to . . . improve policy selection and implementation. It is also an illustration of the contributions that we can make to policy formulation and analysis."

Note: Simulation analysis for liver transplants continues under other auspices. The levels of liver criticality have been expanded from 4 to 17, and the waiting list continues to grow. Source: Pritsker, 1998.

relatively straightforward (at least on a conceptual level) when the entire system is controlled by a single entity with a single well defined objective, they present great difficulties when independent agents with different objectives and constraints interact, as can occur, for example, when a supplier has more than one customer for a particular product. Advanced modeling techniques are just now being applied to these problems, but a great deal more research in this area will be necessary.

Examples of how supply-chain management models work follow. In the late 1980s, American Airlines used an integer linear programming model to assign crews for more than 2,300 flights per day to more than 150 different cities using 500 jet aircraft. The mathematical model was sufficiently detailed that one could examine the effects on the system of allocating resources in different ways. As a result of the modeling effort, the airline made decisions regarding fleet planning, crew-base planning, and schedule development that resulted in a 0.5 percent reduction in operating cost and a $75 million increase in revenue in 1988 (Abara, 1989). Vanderbilt University Medical Center used a supply-chain management process to redesign its perioperative services. This project reduced costs by $2.3 million and improved the quality of care by ensuring that appropriate clinical supplies were delivered during the perioperative period (Feistritzer and Keck, 2000). The Deaconess Hospital of Evansville, Indiana, used a supply-chain management tool to improve its drug distribution in the operating room; savings totaled $115,000 in the first year (Thomas et al., 2000). It has been estimated that the health care industry could save more than $11 billion a year with supply-chain management techniques (McKesson, 2002).

Tools that can be used to examine the system at a higher level of abstraction are just evolving (Pierskalla, 2004; Uszoy, in this volume). These tools will support the modeling of large, complex systems involving interactions among many, possibly thousands, of agents with specific objectives and constraints. However, developers of modeling techniques at this level have encountered a number of difficulties. First, because of the sheer size and complexity of the systems, the efforts involved in developing and documenting models are very time consuming. In addition, data that provide realistic estimates of critical parameters to populate these models are often hard to obtain, if they are available at all. For example, considering the number of health care providers a patient deals with over a lifetime, data will have to be collected systematically over many years. Most existing tools for such modeling have significant drawbacks that have only recently begun to be understood and addressed.

Economic and Econometric Models

The economic and econometric models described below primarily use statistical techniques to elucidate causal relationships among system variables; these models are generally based on historical data and can have different levels of predictive power. Models based exclusively on time series, in which the only independent variable considered is time, essentially assume that past history is representative of the future. Models such as data-envelopment analysis that try to develop causal relationships between system-performance measures and independent variables other than time are often more enlightening but require much more detailed data.

In the context of health care delivery, these models might be used to determine the needs of certain segments of a population based on their economic situation, for example, or the relationship between different types of preventive treatments for a disease and the progression of the disease over patients' lifetimes. Extensive studies of this kind are already widely used in various aspects of health care, such as the approval of new drugs and diagnostic tests by the Food and Drug Administration (Ness et al., 2003; O'Neill and Dexter, 2004; Ozcan et al., 2004). More than a decade ago, the Commonwealth of Australia passed into law guidelines requiring an economic assessment of new drug applications for its national formulary (Freund et al., 1992).

Game Theory and Contracts. Game theory examines how agents with different agendas behave when they interact. The game-theory framework for addressing these interactions has recently been used in a number of simple models of supply-chain management. Extensive research has also been done on different types of contracts between parties that can provide incentives for actors to behave in ways that benefit the overall system (Tsay and Nahmias, 1998).

A significant difficulty with these models is that their solutions generally pertain to the long-run steady state of the system. Not much has been done by way of studying how well these techniques work in transient regimes, for example, when the constituent members of a patient's care team change over time. Many of these models also assume perfect information sharing, which is unlikely in practice, and researchers are beginning to examine the effects of different information-sharing protocols, as can occur among care providers in a distributed network of providers or when patients must undergo emergency treatment by someone other than their primary caregivers. In short, a great deal of research remains to be done in this area.

Systems-Dynamics Models. Based on pioneering work by Forrester (1961), systems-dynamics models define specific input-output relationships for system components and use them to simulate the operation of a system, basically using techniques derived from the numerical solution of systems of differential equations. These techniques have been used to solve business problems for many years (Sterman, 2000) and can be used to model large, complex systems. However, they require accurate definitions of input-output relationships because feedback loops with gain and loss coefficients are used to capture system behavior. If these parameters are not estimated correctly, model results can be substantially wrong.

Nevertheless, systems-dynamics models can be powerful tools for gaining a high-level understanding of the behavior of large systems, as has been demonstrated by their prediction of the "bullwhip effect" in supply chains, whereby the variability of orders placed by different parties is amplified at each stage of the supply chain, ultimately causing huge swings for the manufacturer (who is "whipped" about). For example, because of variability in orders for replenishing stock (e.g., medicines in pharmacies), manufacturers must make assumptions regarding future needs, which can lead to either undersupply or oversupply that can have serious economic consequences for the manufacturer. WalMart, a mass retailer with a large network of stores, has minimized the bullwhip effect in its supply chain by sending point-of-sales data directly to manufacturers. System-dynamics modeling has been used to analyze emergency care systems and other aspects of health care delivery (Lattimer et al., 2004).

Measuring and Monitoring Productivity. Despite an ambitious, well defined quality agenda, there has been little direct interaction between the engineering community and the health care community in the development of productivity measures and monitoring systems. Until recently, the measurement of productivity in the health care sector has been seriously hampered by a limited understanding of the relationships between inputs, outputs, and outcomes for different patient populations. For the most part, health care providers are trained to focus on the unique characteristics and needs of individual patients; they have very little training or perspective on the characteristics (and needs) of patient populations.

The advance of evidence-based medicine and disease management, which focus on patient populations, is encouraging the development of more uniform/standardized output- and outcome-based performance measures based on the response of defined patient populations to best-practice, "standardized" interventions. For example, for patient populations with x condition (and y degree of severity), there is a best-practice treatment (i.e., the most evidence-based, safest, timeliest, most patient centered treatment) that yields the best outcome (i.e., the most positive change in health state) for the lowest cost (i.e., the most efficient use of inputs and infrastructure).

Modeling and simulation of care delivery processes and systems can help care provider teams and organizations better understand, test, and optimize the processes/systems that support best-practice use of inputs (e.g., people, resources, facilities, equipment, information on patient conditions, evidence-based medicine) to achieve "best" outputs that contribute to best patient outcomes. Over time, the progress of automation and the widespread implementation of information/communications systems in health care delivery and advances in the fields of genomic/proteomics should enable the capture of more detailed input, patient population, process, and outcomes data. This will lead to a more sophisticated understanding and better measurements of the quality and productivity performance of health care delivery at all levels of the system and facilitate the application of more sophisticated analytical and predictive systems tools.

At the present time, the health care system, like many other service industries, does not have good measures of productivity. Although the efficiency of a given unit can often be determined, measuring the efficiency and productivity of a system is much more difficult. With the help of a number of the systems tools described above, performance metrics can be established and the impact of various changes on those metrics can be estimated. Additional research on the measurement of productivity would be of great benefit to the health care community.

Financial-Engineering Tools for Risk Management

The effective operation of any system requires management of risks. In health care, risk management is critical because of the substantial personal risks for individual patients and the financial and reputational risks for providers, insurers, and purchasers of health care. Risk-management tools can substantially improve the delivery of health care by improving the financing of operations and the allocation of resources, reducing individual exposures to extreme risks, and creating incentives for improving processes. Tools to assist in decision making in the presence of risks are as useful to individual patients and care teams as they are to organizations and the regulatory agencies and other actors in the larger environment.

In this section, risks are identified and general processes of risk management and financial engineering are described. This is followed by a description of financial-engineering tools that could have significant benefits for the health care delivery system at the organizational and environmental levels of the system.

In this report, *risk* is defined broadly as the chance of injury, damage, or loss, and the focus is on reducing variations that lead to extreme risks. The goal of risk management is to reduce risk to the patient, caregiver, or organization by ensuring predictability in the use of resources within the constraints of a fixed expenditure of funds.

Effective risk management requires that the kinds of risk be differentiated. In health care, individual risks, or patient risks, are potential compromises to the health of an individual caused by some action of the system. Other kinds of risk involve potential losses at higher levels of the health care system. Care team members face occupational risks, such as exposure to disease, physical duties, and workplace hazards (e.g., exposure to toxic substances, radiation, and equipment malfunctions). Health care organizations also face a variety of risks (McDonough et al., 2004):

- operational risk, which includes all risks associated with the delivery of services
- competitor risk, such as the potential of losing market share to competitors
- financial risk, such as the risk of nonpayment or reduced payment for services or the risk of significant financial liability
- environmental risk, such as the risk of damage by forces external to the organization
- model risk, that is, the risk that the models used for evaluating other types of risk are not accurate

Risks at the political-economic environmental level are incurred not only by individual organizations, but can also arise from interactions among organizations, the lack of adaptability of organizations, and the misalignment of individual and societal objectives.

Risk management in the health care system involves the analysis and assessment of risks, as well as the development of strategies to reduce risk, protect against losses, and ensure that risks transferred from one agent to another are compensated fairly. Risk management generally answers the following questions:

- What can create a loss?
- How often, how severe, and when can losses occur?
- Which losses are manageable?
- How can risks be transferred elsewhere?
- What is fair compensation for assuming or releasing risks?
- How does risk affect the overall strategy of the organization?

In a general corporate context, risk management can lead to more productive employees; less volatility in revenue and cost changes; better coordination among organizational units, as well as with suppliers and customers; more effective purchases and sales of risk-based products; and the development of organizational structures that achieve risk-management goals.

One of the key tools for risk management is financial engineering, the application of mathematical and computational tools to financial issues (see Mulvey, in this volume). Financial engineering includes modeling and predicting markets, evaluating options and other financial derivatives, allocating assets and liabilities, trading in financial markets, determining policies for efficient market development, and providing quantitative and information services for financial markets. The overall goal of most financial engineering is to increase return on *resources invested* (a measure of performance or effectiveness) while reducing risk.

An increase in return on investment and a simultaneous reduction in risk ultimately increases efficiency. The objective is to increase the output for a given amount of input, as well as to control the reliability, predictability, and consistency of the process that creates these outputs. Viewed as a mechanism for improving efficiency, financial engineering is a product of the traditional fields of industrial engineering and operations research, for which the overall goal is to produce a system that yields the best possible product or process in terms of quality, customer/patient value, low cost, and timely response.

The following sections describe three major areas of financial engineering that are most relevant to the risk analysis/management needs of health care organizations and environmental level actors.

Predicting and Assessing Uncertain Outcomes: Stochastic Analysis and Value-at-Risk

To manage risk, it must first be quantified, analyzed, predicted, and forecast. Some analyses assume existing conditions and rely on statistical descriptors of the frequency and extent of previous outcomes. Statistical analysis focuses on what has happened in the past and how it relates to an entire population. Stochastic analysis, the main type of analysis in financial engineering, infers current or future behavior for systems with random outcomes that follow assumed, observed, or approximated distributions. Stochastic analysis is also the tool used in predicting and quantifying risk.

The financial-engineering concept of value-at-risk (VaR) is a widely used tool of stochastic analysis. VaR is used to measure the worst expected loss over a given time interval under normal market conditions at a given confidence level (Jorion, 1997). For example, a bank with a billion-dollar portfolio might state that its daily VaR is $10 million at the 99 percent confidence level. This means there is only one chance in 100, under normal market conditions, that the bank will experience a loss of more than $10 million in a day. The VaR summarizes the bank's exposure to market risk and the probability of an adverse move. If managers and shareholders are uncomfortable with the level of risk, the process used to calculate the VaR can be used to decide where risk should be reduced.

VaR has become a standard measure for the banking industry and a required measure in regulatory compliance for capital requirements. Because VaR captures potential loss and likelihood, it has also become a common measure for firms outside the banking industry and may become a general standard in risk management.

A basic form of VaR estimation is to assume a probability distribution for the values of risky assets. For a bank that holds stocks, for example, the distribution might be a form of multivariate-normal or log-normal distribution. A typical VaR analysis would then form an estimate of the parameters of this distribution and the mean, variances, and covariances of the stock returns over a given period of time. Generally, these estimates are based on statistical analyses of stock returns (perhaps with corrections for current conditions). Once the parameters have been determined, the overall value distribution of the portfolio can be found. VaR is the difference between the first percentile of the cumulative distribution and the current value of the portfolio.

VaR also has useful characteristics for health care analyses. Besides being used for financial management in health care, VaR can also be used to assess potential losses for many groups of insured patients in a given period. Cash requirements for health care organizations can be estimated and the value of assuming and transferring risks can be assessed.

VaR is just one financial-engineering tool that may be of benefit to health care. Other tools that might be relevant include credit assessments of individuals and organizations, pricing of services, pricing of risks that exceed given levels (i.e., derivative pricing), and valuations of combined risks for engaging in multiple markets (e.g., worker compensation, health insurance, and life-risk insurance).

Optimization Tools for Individual Decision Making

Financial engineering tools are not only descriptive (e.g., stochastic and statistical analyses), but also prescriptive. Thus, they can provide a basis for making decisions to yield best results. Decision making under uncertainty (also known as stochastic programming), an essential aspect of operations research, is based on optimization tools that can compute best values for variables in mathematical representations of the decision process and measure outcomes (objectives). Optimization tools in this context rely on the stochastic analysis of the effects of uncertainty and the relationship between those effects and the decisions represented in the mathematical model.

Optimization under uncertainty has had a wide range of applications in the financial industry, as well as in manufacturing, several other major services industries (e.g., telecommunication, transportation, and energy), and many aspects of the health care industry (e.g., radiation treatment, cancer diagnosis, and combined drug therapies). In the financial industry, these tools are often used to optimize portfolios by assigning weight to each characteristic of each asset to predict a certain return with the least risk. (In 1990, Markowitz, Miller, and Sharpe were awarded the Nobel Memorial Prize in economics for their work on portfolio optimization theory). Recent portfolio optimizations include asset-liability management (i.e., the coordination of assets and liabilities over time).

Portfolio optimization and asset-liability management have direct implications for health care. For example, a health care insurance organization can use these tools to determine optimal allocations of risks in terms of geographic regions, patient demographics, and investment capital to meet the needs of insured individuals. An insurance organization can also assess the value of expanding insurance to cover areas, such as life, and the incremental reductions in capital needs as a result of risk pooling.

Besides allocating liabilities and assets, a health care organization might use financial-engineering optimization tools to price services to determine the most efficient distribution of resources. Determining optimal prices, often called revenue management or yield management, is a common practice in the airline industry. In general, the goal is to determine allocations of scarce resources (e.g., passenger seats) that can be made available at different prices. In health care, revenue management might be used, for example, to schedule elective procedures, bundle services associated with different diagnoses or the management of chronic conditions, and determine priorities for scarce resources, such as diagnostic equipment, operating rooms, and critical care facilities. Asset-liability management and revenue management are only a sampling of optimization-based tools in financial engineering and risk management. Besides the direct implications for health care suggested above, they may also have less obvious applications that will require additional research.

Market Models

In general, the issues of moral hazard and adverse selection (i.e., the incentive to cheat or conceal information in the absence of penalties for doing so) present greater difficulties in the health care context than in financial services, and addressing these issues will require modeling of an organization's decisions as well as of individual patients' decisions. In these cases, the models must go beyond individual decision making to distributed decision making.

Distributed Decision Making and Agency Theory

The overall performance of the health care system is determined by many decision makers—patients, providers, insurers, and payers. Individual optimization tools may determine the best outcome for a single agent in the system, but the collection of actions by these individuals may not lead to the best outcome for the performance of the entire system. Analyses of the overall system may include models of the market and the effect of each agent's actions on the efficiency of the results.

Market models that combine optimal decisions for individual agents combine the results of individual decisions and generally iterate among decision makers to find an overall system equilibrium in which no agent has an incentive to change his or her decision. The result is a model of reality that can be used to determine the effects of different market structures, regulations, and external incentives.

One economic sector that has benefited from distributed decision-making models is the energy industry, which changed from a regulated monopoly (or collection of regulated monopolies) to a variety of forms of open competition in commodities, such as natural gas and electricity. Distributed-decision models have been used to assess the value of market mechanisms relative to a central system to determine resource allocations that minimize overall societal cost. If an individual agent's behavior does not contribute to the socially optimal outcome, the difference is often called the agency cost. Such costs arise, for example, in decisions by corporate executives who represent shareholders to the detriment of bondholders. Agency theory quantifies these costs and analyzes the value of alternative contracts and procedures to reduce them.

Distributed-decision models could be used to analyze the health care system, which has a multiplicity of independent agents. The impact of varying patient costs, insurance coverage, and care convenience, for example, can be incorporated into an overall system model to determine optimal decision processes for all agents. The results of these analyses could be used to determine tax policies, Medicare and Medicaid payments, and insurance regulations and their impact on the overall efficiency of the health care system. Because of the enormous size of the health care system and the wide variety of interests and objectives of its participants, analyses would be challenging. This is another area where research will be necessary.

Knowledge Discovery in Databases

In addition to modeling the system, the large amounts of data that are collected about products, customers, and markets and entered into databases can be accessed to provide information about the location of sales, the temporal variability of sales, returned products, and other detailed information. Large databases also often contain embedded knowledge that goes beyond the obvious. Customer surveys often ask questions that seem unrelated to the purchase of a particular item, and that information may be a rich source of insight. If, for example, a company determines that a large fraction of a group of customers regularly purchases both its product A and another manufacturer's product B, the company can use this knowledge to reach selected potential customers or sharpen the focus of an advertising campaign. If a database reveals customer loyalty to a particular manufacturer, that loyalty can become a key marketing objective.

Large databases can provide a basis for addressing system-wide issues in health care. Information in databases can reveal relationships that are not obvious from an examination of a smaller number of instances. The detailed medical history of a large group of patients can reveal interactions among drugs or the epidemiological role of certain drugs in specific diseases. Mitchell (1997) has reported that data mining successfully predicted that women who exhibited a particular group of symptoms had a high risk of requiring emergency C-sections. McCarthy (1997) describes how Merck-Medco Managed Care has used data mining to help identify less expensive drug treatments that are equally effective for specific patients. By examining a large Medicaid database, Ray et al. (2004) found an unrecognized risk of sudden cardiac arrest from a commonly prescribed antibiotic used in combination with other drugs or substances that inhibit the breakdown of the antibiotic. In these examples, information in a database can replace anecdotal observations with a large number of examples. Databases can also be explored to forecast health care costs, plan system management, and set prices for services.

Information from databases created for different purposes (e.g., financial reporting and patient history) must usually be modified before it can be analyzed. Pertinent information from different databases must be grouped together, vacant fields removed or average values inserted, duplicated files eliminated to ensure statistical integrity, and accuracy of the data confirmed. These steps can be both time consuming and difficult.

Data Mining

Four different types of information can be extracted from databases using computer techniques:

- classifications (e.g., characteristics that suggest a high probability that a patient will have a stroke before age 55)
- estimations (e.g., if the rate of change in potassium exceeds some limit, a patient may be at increased risk for an arrhythmia)
- variability (e.g., variations in practitioner-to-practitioner procedures)
- predictions (e.g., the likely number of deaths from the flu virus in the winter of 2005)

Once a set of independent variables is identified, the analysis can then continue to determine the relationship to a dependent variable:

- Is a patient with symptoms A and B likely to develop symptom C?
- What is the efficacy of drug D for the treatment of symptom E?
- Is there evidence that patients taking drugs G and H are more or less likely to develop a particular side effect?
- Is the tendency more pronounced for patients over 60?

All of the examples above can be called supervised learning strategies. Questions are posed, and the computer searches the database to determine whether relationships exist or can be quantified for specific variables.

Another approach is to instruct the computer to search for clusters of attributes that show either positive or negative correlations, so-called unsupervised clustering. This technique may be useful for identifying atypical instances. For example, data points representing outliers may be particularly useful for identifying undesirable reactions to certain combinations of drug treatment that could reveal relatively improbable, but very troublesome, events. Clearly, there is a need for better data mining of multiple drug interactions, tracing of adverse events, and updating of analyses as new drugs come on the market.

Predictive Modeling

If a causal relationship has been established between sets of variables by data mining, and if the statistical significance of these relationships is high, a predictive model can be constructed to predict the consequence of various actions. For example, a model might state that a patient with symptoms X, Y, and Z who is treated with drugs A, B, and C will have a high probability of specific reactions. In principle, the relative importance of each variable must be known for the model to be effective. In practice, however, if *all* of the principal variables are included in the model, it is often a fair assumption that they have equal influence on the final output. Obviously, a large amount of data is necessary to find enough patients with the three identified symptoms and the three specific drugs to ensure the statistical significance of the results. The variability in inputs and outputs to the model and the number and independence of the observations are critical to determining the statistical significance of predictions.

Neural Networks

In the absence of large comprehensive databases, neural networks have been used to achieve the same purpose as predictive modeling. Once a relationship has been observed among the three symptoms X, Y, and Z and the drugs A, B, and C, the problem is to determine the strength of the interactions. In contrast to the assumption of equal influence of all of the dependent variables, the assumption here is that they are not equal.

A neural network consists of several layers, each of which contains a number of nodes. Each node in the first layer is connected to all of the nodes in the next layer. This is repeated for subsequent layers. The number of nodes in the first layer is equal to the number of independent variables; and values for the attributes of the independent variables are entered into the nodes in the first layer. Each node connection is then weighted.

Based on the values of the input variables, the connections in the network, and the weights assigned to the nodes, the output values for the dependent variables can be calculated. The calculated outputs are then compared with known values for the dependent variables determined from the database. If the output values and known values differ, the weights for nodes in the network are adjusted. This process, called network learning, continues until the output of the network reflects the output that is known for particular data inputs. In use, the "learned" weights are kept fixed and the values of the input variables are changed thereby allowing

an examination of the impact of different strengths for the independent variables.

Neural networks and related "learning" methods have been developed for use in aspects of health care where the amount and kind of data available require unconventional approaches. Examples include prediction and control in neurosurgical intensive care, decision support in acute abdominal pain, automatic detection of emphysema, diagnosis of acute appendicitis, and predicting clinical outcomes for neuroblastoma patients (Eich et al., 1997; Friman et al., 2002; Pesonen, 1997; Swiercz et al., 1998; Wei et al., 2004).

SYSTEMS-CONTROL TOOLS

Systems-control tools are primarily used to ensure that processes are operating within their prescribed limits, thereby reducing errors and improving the use of resources. Controlling systems requires a clear understanding of performance expectations and the operating parameters that affect the achievement of those expectations. Control, therefore, depends on measuring parameters and adjusting them to achieve the desired operating levels. Robust control systems require that process and outcome data be collected and made accessible in real time so that operators can make timely and appropriate decisions that will improve system quality and increase productivity. Obviously, some of the tools discussed in the sections on design and analysis tools are also applicable to systems control (e.g., FMEA can be used to identify key process variables).

The control of a complex system must be based on a comprehensive understanding of interactions among the elements in the system and taking actions necessary to ensure smooth operation. Because health care delivery depends largely on human intervention, the control of the system depends on the proper allocation of critical manpower. Although systems-control tools are most often used at the care team and organizational levels, the principles underlying systems control can also be relevant to individual patients actively participating in their own treatment (e.g., to ensure the regular administration of drugs or treatment or the measurement of vital signs) (Table 3-5).

Statistical Process Control

With statistical process control (SPC), a provider of a given procedure can know if that procedure is within acceptable limits, and, if not, whether corrective actions should be taken. Effective clinical practice depends on the correct interpretation of data, whether the data relate to a patient's blood glucose level or the time between a patient's heart attack and the administration of thrombolytics. Data can measure the quality and outcome of an action most effectively when it is displayed over time. The most basic method of displaying data over time is the run chart, in which data points are plotted in a graph against two variables

TABLE 3-5 Systems-Control Tools

Tool/Research Area	Patient	Team	Organization	Environment
Statistical process control	X	X	X	
Scheduling		X	X	

represented on the X and Y axes (Figure 3-1). The goal line across the bottom is added as a vantage point from which to judge performance.

A clinician attempting to determine whether a patient's blood glucose level is under control (or stable) over time by direct sampling is confronted with the problem of determining how an individual result should be interpreted. Because a single observation is subject to some variability, a single measurement that differs significantly from the mean may signal a problem with the patient, or it may be the result of a statistical fluctuation. Determining which of these is correct could require a large number of observations.

The purpose of SPC is to allow a clinician to determine the status of the variable—with a limited number of measurements under the circumstance that the variable is subject to random fluctuations. Many patient variables must be managed over time, such as blood glucose level, blood pressure, and prothrombin time. SPC can be a critical tool for helping a clinician analyze data quickly (1) to determine if the process being measured is under control, that is, if fluctuations are the result of random events or a systematic change, and (2) to ensure that the process of care can lead to the desired outcome, such as stable blood coagulation levels within the *specifications* established by best practices. Although these two functions are related, it is important to note that *a process can be under control but still lead to an undesired outcome.*

For instance, blood glucose levels may be very stable at a high level, say 250, where it could be said to be under control but could still lead to an inappropriate patient outcome.

Control Chart

The control chart provides a way of detecting whether a process is under control. A limited number of measurements are made over time, and the mean and range are then calculated (Figure 3-2). The acceptable variation in the process is designated by an upper control limit (UCL) and a lower control limit (LCL), which are calculated based on the range and the mean of the measurements. The UCL is generally three standard deviations above the mean, and the LCL is essentially three standard deviations below the mean.

When data vary within that range, the variation is typically due to common causes. Data points outside the control limits signal a special cause and indicate the likelihood that something in the care process has fundamentally changed. Sometimes the change is intended by the clinician—for example, a change in dosage that dramatically lowers a patient's blood pressure or body temperature. The control chart in Figure 3-2 shows the percentage of INRs (a measure of blood coagulation) within 0.5 of the desired range. Fluctuations are between the UCL and LCL, and no points fall outside that range. Therefore, these variations appear to be

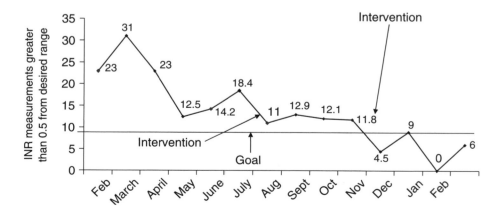

FIGURE 3-1 A run chart showing blood coagulation levels as a function of time. Source: IHI, 2003.

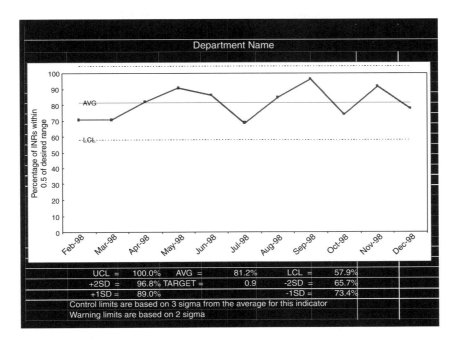

FIGURE 3-2 Control chart showing the percentage of INRs (a measure of blood coagulation) within 0.5 of the desired range. Source: IHI, 2003.

from common causes, and the process of care appears to be stable. This may or may not be the result that was planned. For example, if the goal is for INRs to be within 0.5 of the desired range for 90 percent of patients, the process of care would have to be improved.

Scheduling

Optimizing the scheduling of personnel (e.g., the nursing staff) is critical to the performance of a system. Scheduling is basically an operations method of matching supply and demand to achieve desired goals or objectives. Tools are available to accomplish this, even when the available resources are limited. Scheduling can help a system make the best use of its personnel, facilities, and inventories. Scheduling can also help "smooth out" demands, such as inpatient arrivals, outpatient arrivals, requests for testing, and so on.

Optimal, or even efficient, scheduling is one way manufacturing and service industries reduce costs and at the same time improve quality and safety. Effective scheduling has several basic requirements:

- a thorough understanding of work processes, work, workload, and work flow
- a complete analysis of the specific steps and sequences of work

- an assessment of available technologies and the creation of new technologies to reduce costs and/or improve quality
- a good forecast of future demands
- appropriate sizing of staff, inventories, and facilities to meet demands
- the smoothing out of variations in demand and work processes
- the avoidance of congestion and bottlenecks

Scheduling models have been used in several areas of health care delivery:

- inpatient scheduling in acute and long-term care settings
- outpatient and clinic scheduling
- workforce scheduling in hospitals, home health care, long-term care facilities, and clinics
- ambulance and emergency-vehicle scheduling
- scheduling for planning and acquisition of facilities and technology capacity
- scheduling for pharmacy, laboratory, radiology, housekeeping, food services, and other departments in an institution

Costs can be reduced and quality and safety improved through proper scheduling of patients, personnel, equipment, facilities inventories, and other assets. Before scheduling can begin, however, key processes must be analyzed and optimized, and work, workload, and forecasted demands must be measured.

Forecasting Demand

Forecasts require descriptions of past levels of demand by categories/products and projections of future demands. In some cases, a simple average of past demands on a system may be used as a forecast. In other cases, probability distributions of past events are used to predict the nature of future events. For hospitals, demands may change in cyclical, seasonal, or just random patterns; changes may be in hourly, daily, weekly, or monthly demands for hospital beds, operating rooms, or emergency care. Although random fluctuations in demand are unavoidable, trends and/or cycles or patterns of demand can be relatively predictable.

Assessing Workforce Size

Assessing workforce size is a complex process that involves: (1) multiple categories of patients with different requirements for care; (2) service standards in patient care; (3) multiple levels of nursing skills; and (4) variability in times per day of patient care and variability in numbers of patients.

Setting Service Standards

In manufacturing, service standards involve on-time delivery, minimization of defective products, and warranties and guarantees. In non-health service industries, service standards usually involve providing service at acceptable levels of quality for a given price. In health care, some standards can be set easily, such as correct medications at appropriate times. Other standards, such as the type and frequency of interventions to prevent disease or improve health and the quality of life, may be difficult to set.

Assessing Workforce Size-and-Skill Mix

In assessing workforce size, work must be organized to meet an average requirement, designed to accommodate natural variations from the average, and designed to ensure that the necessary number and mix of people is available to provide the desired level of service. One can easily estimate the mean and standard deviation of demand, but capacity decisions based on average demand do not account for demand that is higher or lower than average. Failing to satisfy requirements or having excess capacity can be very costly.

Personnel Scheduling

In many ways, planning and scheduling health care personnel is conceptually similar to scheduling for personnel in other sectors. In some important ways, however, the

problems in health care are more complex (Mullinax and Lawley, 2002). First, interrelations among highly trained and skilled personnel who must be available at appropriate times for different patients must be scheduled. Second, it is frequently difficult to measure quality of work, especially in terms of successful patient outcomes (see Box 3-4).

Hershey et al. (1981) conceptualized the staffing process for nursing as a hierarchy with three decision levels (corrective allocations, shift scheduling, and workforce planning) operating over different time horizons and at different levels of precision. Corrective allocations are made daily, shift schedules are the days-on/days-off work schedules for each nurse for four to eight weeks ahead, and workforce plans are quarterly, semiannual, or annual plans of nursing needs by skill level. Because of time lags, workforce planning must be done early to meet anticipated long-term fluctuations in demand and supply.

Effective shift scheduling (i.e., scheduling that meets the health care needs of patients and satisfies the preferences of nurses at minimal cost) is a complex problem that has attracted the interest of operations researchers. The earliest and simplest scheduling model, the cyclic schedule, repeats a fixed pattern of days on and off for each nurse indefinitely into the future but cannot make adjustments for forecasted changes in workload, extended absences, or the scheduling preferences of individual nurses. Rigid schedules place heavy demands on the corrective allocations and workforce planning levels to avoid excessive staffing (Hershey et al., 1981). In flexible scheduling, the preferences of staff are considered in scheduling decisions (Miller et al., 1976; Warner, 1976). More complicated mathematical programs (e.g., simulation and mixed-integer program techniques) have been used to schedule other personnel (Tzukert and Cohen, 1985; Vassilacopoulos, 1985).

Improving Hospital Flow

Busy emergency departments must handle three inflows of patients: (1) patients who need emergency service but do not require admission to the hospital; (2) patients who need emergency services and do require admission; and (3) patients who do not need emergency care but use the emergency room as their primary source of health care. When the emergency room is the patient's primary destination and admission to the hospital is not required, segmentation and queuing methods, as described previously, can be extremely helpful in shortening waiting times and delays.

Historically, groups 1 and 3 have been at the mercy of group 2. From 1997 through 2000, the Institute for Healthcare Improvement worked with emergency departments at 91 hospitals, representing a total of 2.6 million visits per year, to reduce waiting times and delays and increase patient satisfaction (IHI, 2003). The hospitals experimented with a fast track for patients who met specified criteria. Testing and measurement showed that 83 percent of all patients use the

BOX 3-4
Nursing Assignments in a Neonatal Intensive Care Nursery

Intensive care nurseries provide health care for critically ill newborn infants. During a typical shift, infants range from those that need only occasional care to those that require constant attention. At the beginning of each shift, the head nurse groups the patients for assignment to staff nurses. Typically each nurse cares for one group of infants throughout the shift. Because of the large variations in infant conditions and several complicating constraints, developing balanced nurse workloads intuitively is difficult. A math program was developed to ensure a balanced workload.

Balanced workloads are important in neonatal intensive care for several reasons. First, and perhaps most important, every nurse needs time to talk with parents and concerned relatives. If a nurse is overburdened, he or she may be unable to perform this essential function. In addition, when workloads are balanced, fewer nurses are required to care for the same group of patients.

The first step in the development of the program was to create a system to quantify the nursing workload of each patient based on neonatal acuity. With the help of several charge nurses, a comprehensive list of care procedures was developed. The procedures were grouped into 14 categories (see table below).

1. Monitoring respiratory status	5. Taking X-rays	9. Administering chest physiotherapy	13. Performing miscellaneous tasks
2. Performing labwork	6. Checking weight	10. Caring for wounds	14. Dealing with unstable patients
3. Administering feedings	7. Administering medications	11. Changing dressings	
4. Checking vital signs	8. Performing suctioning	12. Intravenous feedings	

Next, a scoring mechanism was developed. Each item on the list was assigned an acuity measure based on the number of times the procedure was performed in a 24-hour period. Each infant was then given a score for each procedure. The cumulative score reflected the amount of nursing care the infant required. The acuity scoring system was then submitted to a panel of neonatal nurses for validation of the content and testing of rater reliability.

The integer linear program based on the scoring system assigns patients to nurses while balancing workloads. The model finds the most balanced workload within a number of constraints: every infant could be assigned to only one nurse; no nurse could be assigned more than two or three patients (depending on state regulations); no nurse could be given a workload that exceeded a specified maximum; and one or two nurses ("admitting" nurses) were assigned smaller initial workloads but then were responsible for new patients that arrived during the shift. The model can also accommodate other considerations. For example, a charge nurse might specify a partial assignment and let the model complete it. This could be important when it is desirable for a nurse to care for the same patient during several shifts.

Ten case studies from a major university hospital were used to benchmark the performance of the model against current practice (see figure). Each case study represents a real patient-to-nurse assignment by a charge nurse in a critical care nursery. The model generated an alternative assignment and then compared the workload imbalance. For example, in Case 9, the assignment by the charge nurse had an imbalance of 79. This means that the nurse with the heaviest workload had to carry out 79 more procedures than the nurse with the lightest workload (not counting admitting nurses). For the same set of patients and nurses, the model generated an assignment with an imbalance of 5, a very significant improvement. In several cases, the model revealed that too many nurses had been scheduled for a shift.

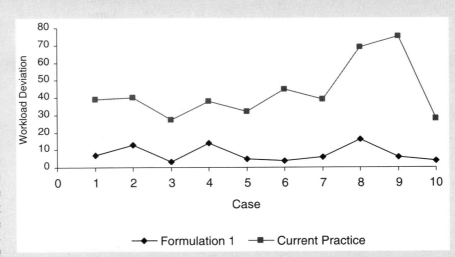

The developers of this model were aware of the common belief of many medical practitioners that quantitative engineering approaches dehumanize health care delivery. By developing a method of assigning workloads fairly and ensuring that nurses' workloads were manageable, this approach, although quantitative, could actually make health care delivery more effective. Properly balanced workloads ensure that nurses have an appropriate amount of work and sufficient time to see to essential human intangibles.

Source: Adapted from Mullinax and Lawley, 2002.

emergency departments between 9:00 a.m. and 1:00 a.m. A fast track that allowed 46 percent of these patients to be seen resulted in an improvement of up to 30 percent in lengths of stay and patient volume.

The remaining 17 percent of patients who required admission to the hospital presented the greatest challenge to hospital flow. Most often, emergency departments divert some of these patients to other hospitals because their hospitals do not have the space to move patients forward (Committee on Government Reform, 2001; GAO, 2003). Moreover, critical shortages in intensive-care beds have led to an increasing number of ambulance diversions and prolonged stays in emergency departments (Besinger and Stapczynski, 1997; Goldberg, 2000).

Addressing this problem requires a system-wide approach that includes the flow of inpatient beds. Otherwise, techniques to manage emergency department flow will have a limited effect on hospital diversion rates and will not address the problem of patients being "boarded" in emergency departments.

Queuing methods that are effective for emergency department arrivals are also ideal for unscheduled patients. They are not as appropriate for scheduled patients. Health care organizations must deal with both scheduled and unscheduled patients. Queuing theory would suggest, therefore, that separate tracks be developed for scheduled and unscheduled patients. For instance, one primary-care clinic, St. John's Regional Health Center in Springfield, Missouri, created separate slots for scheduled and unscheduled patients by setting aside one operating room for unscheduled emergent cases. With this simple maneuver, they increased the number of surgical cases handled during normal business hours by 5.1 percent and reduced after-hours procedures by 45 percent. As a result, surgeons realized a 4.6 percent increase in revenue (IHI, 2003).

Patient Scheduling

Outpatients

Scheduling of patients in clinics for outpatient services is one of the earliest documented uses of operations research to improve health care delivery. Bailey (1975) applied queuing theory to equalize patients' waiting times in hospital outpatient departments based on original work done in 1952. He observed that many outpatient clinics are essentially a single queue with single or multiple servers. The problem then becomes creating an appointment system that minimizes patient waiting time and keeps servers busy.

The three most commonly used scheduling systems involve variations on block scheduling, modified block scheduling, and individual scheduling. In block scheduling, all patients are scheduled for one appointment time, for instance, 9:00 a.m. or 1:00 p.m. They are then served on a first-come, first-served basis. In modified block scheduling,

the day is divided into smaller blocks (e.g., the beginning of each hour), and smaller blocks of patients are scheduled for those times, which decreases patient waiting time. By contrast, in individual scheduling systems, which are commonly used in the United States, patients are scheduled for specific times throughout the day, often depending on staff availability.

The extensive literature on outpatient scheduling began in the 1950s and peaked in the 1960s and 1970s. Because many studies were based on queuing or simulation, parametric distributions were determined for patient service times. Scheduling schemes to reduce patient waiting time without increasing physician idle time were analyzed using these distributions as inputs (Callahan and Redmon, 1987; Fries and Marathe, 1981; O'Keefe, 1985; Vissers and Wijngaard, 1979).

Inpatients

Inpatient scheduling has three major dimensions: (1) scheduling of elective admissions and emergency admissions into appropriate units of the hospital each day; (2) daily scheduling of inpatients to appropriate care units in the hospital for treatment or diagnosis; and (3) scheduling discharges of patients to their homes or other institutions. Clearly, these scheduling activities are linked and depend on many characteristics of the patients and the hospital. The models used for inpatient scheduling are more complex and require more data and better information systems than models for outpatients. Many different methodologies might be used based on queuing models.

For scheduling admissions, queuing and simulation models are most often used. Early examples include a model of a five-operating room, 12-bed, postanesthesia care unit (Kuzdrall et al., 1981). Trivedi (1980) describes a stochastic model of patient discharges that could be used to help regulate elective admissions and meet occupancy goals. Other authors who have addressed this topic are Cohen et al. (1980); Green (2004); Hershey et al. (1981); Kao (1974); Kostner and Shachtman (1981); and Weiss et al. (1982).

Improving Overall Organizational Performance

In addition to the tools described above, businesses, companies, and industries have found a number of other ways to improve their performance and the quality of their products and services. Three examples are described below.

The Baldrige National Quality Program

The Malcolm Baldrige National Quality Award was created in 1987 to improve U.S. industrial competitiveness and encourage the pursuit of quality in all sectors of the economy. The Baldrige National Quality Program, a public-private partnership, presents awards to large manufacturing companies, small businesses, service organizations, educational organizations, and health care providers that demonstrate major improvements in the quality of their products or services by reengineering processes, adopting continuous improvement approaches, involving employees in decision making, analyzing the operation of all elements of the enterprise, and measuring and controlling operations to optimize performance. In comparing the overall performance of units that have won this award with their competition, it is clear that quality has been improved in many economic sectors. The national recognition of the Baldrige award has motivated many organizations to improve their performance and the quality of their products and services (NIST, 2005).

Toyota Production System

In the early 1950s, Toyota introduced a variety of procedures that ultimately became known as the Toyota Production System. The system is designed to bring problems to light, resolve them, and improve the overall system to ensure that problems are not repeated. With this combination of procedures and processes, Toyota has become the leader in production efficiency and a producer of very high quality products. Toyota's ultimate goal is "defect-free operations" (Spear and Bowen, 1999). The reduction of waste, just-in-time inventory control, and the empowerment of individuals to contribute to continuous improvement in performance are just some aspects of Toyota's system that are applicable to health care delivery (see Bowen in this volume and Monden, 1983).

Six Sigma Method

The quality of a final product or process depends on many factors, including the complexity of the product and the controls in place at each step of production. Motorola introduced the concept of Six Sigma quality with the objective of creating a manufacturing operation that generates only two defective parts per billion; a defective part is defined as one with performance outside its design specifications. However, because the mean value for the key parameter that characterizes the operating system frequently drifts, the number of defective parts in practice is generally assumed to be approximately 3 to 4 parts per million (Harry, 1988).

Full-time Six Sigma project managers are given formal classroom training in process analysis and statistical methods and are mentored by experts in the Six Sigma method. In some cases, they have focused on specific departments or processes, and, in other cases, the method has been used on an enterprise-wide basis to achieve a cultural transformation (Pexton, 2005).

Applicability to the Health Care System

The quality improvement programs described above, which use a range of systems-engineering tools and innovative management practices, were developed more than two decades ago largely for the manufacturing sector. Only very recently have they begun to be used to improve performance in the health care sector. Nevertheless, the adoption of these and related tools and strategies by a small but growing number of health care provider organizations has demonstrated their potential for improving all six dimensions of health care quality as defined by IOM.

A recent study by the Pittsburgh Regional Health Initiative describes a systems approach to redesigning work systems. In one study, the goal was to eliminate central-line-associated bloodstream infections using techniques like those practiced at Toyota. By using simple tools and devices, the number of infections transmitted was significantly reduced, and general procedures were subsequently changed accordingly (Shannon et al., in progress).

Many of the most common challenges addressed by the Six Sigma method are the same as the challenges facing health care (e.g., safety, technology optimization, market growth, resource utilization, length of stay, and throughput). Defects in health care might be the number of two-year-olds not completely immunized (per million two-year-olds in the population), the number of pregnant women who do not receive prenatal care in the first trimester (per million pregnancies), or the number of patients with clinical depression who are not diagnosed (per million patients with depression) (Chassin, 1998).

A number of approaches have been undertaken by medical professionals in recent decades to apply systems thinking to the problems of safety and quality, including actions to change the behavior of health professionals and patients (e.g., making changes in strategies and the division of labor) to improve system performance. For example, the Chronic Care Model developed by Dr. Ed Wagner of the Group Health Cooperative of Puget Sound identifies six areas of interconnected activity necessary for the management of patients with chronic disease. The model encourages interactions between care provider teams and chronic care patients and their families, who are trained and equipped to participate actively in the care delivery process (see Box 3-5). Batalden et al. (2003a,b) have documented and promoted "success characteristics" of clinical microsystems—small, functional, frontline units that provide most health care to most people (see also Godfrey et al., 2003; Huber et al., 2003; Kosnik and Espinosa, 2003; Mohr et al., 2003; Nelson et al., 2002, 2003; Wasson et al., 2003).

The Institute for Healthcare Improvement (IHI) has engaged large numbers of individuals and institutions in carrying out change focusing on improving many levels of the present system and using some of the systems tools described above (Box 3-6). Although achieving some of their goals has proven to be difficult, many important lessons have been learned, and significant efforts have been made to disseminate these lessons.

BOX 3-5
The Chronic Care Model

The Chronic Care Model, developed by Dr. Ed Wagner, director of the MacColl Institute for Healthcare Innovation at the Group Health Cooperative of Puget Sound, is based on the premise that good outcomes in health care (e.g., better clinical control, more self-confidence and a better quality of life for patients, lower costs, etc.) require productive interactions between prepared, proactive provider teams and active patients, families, or caregivers who are ready to participate in their care. To make those productive interactions happen, the model identifies six fundamental areas of interconnected activity and support that encourage high-quality management of patients with chronic diseases.

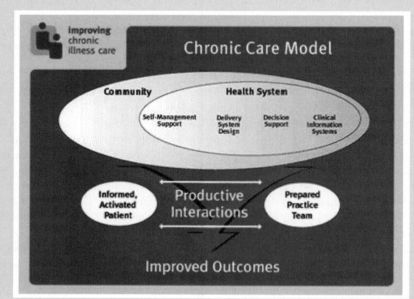

These six qualities should be the hallmarks of health care delivery systems:

1. **Self-management support** involves empowering patients through motivational interviewing and integrating assessment, tailoring, problem solving, and goal setting into everyday care.
2. **Delivery system design** addresses the questions of who should be on a care team, what kind of interaction each member of the team should have with the patient (e.g., delivering the services that are known to work, such as case management, group visits, planned visits, and follow-up), how team members should interact with each other, and how patients should telephone or e-mail caregivers.
3. **Decision support** provides health care professionals with guidelines to ensure that best-practice, evidence-based health care is delivered.
4. **Clinical information systems** provide a means of making the information about an entire patient population (a registry) available to the patient and provider when it is needed.
5. **The health care organization,** which subsumes and supports the office practice, determines senior leaders' goals for health care quality and how the business plan makes the goals actionable.
6. **The community,** within which the whole health care system exists, provides resources and policies that influence the patient's interactions with the extended care delivery system.

Source: Davis, 2005. Originally published in Wagner, 1998.

APPLYING SYSTEMS TOOLS TO HEALTH CARE DELIVERY

The systems tools described in this chapter can be applied to all four levels of the health care system, with the caveat that they must be adapted to the specific conditions and circumstances of this unique patient-centered environment.

Patient Level

In the past, systems tools have not been widely applied to individual patients, but they should be. The ultimate purpose of using these tools should be to improve patient care and ensure that the system is responsive to patients' needs and wishes. Concurrent engineering tools like QFD can be used most effectively in the design/redesign of care delivery systems in the hospital and ambulatory clinics and, as information/communications technologies advance, in virtual settings, such as patients' homes. Human-factors expertise focused on care provider-patient relationships can help modify care instructions to ensure that they are meaningful to patients and encourage patients to participate in care processes. Indeed, human-factors engineering will be critical in moving toward remote care delivery and viable self-care systems,

---

BOX 3-6
Institute for Healthcare Improvement

The Institute for Healthcare Improvement (IHI), a not-for-profit research center, was established in 1991 by Dr. Donald Berwick for the purpose of improving the quality and efficiency of health care. IHI's 15-member board of directors is drawn from leading health care institutions and the academic community. IHI researchers identify specific problems and bring together multidisciplinary teams of experts from across the country to work on them. IHI then creates a collaborative group of 30 to 50 health care institutions that agree to implement the new processes and share their findings. Each collaborative project lasts from nine months to three years.

Problem areas tackled by IHI groups have included: reducing medication errors; reducing waiting times in emergency rooms; reducing surgical infection rates; improving the performance of supply chains; and reducing ventilator-induced pneumonia. IHI has had considerable success, both nationally and internationally, and now has an annual operating budget or more than $30 million, most of it from the health care industry. More than 200 faculty members from different academic institutions lead the project teams, and a network of more than 175 health care institutions are working together to solve specific problems. Because the projects are funded by the participating institutions, they have a vested interest in implementing the new ideas and procedures that are developed. The annual IHI National Forum now attracts more than 4,000 attendees.

Source: IHI, 2005.

---

ensuring the usability and reliability of information/communications systems and other systems patients will have to use for professionally guided, self-instructed care in their homes, and maintaining communications and relationships of trust with care providers.

Modeling and simulation tools can be used to improve patient access to care providers (e.g., more efficient scheduling of appointments), reduce patient waiting times in care centers, and ensure that laboratory test results are available on demand. Patients will also benefit directly from improved scheduling of personnel, from the development of predictive models for treating particular diseases, and from improved regimes for administering medication.

The use of systems tools at the patient level will require detailed data on patient flows, delay times, and service times by caregivers, laboratories, support staff, and so on. Some of these data can be collected from computer records, but much of it will require individual measurements of, for example, time spent in accomplishing various tasks. Significant differences among facilities will require that data be collected for particular environments. One advantage of systems tools is that they are sufficiently general that they can be applied in very diverse environments.

Frontline Care Team Level

In this section, we highlight the benefits of these same tools for caregiver teams. Benefits to caregivers and patients lead, in turn, to benefits for organizations and the overall health care environment by improving the efficiency of operations throughout the entire system. A health care system designed to meet the needs and wants of both patients and caregiver teams can provide a smoothly operating environment that is best for both caregivers and patients.

Human factors might be used to assess the effectiveness of cross-checks among care groups. Analyses that can reveal where a system can fail, either by predicting errors or by identifying inefficiencies, generally depend more on interactions among individuals who work in the system and understand all of its aspects and components than on large amounts of data. However, modeling and simulation tools do require good data. These tools can focus on improving the clinical and administrative operation of a practice, including the scheduling of personnel, the allocation of physical resources, and the reduction or elimination of tasks that require substantial time but may be of limited value to the team or the patient. Simulation of an operating room can improve the organization of facilities, personnel, and supplies to ensure the highest level of safety and effectiveness. The simulation of nurses' stations can ensure that supplies are available when needed and that support is provided to reduce unnecessary tasks. These analyses can also identify ways of automating some tasks and reducing unnecessary repetitions of tasks (e.g., data entries).

Modeling and simulation of back-office operations can help reduce the time spent by physicians and nurses in data recording and improve communications with patients. The proper scheduling of team members can reduce overload and improve the quality of the workplace for the team as a whole. The data for some of these analyses must be collected locally through detailed observations. These data can then be supplemented with data from a comprehensive information technology system designed to provide detailed records of events, personnel, and resources.

Enterprise-management tools address interactions between the caregiver team and the enterprise. Supply-chain management is intended to reduce inventory and ensure that needed supplies are available when required. It can also reduce inventory costs without compromising the availability of the means and personnel to handle emergencies. The significant data necessary for these analyses can involve a number of operating units of the system. Experience in other industries suggests that these data needs can only be provided by an information system that connects all elements of the enterprise.

Game-theory tools, contracts, and system-dynamic models can enable caregiver teams to explore "what-if" questions to predict the consequences of taking very different actions, such as the consequences of a major emergency or different ways of managing and controlling large fluctuations that might be introduced into a local system. For example, what actions should be taken if an emergency room is suddenly overburdened? How should nurses be allocated if only 10 percent are unavailable on a given day? How should priorities be set for using an operating room?

Optimization tools for decision making can help answer the same questions. Longer-term efforts to optimize the care team's efforts can be addressed by predictive, rather than descriptive, models. Predictive models, such as neural networks, require an understanding of the causes and effects of unexpected changes in the operational environment. The data requirements for predictive analyses are complex and require historical knowledge of the operation of the care team, as well as information about the operation of the enterprise, at least as it affects the care team. Large-scale databases on patients, diseases, and treatments are also necessary. Collecting the necessary data for these analyses without a comprehensive information system would be practically impossible. Even if it could be done, the cost would be exorbitant.

Organizational Level

At the organizational level, analyses and other systems approaches become more complex. Analyses and other studies at this level must address interactions among many elements of a system. Questions may relate to cost, overall organizational efficiency, trade-offs among departments, and organizational responses to major emergencies. Human-factors studies might be used to ensure that new software-intensive systems promote continuity of care (e.g., avoid fragmentation and complexity).

Health care provider organizations have the large, complex task of providing all of the support functions for both clinical care (e.g., radiology, laboratories, operating rooms, etc.) and infrastructure (e.g., finance, administration, accounting, etc.). In the current health care system, clinical and infrastructural needs are addressed separately. Although each clinical support function and each infrastructural need requires a high level of reliability and standardization, a truly patient-centered system will require high-performance systems at all levels.

At the organizational level, some of the more traditional engineering approaches (e.g., supply-chain management) are readily applicable. Indeed, some of the larger health care institutions have already adopted them. Systems-engineering techniques are critical to analyzing data and using modeling and simulation strategies to improve outcomes (e.g., interactions among reimbursement policies, regulations, improved care, etc.). All of these tools (i.e., systems tools, analysis, modeling, and simulation) are applicable, not only at this level, but also at the environmental level.

Data needs for these analyses can place a heavy burden on information systems, and data must be available on activities outside the boundaries of the organization (e.g., IPAs, drug suppliers, rehabilitation centers, emergency response units, etc.). To meet these needs, information systems will require interconnectivity of various elements of the overall health care delivery system.

Environmental Level

Questions at this level concern overall trends and system responses, such as regulation and oversight, reimbursement strategies, cost trends for the treatment of various diseases, the supply of caregivers, the availability of evidence-based medical information, research on the development of predictive models, and system responsiveness to major outbreaks of disease. The data requirements for addressing these and other high-level system questions depend on the issue being investigated, but, in general, information must be available from a host of institutions and organizations. To ensure that information from these many sources is available, there must be a comprehensive information system that facilitates communication and encourages information exchange among entities in the health care delivery system.

The use of systems engineering to investigate and improve the overall health care system will reflect an important change in the way reforms and changes are approached and a movement away from the old, entrenched cultures that have characterized the system historically. The hope is that systems-engineering tools can bring these deeply entrenched structures to the surface where they can be investigated and evaluated in terms of the needs of a twenty-first century health care delivery system.

Up to now, most health care professionals have not understood the relevance of systems-engineering tools to the safety and quality of patient-centered care. One of the objectives of this report is to encourage a conversation on this subject between the engineering community and health care professionals at all levels. Working together, these two communities can take advantage of the benefits of systems-engineering tools to manage and optimize costs; ensure high-quality, timely production processes; improve the safety and quality of care; and, ultimately, provide a truly patient-centered health care delivery system.

BARRIERS TO IMPLEMENTATION

Significant barriers to the widespread diffusion and implementation of systems-engineering tools in health care include impediments related to inadequate information technology and economic, policy, organizational, and educational barriers.

Inadequate Information and Information Technology

In general, at the tactical or local level, data gathering and processing and associated informational needs do not present significant technical or cost barriers to the adoption of systems-engineering tools (e.g., SPC, discrete-event simulation, queuing methods). By contrast, there are significant structural, technical, and cost-related barriers at the organization, multi-organization, and environmental levels to the strategic implementation of tools for modeling and simulation, enterprise management, financial engineering and risk analysis, and knowledge discovery in databases. The use of these tools requires integrated clinical, administrative, and financial information systems (e.g., clinical data repositories, etc.) that are expensive to install and maintain, and only a relatively small number of large integrated provider organizations or networks (e.g., Veterans Health Administration, Kaiser-Permanente, Mayo Clinic, Group Health Cooperative of Puget Sound, etc.) have such information systems in place.

Without access to integrated clinical information systems, it is extremely difficult for small, independent elements of highly distributed, loosely connected care provider networks to take advantage of tactical systems tools and virtually impossible for them to take advantage of enterprise-management and other systems-analysis tools. In principle, with the advance of computerization and automation in health care delivery, the cost of capturing relevant data for design, analysis, and control of processes and systems should come down. However, the health care system does not have interoperability standards for information/communication systems that would make it possible to connect the myriad pieces of the fragmented, distributed delivery system. This absence of interoperability presents a formidable barrier to the use of strategic, data-intensive systems tools at the organizational and environment levels. (Information/communications-related challenges to patient-centered, high-performance health care delivery are addressed at greater length in Chapter 4.)

Policy and Market Barriers

In the present system, reimbursement practices and rules, regulatory frameworks, and the lack of support for research continue to discourage the development, adaptation, and use of systems-engineering tools to improve the performance of the health care delivery system. The current "market" for health care services does not reward care providers who improve the quality of their processes and outcomes through investments in systems engineering, information/communications technologies, or other innovations (Hellinger, 1998; Leape, 2004; Leatherman et al., 2003; Miller and Luft, 1994, 2002; Robinson, 2001). The lack of comparative quality and cost data and the corresponding lack of quality/cost transparency in the market for health care services prevent patients from making informed choices on the basis of quality or value (quality/cost) (see Safran, in this volume, and Rosenthal et al., 2004). In the prevailing payment/reimbursement climate, care providers are not reimbursed on the basis of the quality of care they provide (IOM, 2001). Care providers have little incentive to invest in systems tools in support of quality improvement, unless they generate revenue directly or demonstrate immediate improvements in operating efficiency.

In recent years, several experiments with new reimbursement approaches have been tried to change the prevailing practice of reimbursing discrete units by a "reasonable cost" method to include fixed-price reimbursement for a definable bundle of services or a care episode. The object of these changes is to give providers an incentive to improve the effectiveness and efficiency of their processes and procedures. For example, the introduction of diagnostic related groups shifted the reimbursement for hospitalization to a fixed price (adjusted for regional labor costs). Severity-adjusted capitation for patients covered under the new Medicare HMO coverage applies the same principles. Some insurers have experimented with linking reimbursement explicitly to quality measures (for example, selected health care organizations may receive a fixed price for organ transplants based on quality, that is, the success rate of the procedure). These are promising first steps toward changing reimbursement to encourage high-quality, efficient care and a systems approach. However, for the vast majority of care providers, there are no such incentives.

Organizational and Managerial Barriers

Other barriers to the widespread use of systems tools in health care are related to the culture, organization, and management structure of most health care provider organizations and the lack of confidence in systems tools and technologies by those who will be called upon to use them.

As discussed in Chapter 1, cultural, organizational, and policy-related factors (e.g., regulation, licensing, etc.) have contributed to rigid divisions of labor in many areas of health care, which has impeded the widespread use of systems tools and related innovations that are likely to have significant, disruptive effects on organizational structures and work processes at all four levels of the health care system (see

Bohmer this volume and Christensen et al., 2000). Organizational changes are difficult under any circumstances, and inflexibility in roles and responsibilities can increase the difficulties. There is ample documentation of tools and technologies that were poorly integrated with/accommodated by existing processes of care delivery that generated additional work for frontline providers and very little apparent reward (Boodman, 2005; Durieux, 2005; Garg et al., 2005; Wears and Berg, 2005)

Ultimately, the benefits of systems tools and technologies can only be realized if their introduction is carefully managed and the people who must use them are adequately prepared, technically and mentally, to change their work practices and organization. First, as Nelson and colleagues observed in their assessment of successful clinical microsystems and as IHI has demonstrated in its successful collaboratives, management must change its philosophy (IHI, 2005; Nelson et al., 2002). Once management is committed to change, the participation of professional caregivers can be enlisted from the outset in the analysis of processes and systems and in the design and implementation of system improvements. In short, there must be mutual trust between health care management and the health care professionals who work with management.

Educational Barriers

Prevailing approaches to the education and training of health care, engineering, and management professionals also present significant barriers to the implementation and diffusion of systems-engineering tools, information/communications technologies, and associated innovations in the health care sector. Currently, very few health care professionals or administrators are equipped to think analytically about health care delivery as a system. As a result, very few appreciate the relevance, let alone the value, of systems-engineering tools. And of these, only a fraction are equipped to work with systems engineers to tailor and apply them to the needs of the health care delivery system.

Students of engineering and management are much more likely to be trained in systems thinking and the uses and implications of systems-engineering tools and information/communications technologies for the management and optimization of production and delivery systems. However, students in most U.S. engineering and business schools are unlikely to find courses that address operational challenges in the quality and productivity of health care delivery. (Educational barriers to the application of systems engineering to health care delivery and the steps necessary to overcome them are addressed at length in Chapter 5.)

The culture of the health care enterprise will have to undergo a seismic change, a so-called paradigm shift, for systems thinking and the health of populations to become integral factors in health care decision making. Even at that point, it will take a tremendous effort and a great deal of

flexibility for organizations to implement fundamental changes based on the optimization of interactions among all elements of the system. Ultimately, the whole must be greater than the sum of its parts. To date, organizations with corporate structures and management have been most successful in accomplishing this.

FINDINGS

Finding 3-1. The health care delivery system functions not as a system, but as a collection of entities that consider their performance in isolation. Even within a given organization (e.g., a hospital), individual departments are often isolated and behave as functional and operational "silos."

Finding 3-2. A systems view of health care cannot be achieved until the organizational barriers to change are overcome. Management and professionals must be committed to removing silos and focusing on optimizing contributions of professionals at all levels.

Finding 3-3. Systems-engineering tools have been used to improve the quality, efficiency, safety, and/or customer-centeredness of processes, products, and services in a wide range of manufacturing and services industries.

Finding 3-4. Health care has been very slow to embrace systems-engineering tools, even though they have been shown to benefit the small fraction of health care organizations and clinicians that have used them. Most health care providers do not understand how systems engineering can help solve health care delivery problems and improve operating performance. Many do not even know the questions systems tools and techniques might address or how to take advantage of the answers Only when people trained in the use of systems-engineering tools are integral to the health care community will the benefits become fully available.

Finding 3-5. Systems-engineering tools for the design, analysis, and control of complex systems and processes could potentially transform the quality and productivity of health care. Statistical process control, queuing theory, human-factors engineering, discrete-event simulation, QFD, FMEA, modeling and simulation, supply-chain management, and knowledge discovery in databases either have been or can be readily adapted to applications in health care delivery. Other tools, such as enterprise management, financial engineering, and risk analysis, are the subjects of ongoing research and can be expected to be useful for health care in the future.

Finding 3-6. Neither the engineering community nor the health care research community has addressed the delivery aspects of health care adequately. Although clinical applications of new medicines, procedures, and devices have been widespread, improving the processes by which care is delivered has been mostly disregarded. The adaptation and improvement of existing systems tools and the creation of new tools to address health care delivery have not been primary objectives of federal agencies or public or private research institutions.

Finding 3-7. Information/communications systems will be critical to taking advantage of the potential of existing and emerging systems-design, -analysis, and -control tools to transform health care delivery. These tools can provide timely collection, analysis, and sharing of process and outcome data that would benefit all stakeholders in the enterprise. Although such systems are available in other industries, meeting the unique requirements of the health care community will require active research.

Finding 3-8. The current organization, management, and regulation of health care delivery provide few incentives for the use or development of systems-engineering tools that could lead to improvements.

Finding 3-9. The widespread use of systems-engineering tools will require determined efforts on the part of health care providers, the engineering community, federal and state governments, private insurers, large employers, and other stakeholders.

RECOMMENDATIONS

Recommendation 3-1. Private insurers, large employers, and public payers, including the Federal Center for Medicare and Medicaid Services and state Medicare programs, should provide more incentives for health care providers to use systems tools to improve the quality of care and the efficiency of care delivery. Reimbursement systems, both private and public, should expand the scope of reimbursement for care episodes or use other bundling techniques (e.g., disease-related groups, severity-adjusted capitation for Medicare Advantage, fixed payments for transplantation, etc.) to encourage the use of systems-engineering tools. Regulatory barriers should also be removed. As a first step, regulatory waivers could be granted for demonstration projects to validate and publicize the utility of systems tools.

Recommendation 3-2. Outreach and dissemination efforts by public- and private-sector organizations that have used systems-engineering tools in health care delivery (e.g., Veterans Health Administration, Joint Commission on Accreditation of Healthcare Organizations, Agency for Healthcare Research and Quality, Institute for Healthcare Improvement, Leagfrog Group, U.S. Department of Commerce Baldrige National Quality Program, and others) should be expanded, integrated into existing regulatory and accreditation frameworks, and reviewed to determine whether, and if so how, better coordination might make their collective impact stronger.

Recommendation 3-3. The use and diffusion of systems-engineering tools in health care delivery should be promoted by a National Institutes of Health Library of Medicine website that provides patients and clinicians with information about, and access to, systems-engineering tools for health care (a systems-engineering counterpart to the Library of Medicine web-based "clearinghouse" on the status and treatment of diseases and the Agency for Healthcare Research and Quality National Guideline Clearinghouse for evidence-based clinical practice). In addition, federal agencies and private funders should support the development of new curricula, textbooks, instructional software, and other tools to train individual patients and care providers in the use of systems-engineering tools.

Recommendation 3-4. The use of any single systems tool or approach should not be put "on hold" until other tools become available. Some system tools already have extensive tactical or local applications in health care settings. Information-technology-intensive systems tools, however, are just beginning to be used at higher levels of the health care delivery system. Changes must be approached from many directions, with systems engineering tools that are available now and with new tools developed through research. Successes in other industries clearly show that small steps can yield significant results, even while longer term efforts are being pursued.

Recommendation 3-5. Federal research and mission agencies should significantly increase their support for research to advance the application and utility of systems engineering in health care delivery, including research on new systems tools and the adaptation, implementation, and improvement of existing tools for all levels of health care delivery. Promising areas for research include human-factors engineering, modeling and simulation, enterprise management, knowledge discovery in databases, and financial engineering and risk analysis. Research on the organizational, economic, and policy-related barriers to implementation of these and other systems tools should be an integral part of the larger research agenda.

CONCLUSION

Information/communications systems will be critical to the effectiveness of existing and emerging systems-design, -analysis, and -control tools in the transformation of health care delivery. Information/communications systems can provide timely collection, analysis, and sharing of process and outcome data that would benefit all stakeholders in the enterprise. Although these systems are available in other industries, meeting the unique requirements of the health care community will require significant investments and active research. Near-term and long-term challenges in this area are addressed in Chapter 4.

REFERENCES

Abara, J. 1989. Applying integer linear programming to the fleet assignment problem. Interfaces 19(4): 20–28.

Ash, J.S., M. Berg, and E. Coiera. 2004. Some unintended consequences of information technology in health care: the nature of patient care information system-related errors. Journal of the American Medical Informatics Association 11(2): 104–112.

Bailey, N.T.J. 1975. The Mathematical Theory of Infectious Disease and Its Applications. London, U.K.: Charles Griffin and Co. Ltd.

Batalden, P.B., E.C. Nelson, J.J. Mohr, M.M. Godfrey, T.P. Huber, L. Kosnik, and K. Ashling. 2003a. Microsystems in health care: Part 5. How leaders are leading. Joint Commission Journal on Quality and Safety 29(6): 297–308.

Batalden, P.B., E.C. Nelson, W.H. Edwards, M.M. Godfrey, and J.J. Mohr. 2003b. Microsystems in health care: Part 9. Developing small clinical units to attain peak performance. Joint Commission Journal on Quality and Safety 29(11): 575–585.

Bertocci, G.E., M.C. Pierce, E. Deemer, and F. Aguel. 2001. Computer simulation of stair falls to investigate scenarios in child abuse. Archives of Pediatrics and Adolescent Medicine 55(9): 1008–1014.

Besinger, S.J., and J.S. Stapczynski. 1997. Critical care of medical and surgical patients in the ER: length of stay and initiation of intensive care procedures. American Journal of Emergency Medicine 15(7): 654–657.

Boodman, S.G. 2005. Not Quite Fail-Safe; Computerizing Isn't a Panacea for Dangerous Drug Errors, Study Shows. Washington Post, March 22, 2005, p. F.01.

Bogner, M.S., ed. 1994. Human Error in Medicine. Mahwah, N.J.: Erlbaum.

Brandeau, M.L. 2004. Allocating Resources to Control Infectious Diseases. Pp. 443–464 in Operations Research and Health Care: A Handbook of Methods and Applications, edited by M.L. Brandeau, F. Sainfort, and W.P. Pierskalla. Boston, Mass.: Kluwer Academic Publishers.

Brewer, T.F., S.J. Heymann, S.M. Krumplitsch, M.E. Wilson, G.A. Colditz, and H.V. Fineberg. 2001. Strategies to decrease tuberculosis in U.S. homeless populations: a computer simulation model. Journal of the American Medical Association 286(7): 834–842.

Callahan, N.M., and W.K. Redmon. 1987. Effects of problem-based scheduling on patient waiting and staff utilization of time in a pediatric clinic. Journal of Applied Behavior Analysis 20(2): 193–199.

Champion, V., J.L. Foster, and U. Menon. 1997. Tailoring interventions for health behavior change in breast cancer screening. Cancer Practice 5(5): 283–288.

Chandler, A.P. 1990. Scale and Scope: The Dynamics of Industrial Capitalism. New York: Belknap Press.

Chaplin, E., M. Mailey, R. Crosby, D. Gorman, X. Holland, C. Hippe, T. Hoff, D. Nawrocki, S. Pichette, and N. Thota. 1999. Using quality function deployment to capture the voice of the customer and translate it into the voice of the provider. Joint Commission Journal on Quality Improvement 25(6): 300–315.

Chassin, M. 1998. Is healthcare ready for Six Sigma quality? The Milbank Quarterly 76(4): 565–591.

Christensen, C.M., R. Bohmer, and J. Kenagy. 2000. Will disruptive innovations cure health care? Harvard Business Review (September-October): 103–111.

Clark, H.H., and S. Brennan. 1991. Grounding in Communication. Pp. 127–149 in Perspectives on Socially Shared Cognition, edited by L.B. Resnick, J.M. Levine, and S.D. Teasley. Washington, D.C.: American Psychological Association.

Cohen, M.A., J.C. Hershey, and E.N. Weiss. 1980. Analysis of capacity decisions for progressive patient care hospital facilities. Health Services Research 15(2): 145–160.

Committee on Government Reform. 2001. National Preparedness: Ambulance Diversions Impede Access to Emergency Rooms. October 16, 2001. Washington, D.C.: Special Investigations Division, Committee on Government Reform, U.S. House of Representatives.

Cook, R.I., J.S. McDonald, and R. Smalhout. 1989. Human Error in the Operating Room: Identifying Cognitive Lock Up. Cognitive Systems Engineering Laboratory Technical Report 89-TR-07. Columbus, Ohio: Department of Industrial and Systems Engineering, Ohio State University.

Davis, C. 2005. Chronic Conditions Expert Host: Commentary on the Chronic Care Model. Available online at: *http://www.ihi.org/IHI/Topics/ChronicConditions/ExpertHostConnieDavis.htm*.

Dittus, R.S., R.L. Klein, D.J. DeBrota, M. Dame, and J.F. Fitzgerald. 1996. Medical resident work schedules: design and evaluation by simulation modeling. Management Science 42: 891–906.

Duraiswamy, N., R. Welton, and A. Reisman. 1981. Using computer simulation to predict ICU staffing needs. Journal of Nursing Administration 11(2): 39–44

Durieux, P. 2005. Electronic medical alerts—so simple, so complex. New England Journal of Medicine 352(10): 1034–1036.

Eddy, D.M., F.W. Nugent, J.F. Eddy, J. Coller, V. Gilbertsen., L.S. Gottlieb, R. Rice, P. Sherlock, and S. Winawer. 1987. Screening for colorectal cancer in a high-risk population: results of a mathematical model. Gastroenterology 92(3): 682–692.

Eich, H.P., C. Ohmann, K. Lang. 1997. Decision support in acute abdominal pain using an expert system for different knowledge bases. Proceedings of 10th IEEE Symposium on Computer-Based Medical Systems (CBMS'97). Available online at: *http://csdl2.computer.org/persagen/DLAbsToc.jsp?resourcePath=/dl/proceedings/cbms/&toc=http://csdl2.computer.org/comp/proceedings/cbms/1997/7928/00/7928toc.xml&DOI=10.1109/CBMS.1997.596400.*

Feistritzer, N.R., and B.R. Keck. 2000. Perioperative supply chain management. Seminars for Nurse Managers 8(3): 151–157.

Feltovich, P., K. Ford, and R. Hoffman, eds. 1997. Expertise in Context. Cambridge, Mass.: MIT Press.

Fone, D., S. Hollinghurst, M. Temple, A. Round, N. Lester, A. Weightman, R. Roberts, E. Coyle, G. Bevan, and S. Palmer. 2003. Systematic review of the use and value of computer simulation modelling in population health and health care delivery. Journal of Public Health Medicine 25(4): 325–335.

Forrester, J.W. 1961. Industrial Dynamics. New York: John Wiley and Sons, Inc.

Freund, D., D. Evans, D. Henry, and R.S. Dittus. 1992. Implications of the Australian guidelines for the United States. Health Affairs 11(4): 202–206.

Fries, B.E., and V.P. Marathe. 1981. Determination of optimal variable-sized multiple-block appointment systems. Operations Research 29(2): 324–345.

Friman, O., M. Borga, M. Lundberg, U. Tylén, and H. Knutsson. 2002. Recognizing Emphysema: A Neural Network Approach. ICPR'02 Proceedings of 16th International Conference on Pattern Recognition. August, 2002. Available online at: *http://www.imt.liu.se/mi/Publications/Publications/PaperInfo/fbltk02.html*.

Gaba, D.M., M.S. Maxwell, and A. DeAnda. 1987. Anesthetic mishaps: breaking the chain of accident evolution. Anesthesiology 66(5): 670–676.

GAO (General Accountability Office). 2003. Hospital Emergency Departments: Crowded Conditions Vary among Hospitals and Communities. GAO-03-460 March 14, 2003. Washington, D.C.: GAO.

Garg, A.X., N.K.J. Adhikari, H. McDonald; P. Rosas-Arellano, P.J. Devereaux, J. Beyene, J. Sam, R.B. Haynes. 2005. Effects of computerized clinical decision support systems on practitioner performance and patient outcomes: a systematic review. Journal of the American Medical Association 293: 1223–1238.

Gertz, D., and J.P.A. Baptista. 1995. Grow to Be Great: Breaking the Downsizing Cycle. New York: Free Press.

Godfrey, M.M., E.C. Nelson, J.H. Wasson, J.J. Mohr, and P.B. Batalden. 2003. Microsystems in health care: Part 3. Planning patient-centered services. Joint Commission Journal on Quality and Safety 29(4): 159–170.

Goldberg, C. 2000. Emergency crews worry as hospitals say, "no vacancy." New York Times, December 17, 2000, p. A39.

Gorunescu, F., S.I. McClean, and P.H. Millard. 2002. Using a queuing model to help plan bed allocation in a department of geriatric medicine. Health Care Management Science 5(4): 307–312.

Green, L.V. 2004. Hospital Capacity Planning and Management. Pp. 15–42 in Operations Research and Health Care: A Handbook of Methods and Applications, edited by M.L. Brandeau, F. Sainfort, and W.P. Pierskalla. Boston, Mass.: Kluwer Academic. Publishers.

Harry, M.J. 1988. The Nature of Six Sigma Quality. Schaumburg, Ill.: Motorola University Press.

Hashimoto, F., and S. Bell. 1996. Improving outpatient clinic staffing and scheduling with computer simulation. Journal of General Internal Medicine 11(3): 182–184.

Hauser, J.R., and D. Clausing. 1988. The house of quality. Harvard Business Review 3: 63–73.

Hellinger, F.J. 1998. The effect of managed care on quality. Archives of Internal Medicine 158(8): 833–841.

Hendee, W., ed. 1999. Proceedings of Enhancing Patient Safety and Reducing Errors in Health Care. Annenberg Center for Health Sciences, Rancho Mirage, California, November 8–10, 1998. Chicago, Ill. National Patient Safety Foundation.

Hershey, J., W. Pierskalla, and S. Wandel. 1981. Nurse Staffing Management. Pp. 189–220 in Operational Research Applied to Health Services, edited by D. Boldy. London, U.K.: Croom-Helm Ltd.

Hollnagel, E., D.D. Woods, and N. Leveson, eds. 2005. Resilience Engineering: Concepts and Precepts. Aldershot, UK: Ashgate Publishers.

Howard, S.K., D.M. Gaba, K.J. Fish, G.S. Yang, and F.H. Sarnquist. 1992. Anesthesia crisis resource management training: teaching anesthesiologists to handle critical incidents. Aviation, Space, and Environmental Medicine 63(9): 763–770.

Howard, S.K., B.E. Smith, D.M. Gaba, and M.R. Rosekind. 1997. Performance of well-rested vs. highly-fatigued residents: a simulator study. Anesthesiology A-981

Huang, X.M. 1995. A planning model for requirement of emergency beds. IMA Journal of Mathematics Applied in Medicine and Biology 12(3-4): 345–352.

Huber, T.P., M.M. Godfrey, E.C. Nelson, J.J. Mohr, C. Campbell, and P.B. Batalden. 2003. Microsystems in health care: Part 8. Developing people and improving work life: what front-line staff told us. Joint Commission Journal on Quality and Safety 29(10): 512–522.

IHI (Institute for Healthcare Improvement). 2003. Improving flow through perioperative services: a practical application of theory. IHI White Paper. Boston, Mass.: IHI

IHI. 2005. Ideas in Action: How Health Care Organizations Are Connecting the Dots between Concept and Positive Change: 2005 Progress Report. Boston, Mass: IHI. Available online at: *http://www.ihi.org/NR/rdonlyres/4CE48D26-2303-4FCD-9BF5-174EA039E725/0/ProgRep020505.pdf*

IOM (Institute of Medicine). 2001. Crossing the Quality Chasm: A New Health System for the 21st Century. Washington, D.C.: National Academy Press.

JCAHO (Joint Commission on the Accreditation of Healthcare Organizations). 2002. Failure Mode and Effects Analysis in Health Care: Proactive Risk Reduction. Oakbrook Terrace, Ill.: JCAHO.

Johnson, C. 2002. The causes of human error in medicine. Cognition, Technology and Work 4(2): 65–70.

Jorion, P. 1997. Value at risk: the new benchmark for controlling market risk. New York: McGraw-Hill.

Kao, E.P.C. 1974. Modeling the movement of coronary patients within a hospital by semi-Markov process. Operations Research 22(4): 683–699.

Klein, H.A., and J.J. Isaacson. 2003. Making medication instructions usable. Ergonomics in Design 11: 7–11.

Klein, H. A. and Meininger, A. R. 2004. Self-management of medication and diabetes: cognitive control. IEEE Transactions on Systems, Man, and Cybernetics, Part A: Systems and Humans 34(6): 718–725.

Klein, R.L., R.S. Dittus, S.D. Roberts, and J.R. Wilson. 1993. Simulation modeling in health care: an annotated bibliography. Medical Decision Making 13(4): 347–354.

Kosnik, L.K., and J.A. Espinosa. 2003. Microsystems in health care: Part 7. The microsystem as a platform for merging strategic planning and operations. Joint Commission Journal on Quality and Safety 29(9): 452–459.

Kostner, G.T., and R.J. Shachtman. 1981. A Stochastic Model to Measure Patient Effects Stemming from Hospital Acquired Infections. Pp. 1209–1217 in Institute of Statistics Mimeo Series 1364. Chapel Hill, N.C.: University of North Carolina.

Kutzler, D.L., and L. Sevcovic. 1980. Planning a nurse-midwifery caseload by a computer simulated model. Journal of Nurse-Midwifery 25(5): 34–37.

Kuzdrall, P.J., N.K. Kwak, and H.H. Schnitz. 1981. Simulating space requirements and scheduling policies in a hospital surgical suite. Simulation 36(5): 163–171.

Lattimer, V., S. Brailsford, J. Turnbull, P. Tarnaras, H. Smith, S. George, K. Gerard and S. Maslin-Prothero. 2004. Reviewing emergency care systems I: Insights from system dynamics modeling. Emergency Medicine Journal 21: 685–691.

Leape, L.L. 2004. Human factors meets health care: the ultimate challenge. Ergonomics in Design 12(3): 6–12.

Leatherman, S., D. Berwick, D. Iles, L.S. Lewin, F. Davidoff, T. Nolan, and M. Bisognano. 2003. The business case for quality: case studies and an analysis. Health Affairs 22(2): 17–30.

Letterie, G.S. 2002. How virtual reality may enhance training in obstetrics and gynecology. American Journal of Obstetrics and Gynecology 187(3 Suppl): S37–S40.

Levy, D.T., K.M. Cummings, and A. Hyland. 2000. A simulation of the effects of youth initiation policies on overall cigarette use. American Journal of Public Health 90(8): 1311–1314.

Lucas, C.E., K.J. Buechter, R.L. Coscia, J.M. Hurst, J.W. Meredith, J.D. Middleton, C.R. Rinker, D. Tuggle, A.L. Vlahos, and J. Wilberger. 2001. Mathematical modeling to define optimum operating room staffing needs for trauma center. Journal of the American College of Surgeons 192(5): 559–565.

Magazine, M.J. 1977. Scheduling a patient transportation service in a hospital. INFOR 25: 242–254.

Mahadevia, P.J., L.A. Fleisher, K.D. Frick, J. Eng, S.N. Goodman, and N.R. Powe. 2003. Lung cancer screening with helical computed tomography in older adult smokers: a decision and cost-effectiveness analysis. Journal of the American Medical Association 289(3): 313–322.

McCarthy, V. 1997. Strike it rich! Datamation 43(2): 44–50.

McDonough, J.E. 2002. Proactive Hazard Analysis and Health Care Policy. Plymouth Meeting, Pa.: ECRI.

McDonough, J.E., R. Solomon, and L. Petosa. 2004. Quality Improvement and Proactive Hazard Analysis Models: Deciphering a New Tower of Babel. Attachment F. Pp. 471–508 in Patient Safety: Achieving a New Standard of Care. Washington, D.C.: National Academies Press.

McKesson. 2002. Empowering Healthcare. Healthcare Financial Management. Available online at: *http://www.findarticles.com/p/articles/mi_m3257/is_1_56/ai_82067693*.

Miller, H.E., W.P. Pierskalla, and G.J. Rath. 1976. Nurse scheduling using mathematical programming. Operations Research 24: 856–870.

Miller, R.H., and H.S. Luft. 1994. Managed care plan performance since 1980: a literature analysis. Journal of the American Medical Association 271(19): 1512–1519.

Miller, R.H., and H.S. Luft. 2002. HMO plan performance update: an analysis of the literature, 1997–2001. Health Affairs 21(4): 63–86.

Mitchell, T.M. 1997. Does machine learning really work? AI Magazine 18(3): 11–20.

Mohr, J.J., P. Barach, J.P. Cravero, G.T. Blike, M.M. Godfrey, P.B. Batalden, and E.C. Nelson. 2003. Microsystems in health care: Part 6. Designing patient safety into the microsystem. Joint Commission Journal on Quality and Safety 29(8): 401–408.

Monden, Y. 1983. Toyota production system: practical approach to production management. Norcross, Ga.: Industrial Engineering and Management Press, Institute of Industrial Engineers.

Mullinax, C., and M. Lawley. 2002. Assigning patients to nurses in neonatal intensive care. Journal of the Operational Research Society 53(1): 25–35.

Murray, M., and D.M. Berwick. 2003. Advanced access: reducing waiting and delays in primary care. Journal of the American Medical Association 289(8): 1035–1040.

Neilson, A.R., and D.K. Whynes. 1995. Cost-effectiveness of screening for colorectal cancer: a simulation model. IMA Journal of Mathematics Applied in Medicine and Biology 12(3-4): 355–367.

Nelson, E.C., P.B. Batalden, T.P. Huber, J.J. Mohr, M.M. Godfrey, L.A. Headrick, and J.H. Wason. 2002. Microsystems in health care: Part 1. Learning from high-performing front-line clinical units. Joint Commission Journal on Quality Improvement 28(9): 472–493.

Nelson, E.C., P.B. Batalden, K. Homa, M.M. Godfrey, C. Campbell, L.A. Headrick, T.P. Huber, J.J. Mohr, and J.H. Wasson. 2003. Microsystems in health care: Part 2. Creating a rich information environment. Joint Commission Journal on Quality and Safety 29(1): 5–15.

Nemeth, C., Cook, R. I., and Woods, D. D. 2004. Messy details: insights from the study of technical work in healthcare. IEEE Transactions on Systems, Man, and Cybernetics, Part A: Systems and Humans 34(6): 689–692.

Ness, R.M., A. Holmes, R. Klein, and R.S. Dittus. 2000. Cost-utility of one-time colonoscopic screening for colorectal cancer at various ages. American Journal of Gastroenterology 95(7): 1800–1811.

Ness, R.M., R.W. Klein, and R.S. Dittus. 2003. The cost-effectiveness of fecal DNA testing for colorectal cancer. Gastrointestinal Endoscopy 57(5): AB94–AB94.

NIST (National Institute of Standards and Technology). 2005. Baldrige National Quality Program. Available online at: *http://www.quality.nist.gov.*

Norman, D.A. 1988. The Psychology of Everyday Things. New York: Basic Books.

Norman, D.A. 1993. Things That Make Us Smart. Reading, Mass.: Addison-Wesley.

Nyssen, A.S., and V. De Keyser. 1998. Improving training in problem solving skills: analysis of anesthetists' performance in simulated problem situations. Le Travail Humain 61(4): 387–402.

O'Keefe, R.M. 1985. Investigating outpatient departments: implementable policies and qualitative approaches. Journal of the Operational Research Society 36(8): 705–712.

O'Neill, L., and F. Dexter. 2004. Evaluating the Efficiency of Hospitals' Perioperative Services Using DEA. Pp. 147–168 in Operations Research and Health Care: A Handbook of Methods and Applications, edited by M.L. Brandeau, F. Sainfort and W.P. Pierskalla. Boston, Mass.: Kluwer Academic Publishers.

Ozcan, Y.A., E. Merwin, K. Lee, and J.P. Morrissey. 2004. State of the Art Applications in Benchmarking Using DEA: The Case of Mental Health Organizations. Pp. 169–190 in Operations Research and Health Care: A Handbook of Methods and Applications, edited by M.L. Brandeau, F. Sainfort, and W.P. Pierskalla. Boston, Mass.: Kluwer Academic Publishers.

Patterson, E.S., R.I. Cook, and M.L. Render. 2002. Improving patient safety by identifying side effects from introducing bar coding in medication administration. Journal of the American Medical Informatics Association 9(5): 540–553.

Patterson, E.S., R.I. Cook, D.D. Woods, R. Chow, and J.O. Gomes. 2004a. Hand-off strategies in settings with high consequences for failure: lessons for health care operations. International Journal for Quality in Health Care 16(2): 125–132.

Patterson, E. S., R.I. Cook, D.D. Woods, and M.L. Render. 2004b. Examining the complexity behind a medication error: generic patterns in communication. IEEE Transactions on Systems, Man, and Cybernetics, Part A: Systems and Humans 34(6): 749–756.

Pesonen, E. 1997. Is neural network better than statistical methods in diagnosis of acute appendicitis? Studies in Health Technology Information 43: 377–381.

Pexton. 2005. One Piece of the Patient Safety Puzzle: Advantages of the Six Sigma Approach. Patient Safety and Quality Healthcare. January/February. Available online at: *http://www.gehealthcare.com/usen/service/docs/patientsafetypuzzle.pdf.*

Phillips, A.N., M. Youle, M. Johnson, and C. Loveday. 2001. Use of a stochastic model to develop understanding of the impact of different patterns of antiretroviral drug use on resistance development. AIDS 15(17): 2211–2220.

Pierskalla, W.P. 2004. Blood Banking Supply Chain Management. Pp. 103–146 in Operations Research and Health Care: A Handbook of Methods and Applications, edited by M.L. Brandeau, F. Sainfort, and W.P. Pierskalla. Boston, Mass.: Kluwer Academic Publishers.

Pritsker, A.B. 1998. Life and death decisions: organ transplantation allocation policy analysis. OR/MS Today (August): 22–28.

Ray, W.A., K.T. Murray, S. Meredith, S.S. Narasimhulu, K. Hall, and C.M. Stein. 2004. Oral erythromycin and the risk of sudden death from cardiac causes. New England Journal of Medicine 351(11): 1089–1096.

Reichheld, F. 1996. The Loyalty Effect. Boston: Harvard Business School Press.

Reinus, W.R., A. Enyan, P. Flanagan, B. Pim, D.S. Sallee, and J. Segrist. 2000. A proposed scheduling model to improve use of computed tomography facilities. Journal of Medical Systems 24(2): 61–76.

Reisman, A., W. Cull, H. Emmons, B. Dean, C. Lin, J. Rasmussen, R. Darukhanavala, and T. George. 1977. On the design of alternative obstetric anesthesia team configurations. Management Science 23: 545–556.

Robinson, J.C. 2001. Theory and practice in the design of physician payment incentives. Milbank Quarterly 79(2): 149–177.

Rosenthal, M.B., R. Fernandopulle, H.R. Song, and B. Landon. 2004. Paying for quality: providers' incentives for quality improvement. Health Affairs 23(2): 127–141.

Schaefer, A.J., M.D. Bailey, S.M. Shechter, and M.S. Roberts. 2004. Medical Treatment Decisions Using Markov Decision Processes. Pp. 595–614 in Operations Research and Health Care: A Handbook of Methods and Applications, edited by M.L. Brandeau, F. Sainfort, and W.P. Pierskalla. Boston, Mass.: Kluwer Academic Publishers.

Shannon, R.P., D. Frndak, J. Lloyd, N. Grunden, C. Herbert, B. Patel, D. Cummings, A. Shannon, P. O'Neill, and S. Spear. In progress. Eliminating Central Line Infections in Two Intensive Care Units: Results of Real-time Investigation of Individual Problems. Harvard Business School Working Paper. Cambridge, Mass.: Harvard Business School Publishing.

Shina, S.G. 1991. Concurrent Engineering and Design for Manufacture of Electronic Products. Boston, Mass.: Kluwer Academic Publishers.

Siddharthan, K., W.J. Jones, and J.A. Johnson. 1996. A priority queuing model to reduce waiting times in emergency care. International Journal of Health Care Quality Assurance 9(5): 10–16.

Spear, S.J., and H.K. Bowen. 1999. Decoding the DNA of the Toyota production system. Harvard Business Review (Sept.-Oct.): 96–106.

Sterman, J.D. 2000. Business Dynamics: System Thinking and Modeling for a Complex World. New York: Irwin McGraw-Hill.

Sullivan, L.P. 1986. Quality function deployment. Quality Progress 19(6): 39–50.

Sullivan, L.P. 1988. Policy management through quality function deployment. Quality Progress 21(6): 18–20.

Swiercz, M., Z. Mariak, J. Lewko, K. Chojnacki, A. Kozlowski, and P. Piekarski. 1998. Neural network technique for detecting emergency states in neurosurgical patients. Medical and Biological Engineering and Computing 36(6): 717–22. Available online at: *http://www.ncbi.nlm.nih.gov/entrez/query.fcgi?cmd=Retrieve&db=PubMed&list_uids=10367462&dopt=Abstract.*

Teng, T.O., N.D. Osgood, and T.H. Lin. 2001. Public health impact of changes in smoking behavior: results from the Tobacco Policy Model. Medical Care 39(10): 1131–1141.

Thomas, J.A., V. Martin, and S. Frank. 2000. Improving pharmacy supply-chain management in the operating room. Healthcare Financial Management 54(12): 58–61.

Trivedi, V.M. 1980. A stochastic model for predicting discharges: applications for achieving occupancy goals in hospitals. Socio-Economic Planning Sciences 14(5): 209–215.

Tsay, A.A., and S. Nahmias. 1998. Modeling Supply Chain Contracts: A Review. Pp. 299–336 in Quantitative Models for Supply Chain Management, edited by S. Tayur, M. Magazine, and R. Ganeshan. Boston, Mass.: Kluwer Academic Publishers.

Tzukert, A., and M.A. Cohen. 1985. Optimal student-patient assignment in dental education. Journal of Medical Systems 9(5-6): 279–290.

Vassilacopoulos, G. 1985. Allocating doctors to shifts in an accident and emergency department. Journal of the Operational Research Society 36(6): 517–523.

Vissers, J., and J. Wijngaard. 1979. The outpatient appointment system: design of a simulation study. European Journal of Operational Research 3: 459–463.

Wagner, E.H. 1998. Chronic disease management: what will it take to improve care for chronic illness? Effective Clinical Practice 1: 2–4.

Walensky, R.P., S.J. Goldie, P.E. Sax, M.C. Weinstein, A.D. Paltiel, A.D. Kimmel, G.R. Seage, E. Losina, H. Zhang, R. Islam, and K.A. Freedberg. 2002. Treatment of primary HIV infection: projecting outcomes of immediate, interrupted, or delayed therapy. Journal of Acquired Immune Deficiency Syndromes 31(1): 27–37.

Warner, D. 1976. Scheduling nursing personnel according to nursing preference: a mathematical programming approach. Operations Research 24: 842–856.

Wasson, J.H., M.M. Godfrey, E.C. Nelson, J.J. Mohr, and P.B. Batalden.

2003. Microsystems in health care: Part 4. Planning patient-centered care. Joint Commission Journal on Quality and Safety 29(5): 227–237.

Wears, R.L. and M. Berg. 2005. Computer technology and clinical work still waiting for Godot. Journal of the American Medical Association. 293: 1261–1263.

Weeks, W.B., and J.P. Bagian. 2000. Developing a Culture of Safety in the Veterans Health Administration. Effective Clinical Practice. November/December. Available online at: *http://www.acponline.org/journals/ecp/novdec00/weeks.htm#authors.*

Wei J.S., B.T. Greer, F. Westermann, S.M Steinberg., C.G. Son, Q.R. Chen, C.C. Whiteford, S. Bilke, A.L. Krasnoselsky, N. Cenacchi, D. Catchpoole, F. Berthold, M. Schwab, and J. Khan. 2004. Prediction of clinical outcome using gene expression profiling and artificial neural networks for patients with neuroblastoma. Cancer Research 64(19): 6883–6891.

Weiss, E.N., M.A. Cohen, and J.C. Hershey. 1982. An interactive estimation and validation procedure for specification of semi-Markov models with application to hospital patient flow. Operation Research 30(6): 1082–1104.

Winner, R.I., J.P. Pennell, H.E. Bertrand, and M.M.G. Slusarczuk. 1988. The Role of Concurrent Engineering in Weapons System Acquisition. IDA Report R-338. Alexandria, Va.: Institute for Defense Analysis.

Woods, D.D. 2000. Behind Human Error: Human Factors Research to Improve Patient Safety. Washington, D.C.: American Psychological Association.

Xiao, Y., D. Gagliano, M.P. LaMonte, P. Hu, W. Gaasch, R. Gunawadane, and C.F. Mackenzie. 2000. Design and evaluation of real-time mobile telemedicine system for ambulance transport. Journal of High Speed Networks 9: 47–56.

Xiao, Y., and C.F. Mackenzie, eds. 2004. Introduction to the special issue on video-based research in high risk settings: methodology and experience. Cognition, Technology and Work 6(3): 127–130.

4

Information and Communications Systems: The Backbone of the Health Care Delivery System

The preceding chapter describes an array of systems-engineering tools and associated techniques for analyzing, designing, controlling, and improving health care delivery processes and systems. This chapter is focused on the application of information and communications technologies to the delivery of safe, effective, timely, patient-centered, efficient, and equitable health care, a review of progress toward the establishment of a National Health Information Infrastructure (NHII), and a description of the tasks that lie ahead. The committee highlights the complementary nature of information/ communications technologies and systems engineering.

THE CENTRALITY OF INFORMATION TO HEALTH CARE DELIVERY

Information and information exchange are crucial to the delivery of care on all levels of the health care delivery system—the patient, the care team, the health care organization, and the encompassing political-economic environment. To diagnose and treat individual patients effectively, individual care providers and care teams must have access to at least three major types of clinical information—the patient's health record, the rapidly changing medical-evidence base, and provider orders guiding the process of patient care. In addition, they need information on patient preferences and values and important administrative information, such as the status and availability of supporting resources (personnel, hospital beds, etc.).

To integrate these critical information streams, they will also need training/education, decision-support, information-management, and communications tools. For individual patients to participate as informed, "controlling" partners in the design and administration of their own care, they must also have access to much the same kind of information and education, decision-support, and communications tools—in a "patient-accessible/usable" form.

At the organizational level, hospitals and clinics need

clinical, financial, and administrative data/information to measure, assess, control, and improve the quality and productivity of their operations. At the environmental level, federal/state funding and regulatory agencies and research institutions need information on the health status of populations and the quality and productivity/performance of care providers and organizations to execute regulatory oversight, protect and advance the public health (surveillance/monitoring), evaluate new forms of care, accelerate research, and disseminate new medical knowledge/evidence.

As discussed in Chapter 3, information and information exchange are also critical to the tactical and strategic applications of systems-engineering tools at all four levels of the system, especially for strategic applications of enterprise-management tools and risk analysis and management tools at the organizational and environmental levels.

The Information Technology Deficit and Its Proximate Causes

Although information gathering, processing, communication, and management are essential to health care delivery, the health care sector as a whole has historically trailed far behind most other industries in investments in information/ communications technologies (DOC, 1999). Moreover, most health care-related information/communications technologies investments to date have been concentrated on the administrative side of the business, rather than on clinical care. As a result of this prolonged underinvestment, little overall progress has been made toward meeting the information needs of patients, providers, hospitals, clinics, and the broad regulatory, financial, and research environment in which they operate. A number of localized efforts have been made to develop and implement electronic patient records and other clinical applications of information/communications technologies since the 1960s, but little progress has been made in closing the gap.

Many factors have contributed to the information/ communications technology deficit: (1) the atomistic structure of the industry (the prevalence of relatively undercapitalized small businesses/provider groups); (2) payment/reimbursement regimes and the lack of transparency in the market for health care services, both of which have discouraged private-sector investment in information/communications systems; (3) historical weaknesses in the managerial culture for health care; (4) cultural and organizational barriers related to the hierarchical nature and rigid division of labor in health professions; and (5) the relative technical/functional immaturity (until very recently) of available commercial clinical information/communications systems.

FROM ELECTRONIC MEDICAL RECORDS TO A NATIONAL HEALTH INFORMATION INFRASTRUCTURE

The idea of transforming paper medical records into electronic medical records (EMRs) was first considered in the mid-1960s, when early prototype systems were developed. A number of large integrated health care provider organizations were early adopters of EMR systems, including Massachusetts General Hospital (COSTAR) in the 1960s, Indiana University Medical School (Regenstrief Medical Record System) in the early 1970s, and others (Kass-Bartelmes et al., 2002; Lindberg, 1979). However, there was little diffusion of these systems in the next two decades. In 1991 and 1997, IOM issued reports documenting the magnitude and implications of the large information-technology gap in U.S. health care and called for the adoption of EMRs as a first, critical step in moving health care delivery toward information/communications-technology-supported improvements in quality performance achieved in other industries (IOM, 1991, 1997).

Building on these studies, a series of reports by IOM, the National Committee on Vital and Health Statistics (NCVHS), and other organizations in the past five years have documented the profound negative impact of the information/ communications technology deficit on patient safety, the number of medical errors, and the quality and cost of care; every one of these reports calls for the development of a comprehensive health care information infrastructure (e.g., NHII) to help close the gap (IOM, 2000, 2001, 2003, 2004; NCHVS, 2001; NRC, 2000).

In *Information for Health: A Strategy for Building the National Health Information Infrastructure*, NCVHS described the NHII as both infrastructure and a defined set of components linked explicitly to health care delivery processes (NCVHS, 2001). IOM (2004) summarized the NCVHS definition as follows:

The NHII is defined as "a set of technologies, standards, applications, systems, values, and laws that support all facets of individual health, health care, and public health". . . It encompasses an information network based on Internet

protocols, common standards, timely knowledge transfer, and transparent government processes with the capability for information flows across three dimensions: (1) personal health, to support individuals in their own wellness and health care decision making; (2) health care providers, to ensure access to complete and accurate patient data around the clock and to clinical decision support systems; and (3) public health, to address and track public health concerns and health education campaigns.

This stream of reports from IOM, NCVHS, and others catalyzed a number of actions in the private and public sectors intended to lay the groundwork for and build momentum toward realization of the NHII (IOM, 2004; PITAC, 2004; Thompson and Brailer, 2004; Yasnoff et al., 2004). Inspired by the 1999 IOM report, *To Err Is Human*, the Leapfrog Group for Patient Safety, a coalition of large companies established expressly for the purpose of using their market power as major purchasers of health care to encourage care providers to improve the safety, quality, and efficiency of health care. The Leapfrog Group called on all health care provider organizations serving Leapfrog members' employees to use information/communications systems (EMRs and computerized physician order entry [CPOE] systems in particular) (see paper by Milstein in this volume).

In April 2004, progress toward an NHII was given new impetus when President Bush called for national implementation of EMRs and announced the creation of the Office of the National Coordinator for Health Information Technology (ONCHIT) in the U.S. Department of Health and Human Services (DHHS); Dr. David Brailer was appointed the first national coordinator. In July, DHHS released a report outlining a 10-year plan to build an NHII, including the creation of electronic health records (EHRs), for all Americans (Thompson and Brailer, 2004). In November 2004, ONCHIT issued a Request for Information (RFI) for a National Health Information Network (NHIN), soliciting proposals for ways to advance interoperability and standards. As of early 2005, ONCHIT had received more than 500 responses from a wide variety of organizations and collaboratives.

One of the respondents to the RFI, the Interoperability Consortium, an alliance of eight information-technology systems vendors (Accenture, Cisco, CSC, Hewlett-Packard, IBM, Intel, Microsoft, and Oracle), describes the current challenges to interoperability:

Dozens of communities and innovative networks across America have begun implementing information exchange solutions—yet they are following no common pathway, no uniform standards, and have established no basis for eventual information exchange among them or with the important national information networks already in existence. A common framework is needed to guide and maximize the value of the enthusiastic efforts already in the field.

In its preliminary blueprint for NHIN, the Interoperability Consortium (2005) stresses that the NHIN must be part of an agenda for the comprehensive transformation of health care delivery:

> The NHIN should be approached as an IT-enabled clinical transformation initiative that fuses technology and process reengineering in order to achieve its stated objectives of improving quality and decreasing costs. Performance metrics must be established to monitor progress, and incentives should be aligned (and periodically adjusted) to reward actual benefit realization. Conversely, the costs attached to supporting and monitoring the effectiveness of this transformation agenda should be included in the NHIN's total cost of ownership.

To meet these requirements, the NHII/NHIN must be a secure, reliable, and adaptable national infrastructure capable of connecting and supporting highly distributed, varied, independently managed, multi-tiered, intra-institutional, clinical information/communications technology systems and applications. This infrastructure would vastly expand the information gathering, exchange, processing, and application capabilities of stakeholders at all four levels of the health care system.

The Promise of a National Health Information Infrastructure

The NHII would provide a platform for the application of a wide range of proven and emerging information/communications technologies that could have a dramatic impact on health care processes and outcomes. The following discussion explores the promise of an NHII for each level of the health care delivery system.

Patient Level

At the patient level, progress toward an NHII would greatly empower individual patients to assume a much more active, controlling role in decision making and in implementing their own health care (i.e., applications that could help bring about a shift from hospital/clinic-based, clinician-directed care to home-based, clinician-guided self-care). The foundations for this shift have been laid by the emergence of the Internet and the World Wide Web, which have provided patients with unprecedented access to information (albeit of mixed quality) and made possible more continuous, asynchronous communication between patients and care providers.

Progress in systems interoperability and data standards is likely to advance the development of patient remote access to self-care educational tools, individual patient health records, and health care provider and insurer services (scheduling, billing, etc.) (see papers by Gustafson and Halamka in this volume). In time, the NHII would also provide a platform for the implementation of new information/communications systems, such as wireless integrated microsystems (WIMS, sensors combined with microelectronics and wireless interfaces), which would enable the remote capture and continuous communication of a patient's physiological data to care professionals, thereby increasing the likelihood of the timely diagnosis and treatment of illnesses.

An improvement in patients' ability to assume greater control and responsibility for care decisions enabled by information/communications technologies would also advance many of IOM's six aims for patient-centered, quality health care. Information/communications technology systems would give patients access to timely, effective, and convenient care; improve patient compliance with guidance/treatment protocols, including preventive measures; and enable continuous, or at least much more frequent, monitoring of patient conditions by care professionals/care teams. Greater compliance with clinicians' guidance—preventive or palliative—and more timely intervention in case of illness would not only benefit the health of the patient but would also reduce the costs of caring for the patient over time.

Care Team Level

At the care team level, progress toward an NHII would accelerate the development, diffusion, and use of a broad spectrum of information/communications technologies to help care providers capture, tap into, and integrate critical information streams for patient-centered care—the patient's health record, information on the patient's preferences and values, the evolving medical-evidence base, the status of clinical orders, administrative information, and a range of process/system performance data—essentially all of the data and information necessary to diagnose and prescribe treatment, as well as to analyze, control, and optimize the performance of the delivery system and subsystems.

Over the past decade, several core clinical applications have been developed to support the clinical information needs of frontline care teams. These include, EHR systems linking various information resources related to clinical care; CPOE systems, through which physicians enter orders for tests, drugs, and other procedures; decision-support tools that draw on clinical-data repositories, and databases that collect and store patient care information from diverse data sources.

Although the utility and functionality of these first-generation core clinical applications have been severely limited by the absence of comprehensive clinical information systems throughout much of the health care delivery system, progress toward the NHII would lead to the development and implementation of next-generation clinical applications that are more fully integrated and capable of translating clinicians' orders into dynamic, automated execution routines, as well as tracking and notifying clinicians of the status of their patients automatically. These applications could lead to changes in the role of the care team and individual care professionals, enabling them to spend less time executing and verifying the execution of orders and more time focusing on healing relationships with individual patients. Implementation of these technologies would also facilitate continuous learning in the care delivery system.

Organizational Level

At the level of the organization, steps toward an NHII would greatly facilitate the capture, integration, and analysis of clinical, administrative, and financial data for measuring and improving the quality, patient-centeredness, and efficiency of health care. As noted in Chapter 3, integration is essential to the application of data-intensive systems tools for systems design, analysis, and control. Beginning in the 1980s, a select group of health care provider organizations and networks began the integration process by adding clinical-department systems to their billing and administrative systems. It is worth noting that most of these forerunner, integrated systems were used by organizations with corporate-type structures and management (e.g., the Mayo Clinic, Kaiser-Permanente, Veterans Health Administration, and others with salaried physicians and wholly owned hospitals and ancillary functions). Only in the last decade have leading hospitals and integrated institutions begun to leverage their information systems by adapting and deploying systems-engineering tools and techniques to analyze, control, and optimize aspects of their operations.

As NHII (and interoperability and data-interchange standards in particular) advances, more and more health care organizations would be able integrate their clinical, administrative, and financial information systems internally, as well as link their systems with those of insurers, vendors, regulatory bodies, and other elements of the extended health care delivery enterprise. This capacity, in turn, would enable provider organizations to make more extensive global or strategic use of data/information-intensive systems-engineering tools, such as enterprise management, financial engineering for risk management, and knowledge discovery in databases.

Environmental Level

The NHII would lead to significant improvements on the environmental level of the health care delivery system. With advances in interoperability standards and other tools and technologies, the NHII would enable connectivity both within and across levels of the delivery system. This, in turn, would facilitate the aggregation and more timely exchange of useful data between and among providers at the organizational level and elements/stakeholder organizations at the environmental level (i.e., public and private payer organizations [insurers, employers], regulatory bodies, and the research community).

A functioning NHII could provide a rich pool of data to support regulation and oversight of the health care delivery system, population health surveillance, and the continuing development of the clinical knowledge/research database. For example, the NHII could accelerate the flow of health care quality data from providers to the Center for Medicare and Medicaid Services and private insurers, data on evidence-based-medicine trials to the Agency for Healthcare Research and Quality, data on infectious diseases and biohazards to the Centers for Disease Control, and data on post-introduction adverse drug events to the Food and Drug Administration (FDA).

NHII could also accelerate the interfacing of the expanding genomic and phenotypic (clinical) knowledge databases. The application of high-level systems-engineering tools (risk analysis) to these massive linked data sets could support significant advances in "predictive medicine"—mathematical and statistical techniques to identify and treat high-risk patients and to personalize treatment strategies.

Although much of the information/communications technology necessary for the realization of NHII exists today, and will certainly improve in the decade ahead, there will be many challenges to putting it in place. Very serious privacy concerns must be addressed, as well as training issues at all levels of the health care system. There are also serious challenges associated with making information/communications systems reliable enough to ensure that records are not lost. Ensuring reliability will require a very large-scale distributed computing system.

Paper-based systems are still the norm at most hospitals, which are all but "drowning" in paperwork. Clearly, it will take a national effort to develop an infrastructure capable of connecting, integrating, and supporting diverse information systems and applications at facilities nationwide. Although individual functions might still vary from facility to facility, the operating framework used for storing records and the protocols by which information is passed between locations and systems must be standardized.

Indeed, interoperability among diverse information/communications systems and messaging standards will be critical to the realization of an information/communications technology-enabled health care system, a programmable system with the capacity for mass customization to meet the needs of individual patients. At every level of the health care system, the focus should be on the patient, and the goal should be to ensure effective interactions between the patient and doctor or health care delivery team. Developing such a system in the coming decade is not an option. It is an absolute necessity for achieving the IOM vision of a patient-centered, high quality health care system.

The remainder of this chapter is divided into two sections. The first focuses on the current status of major components of the emerging NHII, identifies technical challenges and opportunities, identifies economic and cultural/organizational barriers to implementation, and provides recommendations for building on current momentum. The second focuses on emerging technologies based on wireless communications and microelectronic systems that have the potential to radically change the structure of the health care delivery system and advance the patient-centeredness and quality performance of the system. Although the widespread implementation of emerging technologies represents a longer term agenda than upgrading and/or diffusing existing clinical information/communications technology applications, the NHII has a 10-year time horizon for realization that can accommodate the incorporation of new technologies. Above all, the implementation of NHII must be part of a comprehensive transformation of health care delivery.

FOUNDATIONS OF A NATIONAL HEALTH INFORMATION INFRASTRUCTURE

The components of a national health information infrastructure can be divided into three interrelated categories: (1) health care data standards and technical infrastructure; (2) core clinical applications, including EHRs, CPOE systems, digital sources of medical knowledge, and decision-support tools; and (3) information/communications systems.

Health Care Data Standards and Technical Infrastructure

If health care data are standardized, they become understandable to all users. The IOM report (2004), *Patient Safety*, considered three key groups of standards:

- *Data interchange formats* are standard formats for electronically encoding data elements (including sequencing and error handling). Interchange standards can also include document architectures for structuring data elements as they are exchanged and information models that define relationships among data elements in a message.
- *Terminologies* are the medical terms and concepts used to describe, classify, and code the data elements and data-expression languages and syntax that describe relationships among the terms/concepts.
- *Knowledge representation* refers to standard methods of electronically representing medical literature, clinical guidelines, and other information required for computerized decision support.

For each group of standards, IOM identified critical challenges and described ongoing efforts led and/or funded by the federal government to address them. In the area of data-interchange formats, in which engineering has played an important role, a number of mature standards, recently endorsed by the secretary of DHHS, address some of the required domains:

- administrative data (the X12 standard of the Accrediting Standards Committee, Subcommittee on Insurance, Working Group 12)
- clinical data (Health Level 7)

- medical images (digital imaging and communications in medicine [DICOM])
- prescription data (National Council for Prescription Drug Programs [NCPDP] Script)
- medical device data (Institute for Electrical and Electronics Engineers [IEEE] Standard 1073)

In its data standards "action plan," IOM called for the rapid development of the next version (version 3.0) of the Health Level 7 clinical-data standards "to support increased interoperability of systems and comparability of clinical data, as well as patient safety," and underscored the need for "implementation guides and conformance testing/certification procedures . . . to insure consistent application of the standards in commercial systems" (IOM, 2004).

In the area of medical terminologies, IOM called for the identification of a "core group of well-integrated, nonredundant clinical terminologies . . . needed to serve as the backbone of clinical information and patient safety systems." With respect to knowledge representation, IOM identified a need for standards "for the representation of clinical guidelines and the implementation of automated triggers" (IOM, 2004).

To accelerate the development and adoption of health care data standards, IOM recommended a significant increase in the technical and material support provided by the federal government to ongoing public-private partnerships in this area (IOM, 2004). IOM also put forward a six-point federal government "work plan."[1] As noted above, the establishment of ONCHIT and the subsequent RFI were focused on interoperability and standards for an NHIN, demonstrating the urgency of the clinical information/communications

---

[1]The Institute of Medicine's "Action Plan for Setting Data Standards" includes two specific recommendations in each of three key areas: *Clinical data standards*: ". . . federal government health care programs should incorporate into their contractual and regulatory requirements standards already approved by the secretaries of DHHS, the Veterans Administration, and the Department of Defense . . . [and] AHRQ should provide support for accelerated completion of HL7 version 3.0, specifications for the HL& clinical document architecture and implementation guidelines, and analysis of alternative methods for addressing the need to support patient safety by instituting a unique health identifier for individuals." *Clinical terminologies*: "AHRQ should undertake a study of the core terminologies, supplemental terminologies, and standards mandated by the Health Insurance Portability and Accountability Act to identify areas of overlap and gaps in the terminologies to address patient safety requirements . . . [and] The National Library of Medicine should provide support for the accelerated completion of RxNorm for clinical drugs, and develop high-quality mappings among the core terminologies and supplemental terminologies identified by the CHI and NCVHS." *Knowledge representation*: "The National Library of Medicine should provide support for the development of standards for evidence-based knowledge representation . . . AHRQ, in collaboration with NIH, the FDA, and other agencies should provide support for the development of a generic guideline representation model for use in representing clinical guidelines in a computer-executable format that can be employed in decision support tools" (IOM, 2004).

technology challenge at the national level and the need for renewed efforts to engage the private sector in developing solutions.

To ensure that the emerging NHII can support next-generation clinical information systems and applications, it is critical that research on advanced interface standards and protocols continue apace and that standards-related issues concerning the protection of data integrity, controlled access to data, data security, and the integration of large-scale wireless communications be addressed early on. There is also a pressing need for low-cost tools for standardizing new and legacy digital data without disrupting the clinical work flow (PITAC, 2004). Other industries that had to accommodate conflicting standards (e.g., computer networks and computer graphic design) used translators to allow the best standard to emerge. Stable funding for research in all of these areas will be essential.

These challenges are neither new nor unique to health care. Indeed, engineers, computer scientists, and researchers and practitioners in other disciplines have been working on them for more than a decade to meet the needs of financial services, telecommunications, and national defense. Much of this work has been supported by federal research and mission agencies (NITRD, 2004). Cross-sector research and learning in the area of information/communications technology standards among federal agencies, health care insurers, and health care providers represents a potentially vast source of knowledge and advancement. To realize this potential, the President's Information Technology Advisory Council has called for increased coordination of federally supported research and development related to standards, computer infrastructure, privacy issues, security issues, and other topics relevant to health care through the Networking and Information Technology R&D (NITRD) Program, an 11-agency program that includes NSF, National Institutes of Health, Agency for Health Care Research and Quality, National Institute of Standards and Technology, Defense Advanced Research Projects Agency, U.S. Department of Energy, and others (NITRD, 2004).

Core Clinical Applications

Clinical information systems provide a mechanism for sharing data collected from various sources (e.g., EHRs in care settings that may include personal health record systems maintained by patients or their representatives). Data become available to clinical information systems via direct entry at the point of care, off-line entry through abstraction from other media, such as handwritten notes, and data collected by other systems, such as laboratory systems or monitoring devices. The data can take many forms—including free text, coded data, speech, document imaging, clinical imaging (e.g., x-rays), and video. In the following section, four core components of clinical information systems are described: (1) EHRs; (2) CPOE systems; (3) digital sources

of medical evidence; and (4) decision-support tools. These descriptions are followed by a discussion of human/information systems interface design and software dependability issues.

Electronic Health Records

The electronic capture of patient-specific clinical information is critical to many health care information/communications technology applications. Attention has been focused in the creation of EHRs since the 1960s, and in 1991, IOM set forth a vision and issued a call for nationwide implementation of computer-based patient records that would be paperless and instantly available throughout the health care system in forms readily understandable to physicians and other providers at point of care and specialists, perhaps in a different location (IOM, 1991). However, the rate of progress toward realizing this vision has been glacial.

Only a fraction of hospitals have implemented comprehensive EHR systems, although many have made progress in certain areas, such as computerized reporting of laboratory results (Brailer, 2003). Rates of adoption of EHR systems are higher in ambulatory care settings—probably about 5 to 10 percent of physician's offices—but these systems vary greatly in content and functionality (IOM, 2004). Although some cases of failed EHR systems have been documented, many more examples show cost savings and quality improvements yielded by EHR systems (Clayton in this volume; Littlejohns et al., 2003; Pestotnik et al., 1996; Wang et al. 2003).

EHRs have been instituted in health care settings in the public and private sectors, and a few communities and systems have implemented secure systems for the exchange of data among providers, suppliers, patients, and other authorized users. Among these are the Veterans Health Administration (see Box 4-1) , Mayo Clinic (see Box 4-2), New England Healthcare Electronic Data Interchange Network, Indiana Network for Patient Care, Santa Barbara County Care Data Exchange, Patient Safety Institute's National Benefit Trust Network, and the Markle Foundation Healthcare Collaborative Network (CareScience, 2003; Kolodner and Douglas, 1997; Markle Foundation, 2003; New England Healthcare EDI Network, 2002; Overhage, 2003; Patient Safety Institute, 2002; Zachariah in this volume).

All of these are exceptions to the rule, however. In most hospitals, orders for medications, laboratory tests, and other services are still written on paper, and many hospitals do not even have the capability of delivering laboratory results and other test results in automated form. The same situation prevails in most small practice settings, where little if any progress has been made toward creating electronic records (IOM, 2004).

A patient's EHR must also include long-term data and information about the patient's daily life. This information will be useful not only in the planning and delivery of

BOX 4-1
Veterans Health Information Systems and Technology Architecture

The Veterans Health Information Systems and Technology Architecture (VistA) supports a continuum of care, from intensive care units and other inpatient areas, to outpatient care settings, long-term care settings, and even home care environments. The Veterans Health Administration (VHA) Computerized Patient Record System provides a single interface where health care providers can review and update patients' medical records, as well as place orders for medications, special procedures, x-rays and imaging, nursing care, dietary requirements, and laboratory tests. In this system, 91 percent of all pharmacy orders are placed electronically (elsewhere, the rate is less than 10 percent).

Other components also have also been put in place to ensure better quality, safer, lower cost health care: (1) a health information infrastructure that provides decision support for population health management; (2) an integrated patient record and care system that includes clinical decision support for providers; and (3) a secure "portal" through which patients can receive reliable, accurate health information, access their health records, and interact with their clinicians.

In the VHA next-generation system, "HealtheVet," VistA has evolved from a facility-centric to a patient-centric system. HealtheVet implements standard functions in five areas: health data repository systems, registration systems, provider systems, management and financial systems, and information and educational systems. The most important of these is the health data repository, which creates a longitudinal health care record that includes data from VHA and non-VHA sources; supports research and population analyses; has improved data quality and security; and has facilitated patient access to data and health information.

Since the late 1990s, VHA has shared its health information, and its technology resources (software, expertise, etc.), with other federal agencies through the Health Information Technology Sharing (HITS) Program. In 2001, HITS was expanded to include some nongovernmental and international organizations. Through the recent HealthePeople Initiative, VHA now offers VistA software and expertise to other public- and private-sector organizations that serve the poor and near poor at no cost (or sometimes minimal cost).

Source: Center for Health Transformation, 2005b; VHA, 2005a,b.

BOX 4-2
Automation of Clinical Practice at Mayo Clinic

The Automation of the Clinical Practice (ACP) Project at Mayo Clinic in Jacksonville, Florida, undertaken in 1993, includes computer-based patient records and mechanisms for automated charging and order creation by physicians. The purpose of ACP was to initiate the "paperless" practice of medicine to improve patient safety and physician effectiveness and reduce expenses. The last paper-based record at the clinic was circulated in January 1996. In 2002, 445,000 patient visits were conducted with the computer-based patient record.

The ACP rollout involved all clinical users. The areas now automated include: (1) an electronic medical record (EMR) that includes all clinical documents, ordering, scheduling, and laboratory test results; (2) a fully electronic, filmless radiology department with speech recognition for documents; (3) an automated intensive care unit with EMR integration and bedside medical device interfaced directly to the EMR; and (4) inpatient and outpatient surgery areas that include surgical scheduling, material management, and nursing documentation.

Patient safety initiatives include: orders that automatically generate task lists for nurses, respiratory therapists, etc.; automated fall risk assessment; and Braden skin-scale assessment in the hospital. A medical data warehouse allows free searches of millions of documents in the EMR of patient care and research. An infectious-disease application allows surveillance for bioterrorism and automated monitoring for infection control. Changing to dictated notes decreased physicians' workloads and improved the legibility and turnaround time of medical records. The system provides real-time availability of clinical information, automatic checking for duplicate or redundant orders, simultaneous access to a patient's chart, improved ability to answer ad hoc questions, more timely responses to physicians questions, and a smoother flow of information, giving the physician a more "complete" picture of the patient's condition at the time of the appointment.

The estimated expenditure to date is $21 million. Using extremely conservative data, savings are estimated at $2.8 to $7.1 million annually. Thus, the system had paid for itself by the fourth year in financial savings alone. This does not include the intangible benefits, such as improvements in patient health, savings in doctors' time, and minimizing of errors.

In 2004, the Department of Applied Informatics, a Knowledge Center, was established through a joint venture with the Cerner Corporation. Using total knee arthroplasty (TKA) as its proof-of-concept project, the Knowledge Center is in the process of moving the project into routine activities. In addition, best practices were packaged into a process-management system. The goal was to show how leveraging information technology improves the quality and safety of care. Initial cost savings were more than $1 million/year from improvements in the TKA procedure. The attributes critical to the success of the project were the clinic's culture and long history as a professional learning organization.

Source: Based on Center for Health Transformation, 2005a.

progressive care, but will also provide evidence for assessing different clinical interventions. Systems-engineering tools and techniques are available for modeling and determining the information needs of a "system" that can deliver progressive care and evaluate that system's performance.

Patient-centered health care delivery in the broadest sense must also focus on what the patient really wants from the entire health care community—the best physical and mental function in daily living possible within the constraints of the patient's physical condition. The key word here is "system," that is, coordinated care, including care in the clinic, the hospital, home, rehabilitation facility, skilled nursing facility, long-term care facility, hospice, and perhaps social and societal programs. NHII is a first step toward obtaining data and information necessary for coordinating care in the clinic and hospital.

The management of large databases, which are essential to comprehensive core clinical applications for information/communications systems, remains a critical determinant. Although databases are effectively managed in select locations, efforts must continue to develop secure, dispersed, multiagent databases that can serve both providers and patients effectively and efficiently.

Computerized Physician Order Entry Systems

Using CPOE systems for entering orders for tests, drugs, and other procedures has led to reductions in transcription errors, which have led to demonstrable improvements in patient safety. When CPOE systems are integrated with other core clinical applications, their impact on patient safety is even greater. One component of a CPOE system is computerized decision support. CPOE systems that include data on patient diagnoses, current medications, and history of drug interactions or allergies can significantly reduce prescribing errors (Bates et al., 1998, 1999; Leapfrog Group, 2000).

CPOE systems also improve the quality of care by increasing clinician compliance with standard guidelines of care, thereby reducing variations in care. For example, a 1998 study by Shojania et al. found that CPOE, combined with the use of a vancomycin guideline, reduced the use of this over-prescribed antibiotic by 32 percent. A study of CPOE use at one large academic medical center (Brigham and Women's Hospital) by Teich et al. (2000) estimated that the overall annual cost savings from reductions in drug costs, laboratory tests, and diagnostic studies and the prevention of adverse drug events were roughly $5 to 10 million annually.

Despite many documented benefits of CPOE systems—improvements in the quality of patient care, decreases in medication errors, and decreases in overall costs—they have not been widely implemented. In the only study that has rigorously examined the adoption of CPOE by hospitals in the United States, less than 2 percent of hospitals were found to have CPOE systems completely or partially available and to require that physicians use them (Ash et al., 1998).

Nevertheless, a few success stories have been well documented, notably the Brigham and Women's Hospital in Boston, Massachusetts, and the Regenstrief Medical Record Systems.

Studies indicate that there are multiple barriers to the effective use of CPOE systems, including the lack of education and training of physicians, problems with user-interface designs, concerns about accuracy and reliability, high upfront fixed and ongoing maintenance costs, a lack of leadership commitment, difficulties in coordinating the introduction of new applications among varied care delivery settings and functions, and poor integration of CPOE systems with existing work processes and other information/communications systems, both clinical (e.g., digital sources of evidence, decision-support tools) and administrative (Boodman, 2005; Durieux, 2005; Garg et al., 2005; Sarata, 2002; Tang in this volume; Wears and Berg, 2005).

To address these problems, a template for patients, based on the current database, could be customized by the physician using evidence-based standards as the "orders" for each patient. One of the most frequent causes of errors and failures to carry out planned treatments has been a lack of integration of orders and results. Branching logic based on results can be used to verify that each step in the treatment is accomplished. The system described would not only reduce errors, such as missed handoffs and unnecessary waiting times, it would also interact with enterprise systems for supply-chain management and capacity planning.

Digital Sources of Evidence and Knowledge

Another key component of the health information infrastructure, digital sources of evidence—including bibliographic references, evidence-based clinical guidelines, and comparative databases—is essential for evidence-based practice. Currently, most digital sources of evidence are stand-alone systems that are not integrated into clinical information systems. The challenge for practitioners is to use these sources of evidence in combination with their experience and expertise to make clinical decisions (Bakken, 2001). However, as the medical-evidence base continues to expand exponentially and more and more clinicians accept the validity of best-demonstrated practices for diagnosis and treatment, there is mounting interest in integrating rapidly expanding digital sources of evidence (including genomic and phenotypic [clinical] data) into decision-support tools that can be fully integrated into care processes.

At the same time, fueled by the rapidly expanding medical-evidence base, there is a growing awareness among care professionals of the need for customization of best demonstrated practice rules for almost all patients. In the past five years, a new field has emerged, "predictive medicine" (i.e., the use of mathematical and statistical strategies to mine phenotypic [clinical] databases to identify and treat high-risk patients and to individualize treatment strategies).

Another emerging area is translational medicine, the use of the results of the genome project to predict and customize treatment.

Decision-Support Tools

The standardization of health care data, the development of digital sources of medical evidence and knowledge, and the creation of EHRs will all facilitate the use of decision-support tools, which are key components of clinical information systems. Decision-support tools that are fully integrated into the care process will enable both care providers and patients to access medical knowledge relevant to the patient's care. They may, for example, identify negative interactions between a drug the patient is already taking and an additional drug that might be prescribed.

A necessary platform for decision-support tools is the clinical-data repository, a database that collects and stores patient care information from diverse sources. Clinical-event monitors, which work with clinical-data repositories in support of real-time delivery of care, are usually triggered by clinical events (e.g., a patient visit, a medication order, a new laboratory result), either when data representing the event enter a repository or when a provider uses a clinical information system. The event monitor combines clinical rules, the triggering event, and information present in the repository to generate alerts, reminders, and other messages important to the delivery of care.

For more than 20 years, departmental systems (e.g., laboratory, x-ray) have had internal computerized systems that control operations and report results. But there is no health care process-management system in which all information concerning a patient's history is gathered in one place in standardized text where the appropriateness and strategy of orders for patient care can be checked. Equally important, a health care process-management system would ensure that the result of each step in treatment was entered into the record and communicated to all relevant parties. The collection of data, the consideration of the decision support offered, followed by the ordering and carrying out of the diagnostic and or treatment plan is an iterative process. As results are entered, the next steps in the care process are instituted.

Human-Computer Interfaces

Because the value of computerized clinical systems depends on how well they support care decisions in the service of patients, the development and implementation of information/communications systems that provide support and increase connectivity among health care providers will require "human-factors" research. This area of research, which combines expertise in cognitive and software engineering, behavioral science and cooperative work, and computer and cognitive sciences, focuses on the development of techniques and concepts that facilitate interactions between people and computers (Winograd and Woods, 1997; Woods, 2000).

Usefulness and usability in software-intensive systems cannot be achieved by patching "user-friendly" interfaces onto user-hostile system architectures. Health care computer systems have been administrator-centered or billing-centered systems rather than provider-centered or patient-centered systems. However, software and telecommunications capabilities are being expanded, although slowly, to achieve continuity of care without losing sight of economic and other pressures (Box 4-3).

A recent study concludes that there is an urgent need for more "research and development in innovative and efficient human-machine interfaces that are optimized for use in the health care sector" (PITAC, 2004). Areas for research include hardware interfaces, as well as sociological and psychological aspects of the use of computerized systems by physicians and other health care workers. The human-computer/information systems interface should be a high priority for health care. The study identifies targets for research: "improved medical-domain voice-recognition data conversion systems; improved automated entry of instrument data; and automated methods for converting both new and legacy electronic data to normalized form" (PITAC, 2004).

Software Dependability

In systems in which software is an element in the critical path, a variety of serious problems have plagued organizations, including lack of dependability and/or usability, the high cost of system failure, high maintenance requirements, and difficulties in updating systems. Because software-intensive systems perform valuable functions, the consequences of failure are generally serious. For example, developers may assemble modules, each apparently dependable, but, when they are integrated, problems and weaknesses emerge. Usability failures are also an issue. For example, if there are too many steps in a program for a user to follow or if a program is too complicated, various "work arounds" will be developed, and patient safety or some other critical parameter may be compromised.

In some cases, the initial software-intensive system may be dependable, but changes in use over time may lead to changes in the software that lead, in turn, to unnoticed side effects that can introduce weaknesses in the system. Another type of failure can occur when cost overruns in the development process prevent the project from ever reaching the commercialization stage. In some instances, noncritical software that interacts directly or indirectly with critical functions introduces failures and weaknesses (NRC, 2004; Rae et al., 2003). As these and other forms of software-system failure show, investments in clinical information systems must be complemented by investments in research on software dependability.

BOX 4-3
Designing Computer Systems for Health Care

Software-intensive systems are the norm for all modern high-performance systems. But simply extending the reach of computer technology will not guarantee high performance in a complex setting like health care. Many other factors must be considered: how well the technology supports human decision making, coordinates activities for different parties, cross-checks decisions to avoid failures, and coordinates activities to achieve continuity. A health care information system design that does not address these cognitive, cooperative, organizational aspects of new computer technology could exacerbate problems or introduce new forms of complexity.

When human-factors practitioners and researchers examined typical human interfaces with computer information systems and computerized devices in health care, they found that many devices were too complex and, given the typical workload, required too much training to use (e.g., Cook et al., 1992; Lin et al., 1998; Obradovich and Woods, 1996). Concepts and methods for use-centered design are available and are used every day in software development (Carroll et al., 1992; Flach and Dominguez, 1995; Nielsen, 1993); thus, usability testing should be standard (Rogers et al., 2001). Health care delivery organizations must be educated as informed consumers of computer information systems and shown how these techniques can be used in testing processes (Patterson et al., 2004).

But much more is involved in human-computer interaction than the adoption of basic techniques like usability testing. One way to ensure that a system is useful as well as usable is to make automation a team player with responsible people in the care process. New levels of automation have had many effects in operational settings. Operational experience, research investigations, incidents, and occasional accidents have shown that new, surprising problems can arise. The key requirement is that an information system be designed for fluent, coordinated interaction between the human and machine elements of the system. When automated systems increase the autonomy or authority of machines without providing tools to support cooperation with people, unexpected problems can contribute to incidents and accidents (Sarter et al., 1997). Increased automation requires new forms of feedback and displays that show human users what automated agents are doing and what they will do next relative to the state of the process (Norman, 1990).

Successful designs reverse this relationship. Instead of people checking on the computer, critiquing software can be used relatively unobtrusively to remind, suggest, and broaden the factors considered by human decision makers and improve performance, even when the computer cannot generate a good solution on its own (Guerlain et al., 1999). Investing in the building of partnerships, the creation of demonstration projects, and the dissemination of techniques for health care organizations will ensure that we receive the benefits of computer technology and avoid designs that introduce new errors (Cook et al., 1998).

Summary

The implementation of core clinical applications of information/communications systems has progressed very slowly because of costs, possible disruptions to current operations, problems with overlapping legacy systems, and problems with the use and integration of various systems. Opportunities for improvement (and research) include: better human-computer system interfaces; software to improve the interoperability of systems from various vendors; systems and accompanying business models for spreading costs among multiple users; and software dependability in the context of health care delivery.

COMMUNICATIONS TECHNOLOGIES

The delivery of quality care, especially in a highly fragmented delivery system, requires that both clinicians and patients have access to complete patient information and decision-support tools and that communications among clinicians and between clinicians and patients are effective. The Internet and the World Wide Web have provided patients with unprecedented access to health information and made possible more continuous, asynchronous communication between patients and their care providers. These technologies for asynchronous communication have enabled the development of self-care educational tools/modules, such as University of Wisconsin's Comprehensive Health Enhancement Support System (CHESS), which promotes informed health monitoring and decision making by giving patients access to disease-specific information (see paper by Gustafson in this volume). The case example of CareGroup Healthcare System (see Halamka in this volume) illustrates many of the challenges and opportunities associated with building fixed-line information/communication networks that increase connectivity and information exchange between patients and clinicians, as well as among dispersed elements of the care team.

Meeting the current and emerging communications needs of health care will require a combination of wireless and fixed-line networks. Because of financial constraints, creating different systems for different settings will not be feasible, however. Vendors of hardware and software components of the system will need system transparency, which can only be achieved once standards have been adopted. The challenge will be to generate a robust, but flexible system that can be duplicated in many different circumstances without requiring major modifications; the system must be based on technology that can be rapidly diffused and at low cost. Five technical factors are important in planning for the implementation of communication networks: (1) bandwidth requirements and availability; (2) latency in transmission throughout the network; (3) continuous availability of the network; (4) confidentiality and security of data; and (5) ubiquity of access to the network (NRC, 2000).

Enabling patients to communicate effectively with health care providers without face-to-face meetings will require many improvements in electronic communications. The Internet and World Wide Web provide a framework for communication links, and a few large provider organizations have demonstrated the potential of these technologies. But making them accessible to large populations in a health care community will require experimentation and research (Perlin et al., 2004). Other issues that must be addressed include ensuring the confidentiality and security of transmissions and health care data. In the long term, sensors that register a patient's vital signs and transmit data via wireless links could greatly improve the "connectivity" between patients and health care providers.

Barriers to Change

There is considerable evidence linking the use of advanced clinical information/communications systems to improvements in the quality, safety, and patient-centeredness of care (Breslow in this volume; Casalino et al., 2003; Clayton in this volume; Demakis et al., 2000; Lansky, 2002; Littlejohns et al., 2003; Miller and Bovbjerg, 2002; Wang et al., 2003; Weingarten et al., 2002). One recent estimate of potential savings to the nation's health care system from widespread implementation of clinical information/communications systems concluded that a fully interoperable network of EHRs would yield $77.8 billion a year in net benefits, or roughly 5 percent of the nation's total annual health care spending (Walker et al., 2005). In spite of the demonstrated benefits to society as a whole, however, many barriers stand in the way of widespread implementation of clinical information/communications systems in the United States.

In the preceding discussion of major components of the NHII, a number of technical impediments to implementation of these systems were identified (e.g., lack of interoperability standards, human-factors barriers; patient and caregivers' concerns about usability, reliability, and security; patients' concerns about the privacy of integrated health information, etc.). In addition, there are economic, cultural/organizational, and educational barriers that must by overcome. (Educational barriers are discussed in Chapter 5.)

Economic Barriers

Significant up-front and continuing costs of implementing clinical information/communications systems (e.g., EMRs, CPOE systems, decision-support tools) are particularly burdensome for individual care providers or small provider organizations, that is, the vast majority of care providers. These costs include not only the cost of hardware, software, and technical support, but also the costs of intensive training of patients and care providers in the use of these technologies, as well as costs associated with the adaptation of work processes, the roles of professionals and support staff, and the infrastructure necessary for information/communications systems to be effective components in the delivery of health care.

At the present time, several factors severely undercut the returns health care providers might expect to capture on their investments. First, the lack of technical interoperability standards for information/communications technologies and components and the lack of standard vocabularies have impeded information connectivity within the highly fragmented health care delivery system. This lack of connectivity, in turn, has severely limited improvements in efficiency and quality.

Presently, the scarcity of comparative quality and cost-performance data and the corresponding lack of quality/cost transparency in the market for health care services prevent patients from making informed choices among care providers on the basis of quality or value (quality/cost) (see Safran, this volume; Rosenthal et al., 2004). At the same time, the current "market" for health care services provides little reward to care providers who improve the quality of their processes and outcomes through investments in systems engineering tools, information/communications technologies, or other innovations (Hellinger, 1998; Leape, 2004; Leatherman et al., 2003; Miller and Luft, 1994, 2002; Robinson, 2001).

Another major barrier is the prevailing reimbursement arrangement for health care services, which does not reimburse care providers differentially on the basis of quality of care. Accordingly, providers have little incentive to invest in information/communications systems or process-management tools in support of quality improvement, unless they directly generate revenue or demonstrate immediate improvements in operating efficiency. (Contrast this with incentives for provider organizations to invest in new diagnostic equipment, such as MRI machines, which begin to generate revenue as soon as they are up and running). Moreover, most private and public insurance reimbursement models actively discourage delivery-related applications of information/communications technology by care providers, for example, by refusing to reimburse patient care/consultations delivered via e-mail (Leape, 2004; Leatherman, et al., 2003; Robinson, 2001).

The mandate of the Medicare Modernization Act and efforts by the Leapfrog Group and other buyers, insurers, and accreditation agencies to remove reimbursement- and regulation-related barriers to the use of information/communications systems in health care represent positive developments (CMS, 2004; Milstein in this volume). Nevertheless, the barriers persist. New financing and networking models will be necessary to encourage small businesses, which employ the vast majority of physicians, to take advantage of information/communications technologies without compromising the care of patients who are not computer literate. A number of public-sector and private-sector entities are already working on a cost-effective way to accomplish this (PITAC, 2004; SNL, 1996; Thompson and Brailer, 2004; Yasnoff et al., 2004).

The committee believes that as conceptual and material progress is made in measuring quality and productivity in health care, significant returns on investment at all levels of the health care system will be demonstrated (NRC, 2002; Triplett, 1999, 2001). But developing and validating system options for measuring the impact of information/communications technologies will require much more support from federal agencies (e.g., National Institutes of Health, National Science Foundation, Agency for Healthcare Research and Quality, Veterans Health Administration, and others). In the meantime, although the anticipated quality and productivity returns to the overall system from widespread application of systems engineering, information/communications technology, and related innovations may be great, in the current context, most individual provider organizations are not convinced that they can capture a large enough fraction of the total "social returns" on their private investments to warrant making these investments in the first place.

Cultural and Organizational Barriers

Clearly, many questions remain to be answered about the potential benefits of advanced information/communications systems in the health care industry, and answering these questions will mean overcoming many barriers. The introduction of systems analysis, systems redesign, and new information/communications systems are likely to cause significant disruptions to organizations and the structure of work processes at all four levels of the health care system. In addition, many clinicians have a very limited understanding of the potential uses, impacts, and benefits of advanced information systems for the production and delivery of care. Thus, the benefits of change are not immediately visible, but the costs are. Not surprisingly, then, there has been significant resistance to innovation and changes in work processes and the division of labor among health care professionals.

The cultural and organizational factors that have contributed to a rigid division of labor in many areas of health care often impede the introduction and exploitation of tools, technologies, and other innovations that could improve quality and productivity in health care (see Bohmer, this volume;

Christenson et al., 2000). Ultimately, the benefits offered by many of these tools and technologies can only be realized if management has the authority and/or capacity to persuade care providers to change their work practices and organization. Not surprisingly, the health care provider organizations most advanced in the use of systems tools and information/communications technologies have corporate management structures—all of their health care professionals are employees and are part of a clearly defined managerial hierarchy.

Findings

Finding 4-1. A fully implemented National Health Information Infrastructure would support distributed, independently managed, multi-tiered, intra-institutional information/communications systems and would dramatically improve the collection, exchange, and processing of information on all levels of the health care system.

Finding 4-2. A critical step toward realizing the National Health Information Infrastructure will be the development and widespread adoption of network standards for health care data and software. Research must focus on standards-related issues concerning the integrity of data, controlled access to data, data security, and the integration of large-scale wireless communications. There is also a pressing need for low-cost tools for standardizing new and legacy digital data without disrupting clinical work flows.

Finding 4-3. Interoperability standards for diverse information/communications systems and messaging standards will be critical to the realization of an information/communications technology-enabled health care system that has the capacity for mass customization to meet the needs of individual patients.

Finding 4-4. Progress in systems interoperability and data standards is likely to improve remote access to self-care educational tools, patient health records, and health care provider and insurer services (scheduling, billing, etc.).

Finding 4-5. Cross-sector learning and research on information and communications standards among federal agencies, health care insurers, and health care providers represents a potentially vast source of knowledge and advancement.

Finding 4-6. The Internet and World Wide Web provide a framework for communication links, but making them accessible to large populations in a health care community to promote communication between patients and health care providers will require experimentation and research, particularly to ensure the confidentiality and security of transmissions of health care data.

Finding 4-7. Opportunities for improvement of core clinical applications of information/communications technologies include: better human-computer interfaces; software to improve the interoperability of systems from various vendors; clinical information systems and accompanying business models for spreading costs among multiple users; the development and management of large, multi-agent databases; and software dependability in the context of health care delivery.

Finding 4-8. A National Health Information Infrastructure could provide a platform for the implementation of new information/communications technologies, such as wireless integrated microsystems, which would enable the remote capture and communication of patients' physiological data to care professionals, thereby increasing the likelihood of timely diagnoses and treatments of illnesses. In the long term, sensors that register a patient's vital signs and transmit data via wireless links could greatly improve the "connectivity" between patients and health care providers.

Finding 4-9. Much of the information/communications technology necessary for the development of the NHII, on all four levels of the health care delivery system, exists today. However, many barriers will have to be overcome before it can be implemented.

Finding 4-10. Although considerable evidence shows that advanced clinical information/communications systems lead to improvements in the quality, safety, and patient-centeredness of care, the health care sector as a whole trails far behind most other industries in investments in these systems. Many factors have contributed to this deficit: the atomistic structure of the industry; current payment/reimbursement regimes; the lack of transparency in the market for health care services; weaknesses in the managerial culture; the hierarchical structure and rigid division of labor; and (until very recently) the immaturity of available commercial clinical information/communications systems.

Recommendations

Recommendation 4-1. The committee endorses the recommendations made by the Institute of Medicine Committee on Data Standards for Patient Safety, which called for continued development of health care data standards and a significant increase in the technical and material support provided by the federal government for public-private partnerships in this area.

Recommendation 4-2. The committee endorses the recommendations of the President's Information Technology Advisory Council that call for: (1) application of lessons learned from advances in other fields (e.g., computer infrastructure, privacy issues, and security issues); and (2) increased coordination of federally supported research and development in these areas through the Networking and Information Technology Research and Development Program.

Recommendation 4-3. Research and development in the following areas should be supported:

- human-information/communications technology system interfaces
- voice-recognition systems
- software that improves interoperability and connectivity among systems from different vendors
- systems that spread costs among multiple users
- software dependability in systems critical to health care delivery
- secure, dispersed, multi-agent databases that meet the needs of both providers and patients
- measurement of the impact of information/communications technologies on the quality and productivity of health care

Recommendation 4-4. The committee applauds the U.S. Department of Health and Human Services 10-year plan for the creation of the National Health Information Infrastructure and the high priority given to the creation of standards for the complex network necessary for communications among highly dispersed providers and patients. To ensure that the emerging National Health Information Infrastructure can support current and next-generation clinical information/communications systems and the application of systems tools, research should focus immediately on advanced interface standards and protocols and standards-related issues concerning access, security, and the integration of large-scale wireless communications. Special attention should be given to issues related to large-scale integration. Funding for research in all of these areas will be critical to moving forward.

Recommendation 4-5. The committee recommends that public- and private-sector initiatives to reduce or offset current regulatory, accreditation, and reimbursement-related barriers to more extensive use of information/communications technologies in health care be expanded. These initiatives include efforts to reimburse providers for care episodes or other bundling techniques (e.g., severity-adjusted capitation; disease-related groups, etc.), public and private support of community-based health information network demonstration projects, the Leapfrog Group's purchaser-mediated rewards to providers that use information/communications technologies, and others.

MICROELECTRONIC SYSTEMS AND EMERGING MODES OF COMMUNICATION

The emerging technologies in wireless communications and microelectronic systems described in this section have the potential to advance the patient-centeredness and quality performance of the health care delivery system and to change the structure of care delivery in the process. Microelectronics promises to be a powerful tool for meeting quality and productivity challenges in health care delivery, provided that resources can be marshaled in a rational way. The micro-electronics revolution began in the 1950s with the advent of integrated circuits and has since revolutionized data process-ing, communications, and control. The number of transistors that can be integrated on a silicon chip the size of a finger-nail has increased from about 2,000 on the first micro-processor (1971) to about 200,000,000 today; the speed of these chips has increased more than a thousand-fold. At the same time, the number of bits of memory on a chip has increased by a factor of more than a million, and costs have decreased just as precipitously. Low-cost disk storage is now approaching a density of more than 40 gigabytes per square inch. In short, the processing and storage of data, the creation of information and knowledge based on those data, and the efficacy of decisions have improved exponentially.

Making Every Room an Intensive Care Unit

In the coming decades, as the number of nurses and physicians decreases, monitoring and diagnostics will have to improve dramatically. Efforts to develop sensors using integrated circuit technology has resulted in microelectro-mechanical systems, which can be combined with micro-electronics and wireless interfaces to create wireless integrated microsystems (WIMS) for use in health care delivery. In the near future, WIMS will be merged with sensors with embedded microcomputers and minute wire-less transceivers (a cubic centimeter in size or smaller) that operate at power levels of less than 1 milliwatt, consistent with long-term operation fueled by batteries maintained by energy scavenged from the environment (Wise, 1996, 2002).

These new devices could potentially provide continuous monitoring of critical functions, thereby turning every hos-pital room into an intensive care facility. WIMS devices small enough to be worn comfortably and unobtrusively could communicate with a bedside receiver that communi-cates, in turn, with monitoring stations and a larger health care facility. The system just described would go a long way toward meeting the objective of the Leapfrog Group of having an ICU physician present in every hospital at all times (Leapfrog Group, 2000).

WIMS systems are still scarce, and their performance is limited, but they are emerging. Blood oximeters, heart rate monitors, and temperature sensors could all be components of WIMS; swallowable capsules for viewing the digestive tract are already in use (Fireman, 2004; Pelletier, 2004; Pennazio et al., 2004). Wearable devices that monitor blood pressure (hypertension), breathing patterns (sleep apnea), and other variables will certainly be available in the near future (see Budinger in this volume). The major challenges to their use are interfaces with the body itself.

Swallowable capsules for all kinds of internal viewing and measurements could significantly improve diagnoses of a variety of conditions and thus could improve the quality of health care. DNA analysis chips will bring advances in genetics into the hospital, and even the local doctor's office (Burns et al., 1998; Mastrangelo et al., 1998), and should lead to improvements in both diagnostics and preventive health care. However, the impact of these developments on costs will be indirect. In addition, privacy issues must be addressed before they can be widely used.

WIMS for health care are expected to be technically fea-sible in the coming decade, but to reduce costs, they must be part of a complete *system*. Bedside receivers and wearable monitors might be technical triumphs, but they could also lead to economic disaster for the company that produces them unless they fit into a larger system.

A similar situation has existed for at least 20 years in the process-control industry. Although prototypes of sophisti-cated sensors have been produced, they are still not widely used because controllers that can exploit their features have not yet been developed. In the transportation industry, the entire control system of the automobile engine had to be redesigned to take advantage of microprocessors and elec-tronic sensing. Comparable redesigning of the health care system will be necessary at every level to take advantage of WIMS.

Advancing Patient Self-Care

The application of WIMS technologies in the hospital promises to significantly improve the quality and patient-centeredness of inpatient and ambulatory care. The potential impact of WIMS on home care and the quality of life for senior citizens and chronically ill patients is even greater (Whitten et al., 2003). Moving WIMS technology into the home is being seriously considered by makers of home com-munications equipment. With properly integrated home-based WIMS systems, patients could be monitored on a continuous basis and care professionals alerted automatically when events merit attention. Continuous or at least more frequent home monitoring of the health status of elderly and chronic care patients could notify clinicians of the need for timely therapeutic interventions that could avoid hospital-izations and shorten hospital stays, thus reducing the costs associated with the care of the patient over time (see Budinger in this volume). Moreover, home-based WIMS could facilitate safe home environments and the activities of daily living that are so important for the health of the elderly and chronically ill.

The main technical problems in the development of WIMS are largely related to reliable interfaces between sensors and the body and ensuring that sensors are capable of differentiating between instrumentation artifacts and physiological events. If these problems can be solved and such systems can "piggyback" on existing communication net-works, they could be implemented within the coming decade.

Therapeutic Uses

WIMS may also have therapeutic uses. The development of wireless *implantable* microsystems has been the subject of research for 40 years or more, but, to date, few devices have been developed besides pacemakers. Pacemakers have become increasingly sophisticated electronically, but their interfaces with the body are primarily via electrodes. Nevertheless, they have set the stage for the emergence of new devices in the coming decade. For example, cardiovascular catheters have been used for diagnosing cardiac conditions for many years, and pressure sensors small enough to be mounted directly on catheters have existed for some time (Chau and Wise, 1988; Ji et al., 1992). In fact, catheter-based electronics for improving diagnostic capabilities are long overdue. Another example is stents, which are widely used for treating coronary occlusions and now have chemical coatings to prevent re-stenosis. In the near future, stents may also be used as platforms for instrumentation, such as wireless sensors for monitoring blood pressure or blood flow that could be activated by a radio frequency wand positioned over the chest. Significant challenges remain involving range, accuracy, and size, but such systems may be feasible soon (Collins, 1967; DeHennis and Wise, 2002; Stangel et al., 2001).

Wireless sensors could also be used in intracranial, intraocular (glaucoma), and intra-arterial applications. Miniature biocompatible packages that can exist for many decades in the body are also being developed for long-term use in chronic conditions (Ziaie et al., 1996).

WIMS could also have a dramatic impact on the treatment of conditions involving the central nervous system. More than 90,000 cochlear implants are in use worldwide today, enabling many profoundly deaf and severely hearing-impaired individuals to function normally in a hearing world (House and Berliner, 1991; Spelman, 1999). Even though their performance is still limited and there is some opposition to them in the deaf community, these devices may render most kinds of deafness treatable disorders in the next two decades. In the United States alone, more than 2 million people are profoundly deaf, and 20 million are severely hearing impaired.

There is considerable interest in treating other neurological disorders using WIMS. Visual prostheses have recently received considerable attention but are still at a very early stage of development (Lui, 2002). The same is true of prostheses for severe epilepsy and paralysis. For example, an implanted electrode array might detect the onset of an epileptic seizure and provide local electrical stimulation or drug delivery to prevent the spread of the seizure. Functional neuromuscular stimulation (FNS) is being used to help quadriplegics stand and even walk, and the use of dense electrode arrays to capture control signals directly from the motor cortex has recently enabled primates to control robotic arms (Chapin et al., 1999; Serruya et al., 2002; Taylor et al., 2002) and humans to control cursors in operating a computer interface (Donoghue, 2004). Combining FNS with cortical control could lead to at least limited closed-loop activation of paralyzed limbs (Wise et al., 2004). And the use of deep brain stimulation in the subthalamic nucleus to eliminate the manifestations of Parkinson's disease has yielded impressive results and is now approved for human use (Limousin et al., 1998). Although all of these devices are still at a relatively early stage of development (Table 4-1), some are gaining acceptance now, and many could be in wide use in the next 20 years, which could substantially impact the quality of health care and the costs of rehabilitation.

Barriers

Microsystems implemented as wearable and implantable devices connected to clinical information systems through wireless communications could provide diagnostic data and deliver therapeutic agents for the treatment of a variety of chronic conditions. In fact, WIMS could potentially restructure care delivery in the hospital. There is no question that microdevices can and will significantly improve the daily lives of many people.

TABLE 4-1 Status of Wireless Devices for Treating Neurological Disorders

Disorder	Device	Status of Device	Comments
Deafness	Cochlear implant	In use.	More than 90,000 implanted worldwide.
Blindness	Retinal prosthesis	Early experimental prototypes.	Many projects under way worldwide; some cortical work.
Paralysis	Functional neuromuscular stimulation (FNS); direct cortical control (DCC)	Experimental FNS prototypes; basic DCC demonstrations in primates; first human implants.	Focus of FNS research is on standing, grasping, and walking systems; DCC seeks to capture control signals from the motor cortex.
Severe epilepsy	Implantable electrode arrays	Some human trials; experimental drug delivery devices.	Limited efficacy to date; continuing trials.
Parkinson's disease	Deep brain stimulation	In clinical use.	Very effective suppression of tremors.

The barriers to the realization of this vision are significant, however. For patients to take on greater control and responsibility for their own care, they will have to be educated or able to educate themselves. In addition, patients must continue to have access to trusted sources of advice and counsel.

Changes in the division of labor between patients and care teams implicit in the self-care model will also have a profound impact on the roles, work processes, and division of labor among members of the patient's care team. Current work rules, licensing requirements, staffing requirements, and regulations designed to ensure the safety, reliability, and quality of care in a hospital/clinic/provider-centered delivery system will also present impediments to a shift to the self-care model. Resistance to change, especially if roles, authority, and jobs are threatened, may arise among care professionals and organizations that deliver services both within and outside of hospital setting (e.g., testing labs, etc.). Current reimbursement systems may also present barriers if care providers are not reimbursed for e-visits, patient modules, remote care services, and so on.

The implications of the self-care model for the health care industry are profoundly disruptive. The move toward self-care could be considered threatening to businesses (e.g., testing laboratories, etc.) and individual care providers whose services will be less in demand. The current complex mix of professional licensing, regulation, liability law, and other constructs established to ensure the health care safety and reliability also pose barriers. The current hierarchical culture and rigid division of labor in the health care profession could make the reallocation of responsibilities and changes in the roles of care team members extremely contentious.

Findings

Finding 4-11. Wireless integrated microsystems could have an enormous beneficial impact on the quality and cost of health care, especially home health care. Microsystems implemented as wearable and implantable devices connected to clinical information systems through wireless communications could provide diagnostic data and deliver therapeutic agents for the treatment of a variety of chronic conditions, thereby improving the quality of life for senior citizens and chronically ill patients.

Finding 4-12. The use of wireless integrated microsystems technologies in hospitals and clinics promises significant improvements in the quality and patient-centeredness of inpatient and ambulatory care. Microdevices that could provide continuous monitoring of critical functions could turn every hospital room into an intensive care facility.

Finding 4-13. Wireless integrated microsystems for health care are expected to be technically feasible in the coming decade, but to reduce costs, they must be part of a complete *system*.

Finding 4-14. Significant cultural and organizational barriers will have to be overcome for the full benefit of WIMS to be realized.

Recommendations

Recommendation 4-6. Public- and private-sector support for research on the development of very small, low-power, biocompatible devices will be essential for improving health care delivery.

Recommendation 4-7. Engineering research should be focused on defining an architecture capable of incorporating data from microsystems into the wider health care network and developing interface standards and protocols to implement this larger network. Microsystems research should be focused on the following areas:

- integration, packaging, and miniaturization (to sizes consistent with implantation in the body)
- tissue interfaces and biocompatibility for long-term implantation
- interfaces and approaches to noninvasive (wearable) devices for measuring a broad range of physiological parameters
- low-power, embedded computing systems and wireless interfaces consistent with *in vivo* use
- systems that can transform data reliably and accurately into information and information into knowledge as a basis for treatment decisions

CONCLUSION

Timely, accurate information is critical to the efficient operation of large dispersed systems. Although the health care system has been slow to recognize this, efforts are now under way to rectify the situation. But it is imperative that research, development, demonstration, and training be expanded and accelerated.

Putting together a system that can make use of information microtechnology, nanotechnology, and biotechnology and ensure that applications are widely available and affordable will require coordination at the national level among device manufacturers, clinicians, and hospital systems. A successful health care system would use information/communications technologies in ways that would be largely invisible to patients but would improve care, reduce costs, and provide patient-centered care. However, unless the approach is coordinated, the impact of new technologies could improve health care for a few but increase costs for everyone else and move the overall system even farther away from providing patient-centered care.

REFERENCES

Ash, J.S., R.N. Gorman, and W.R. Hersh. 1998. Physician Order Entry in U.S. Hospitals. Pp. 235–239 in Proceedings/AMIA Annual Symposium. Bethesda, Md.: American Medical Informatics Association.

Bakken, S. 2001. An informatics infrastructure is essential for evidence-based practice. Journal of the American Medical Informatics Association 8(3): 199–201.

Bates, D.W., L.L. Leape, D.J. Cullen, N. Laird, L.A. Petersen, J.M. Teich, E. Burdick, M. Hickey, S. Kleefield, B. Shea, M. Vander Vliet, and D.L. Seger. 1998. Effect of computerized physician order entry and a team intervention on prevention of serious medication errors. Journal of the American Medical Association 280(15): 1311–1316.

Bates, D.W., J.M. Teich, J. Lee, D. Seger, G.J. Kuperman, N. Ma'Luf, D. Boyle, and L. Leape. 1999. The impact of computerized physician order entry on medication error prevention. Journal of the American Medical Informatics Association 6(4): 313–321.

Brailer, D.J. 2003. Use and Adoption of Computer-Based Patient Records in the United States: A Review and Update. PowerPoint presentation to the IOM Committee on Data Standards for Patient Safety, Irvine, California, January 23, 2003.

Boodman, S.G. 2005. Not Quite Fail-Safe; Computerizing Isn't a Panacea for Dangerous Drug Errors, Study Shows. Washington Post, March 22, 2005, p. F.01.

Burns, M.A., B.N. Johnson, S.N. Brahmasandra, K. Handique, J.R. Webster, M. Krishnan, T.S. Sammarco, P.M. Man, D. Jones, D. Heldsinger, C.H. Mastrangelo, and D.T. Burke. 1998. An integrated nanoliter DNA analysis device. Science 282(5388): 484–487.

CareScience. 2003. Santa Barbara County Care Data Exchange. Available online at: *http://www.carescience.com/healthcare_providers/cde/ care_data_exchange_santabarbara_cde.shtml.*

Carroll, J.M., W.A. Kellogg, and M.B. Rosson. 1992. Getting around the task-artifact cycle: how to make claims and design by scenario. ACM Transactions on Information Systems 10(2): 181–212.

Casalino, L., R.R. Gillies, S.M. Shortell, J.A. Schmittdiel, T. Bodenheimer, J.C. Robinson, T. Rundall, N. Oswald, H. Schauffler, and M.C. Wang. 2003. External incentives, information technology, and organized processes to improve health care quality for patients with chronic diseases. Journal of the American Medical Association 289(4): 434–441.

Center for Health Transformation. 2005a. Transforming Examples: Mayo Clinic, Jacksonville, FL. Available online at: *http:// www.healthtransformation.net/Transforming_Examples/ transforming_examples_resource_center/129.cfm.*

Center for Health Transformation. 2005b. Transforming Examples: Veterans Administration Healthcare System—My HealtheVet. Available online at: *http://www.healthtransformation.net/ Transforming_Examples/transforming_examples_resource_center/ 142.cfm.*

Chapin, J.K., K.A. Moxon, R.S. Markowitz, and M.A. Nicolelis. 1999. Real-time control of a robot arm using simultaneously recorded neurons in the motor cortex. Nature Neuroscience 2(7): 664–670.

Chau, H.-L., and K.D. Wise. 1988. An ultraminiature solid-state pressure sensor for a cardiovascular catheter. IEEE Transactions on Electron Devices 35(12): 2355–2362.

Christenson, C.M., R. Bohmer, and J. Kenagy. 2000. Will disruptive innovations cure health care? Harvard Business Review (September-October): 103–111.

CMS (Centers for Medicare and Medicaid Services). 2004. Medicare Modernization Act. Available online at: *http://www.cms.hhs.gov/ medicarereform/.*

Collins, C.C. 1967. Miniature passive pressure transducer for implanting in the eye. IEEE Transactions on Bio-medical Engineering 14(2): 74–83.

Cook, R.I., D.D. Woods, M.B. Howie, J.C. Harrow, and D.M. Gaba. 1992. Unintentional delivery of vasoactive drugs with an electromechanical infusion device. Journal of Cardiothoracic and Vascular Anesthesia 6(2): 238–244.

Cook, R.I., D.D. Woods, and C. Miller. 1998. A Tale of Two Stories: Contrasting Views of Patient Safety. Report from a Workshop on Assembling the Scientific Basis for Progress on Patient Safety. Chicago, Ill.: National Patient Safety Foundation.

DeHennis, A., and K.D. Wise. 2002. A Double-Sided Single-Chip Wireless Pressure Sensor. Pp. 252–255 in Digest of the IEEE MEMS Conference, Las Vegas, Nevada. New York: IEEE.

Demakis, J.G., C. Beauchamp, W.L. Cull, R. Denwood, S.A. Eisen, R. Lofgren, K. Nichol, J. Woolliscroft, and W.G. Henderson. 2000. Improving residents' compliance with standards of ambulatory care: results from the VA cooperative study on computerized reminders. JAMA 284(11): 1411–1416.

DOC (U.S. Department of Commerce). 1999. The Emerging Digital Economy II: Appendices. Washington, D.C.: DOC.

Donoghue, J.P. 2004. Presentation at Neural Interfaces Workshop, Bethesda, Maryland, November 15–17, 2004.

Durieux, P. 2005. Electronic medical alerts—so simple, so complex. New England Journal of Medicine 352(10): 1034-1036.

Fireman, Z. 2004. The light from the beginning to the end of the tunnel. Gastroenterology 126(3): 914–919.

Flach, J.M., and C.O. Dominguez. 1995. Use-centered design. Ergonomics in Design 3(3): 19–24.

Garg, A.X., N.K.J. Adhikari, H. McDonald; P. Rosas-Arellano, P.J. Devereaux, J. Beyene, J. Sam, R.B. Haynes. 2005. Effects of computerized clinical decision support systems on practitioner performance and patient outcomes: a systematic review. Journal of the American Medical Association 293: 1223–1238.

Guerlain, S., P.J. Smith, J.H. Obradovich, S. Rudmann, P. Strohm, J.W. Smith, J. Svirbely, and L. Sachs. 1999. Interactive critiquing as a form of decision support: an empirical evaluation. Human Factors 41(1): 72–89.

Hellinger, F.J. 1998. The effect of managed care on quality. Archives of Internal Medicine 158: 833–841.

House, W.F., and K.I. Berliner. 1991. Cochlear Implants: From Idea to Clinical Practice. Pp. 9–33 in Cochlear Implants: A Practical Guide, edited by H. Cooper. San Diego, Calif.: Singular Publishing Group, Inc.

Interoperability Consortium. 2005. Development and Adoption of a National Health Information Network: Response to ONCHIT's RFI. January 18, 2005.

IOM (Institute of Medicine). 1991. The Computer-Based Patient Record: An Essential Technology for Health Care. Washington, D.C.: National Academy Press.

IOM. 1997. The Computer-Based Patient Record: An Essential Technology for Health Care. Revised edition. Washington, D.C.: National Academy Press.

IOM. 2000. To Err Is Human: Building a Safer Health System, edited by L.T. Kohn, J.M. Corrigan, and M.S. Donaldson. Washington, D.C.: National Academy Press.

IOM. 2001. Crossing the Quality Chasm: A New Health System for the 21st Century. Washington, D.C.: National Academy Press.

IOM. 2003. Key Capabilities of an Electronic Health Record System. Washington, D.C.: National Academies Press.

IOM. 2004. Patient Safety: Achieving a New Standard of Care. Washington, D.C.: National Academies Press.

Ji, J., S.T. Cho, Y. Zhang, K. Najafi, and K.D. Wise. 1992. An ultraminiature CMOS pressure sensor for a multiplexed cardiovascular catheter. IEEE Transactions on Electron Devices 39(10): 2260–2267.

Kass-Bartelmes, B.L., E. Ortiz, and M.K. Rutherford. 2002. Using informatics for better and safer health care. Research in Action Issue 6. AHRQ Pub. No. 02-0031. Rockville, Md.: Agency for Healthcare Research and Quality.

Kolodner, R.M., and J.V. Douglas, eds. 1997. Computerized Large Integrated Health Networks: The VA Success. New York: Springer-Verlag.

Lansky, D. 2002. Improving quality through public disclosure of performance information. Health Affairs (Millwood) 21: 52-62.

Leape, L.L. 2004. Human factors meets health care: the ultimate challenge. Ergonomics in Design (summer): 6–12.

Leapfrog Group. 2000. Leapfrog Patient Safety Standards: The Potential Benefit of Universal Adoption. Available online at: *http://www.leapfroggroup.org*.

Leatherman, S., D. Berwick, D. Iles, L.S. Lwein, F. Davidoff, T. Nolan, and M. Bisognano. 2003. The business case for quality: case studies and an analysis. Health Affairs 22(2): 17–30.

Limousin, P., P. Krack, P. Pollack, A. Benazzouz, C. Ardouin, D. Hoffmann, and A.L. Benabid. 1998. Electrical stimulation of the subthalamic nucleus in advanced Parkinson's Disease. New England Journal of Medicine 339(16): 1105–1111.

Lin, L., R. Isla, K. Doniz, H. Harkness, K.J. Vicente, and D.J. Doyle. 1998. Applying human factors to the design of medical equipment: patient-controlled analgesia. Journal of Clinical Monitoring and Computing 14(4): 253–263.

Lindberg, D.A.B. 1979. The Development and Diffusion of a Medical Technology: Medical Information Systems. Pp. 201–239 in Medical Technology and the Health Care System: A Study of the Diffusion of an Equipment-Embodied Technology. Washington, D.C.: National Academy of Sciences.

Littlejohns, P., J.C. Wyatt, and L. Garvican. 2003. Evaluating computerised health information systems: hard lessons still to be learnt. British Medical Journal 326(7394): 860–863.

Lui, W. 2002. Retinal Implant: Bridging Engineering and Medicine. Pp. 492–495 in Digest of the IEEE International Electron Devices Meeting, San Francisco, California, December 2002. New York: IEEE.

Markle Foundation. 2003. Connecting for Health Unites over 100 Organizations to Bring American Healthcare System into Information Age. Press release. Available online at: *http://www.markle.org/resources/press_center/press_releases/2003/press_release_06052003.php*.

Mastrangelo, C.H., M.A. Burns, and D.T. Burke. 1998. Microfabricated devices for genetic diagnostics. Proceedings of the IEEE 86(8): 1769–1787.

Miller, R.H., and R.R. Bovbjerg. 2002. Efforts to improve patient safety in large, capitated medical groups: description and conceptual model. Journal of Health Politics, Policy and Law 27(3): 401–440.

Miller, R.H., and H.S. Luft. 1994. Managed care plan performance since 1980: a literature analysis. Journal of the American Medical Association 271(19): 1512–1519.

Miller, R.H., and H.S. Luft. 2002. HMO plan performance update: an analysis of the literature, 1997–2001. Health Affairs 21(4): 63–86.

NCHVS (National Committee on Vital and Health Statistics). 2001. Information for Health: A Strategy for Building the National Health Information Infrastructure. Washington, D.C.: U.S. Department of Health and Human Services. Available online at: *http://ncvhs.hhs.gov/nhiilayo.pdf*.

New England Healthcare EDI Network. 2002. About NEHEN. Available online at: *http://www.nehen.net/*.

Nielsen, J. 1993. Usability Engineering. Boston, Mass.: Boston Academic Press.

NITRD (National Coordination Office for Information Technology Research and Development). 2004. Revolutionizing Health Care Through Information Technology. Arlington, Va.: NITRD. Available online at: *http://www.itrd.gov/pitac/reports/20040721_hit_report.pdf*.

Norman, D.A. 1990. The "problem" of automation: inappropriate feedback and interaction, not "over-automation." Philosophical Transactions of the Royal Society of London B327: 585–593.

NRC (National Research Council). 2000. Networking Health: Prescriptions for the Internet. Washington, D.C.: National Academy Press.

NRC. 2002. At What Price?: Conceptualizing and Measuring Cost-of-Living and Price Indexes, edited by C.L. Schultze and C. Mackie. Washington, D.C.: National Academy Press.

NRC. 2004. Summary of a Workshop on Software Certification and Dependability. Washington, D.C.: National Academies Press.

Obradovich, J.H., and D.D. Woods. 1996. Users as designers: how people

cope with poor HCI design in computer-based medical devices. Human Factors 38(4): 574–592.

Overhage, J.M. 2003. Improving Patient Safety in Chronic Diseases Using Electronic Medical Records. PowerPoint presentation to the IOM Committee on Data Standards for Patient Safety, Washington, D.C., April 1, 2003.

Patient Safety Institute. 2002. Presentation to the 5th National HIPAA Summit—Beyond HIPAA: Clinical Data Standards and the Creation of an Interconnected Electronic Health Information Infrastructure. Available online at: *http://www.ehcca.com/presentations/HIPAA5/walker.pdf*.

Patterson, E.S., M.L. Rogers, and M.L. Render. 2004. Fifteen best practice recommendations to improve the effectiveness of bar code medication administration. Joint Commission Journal on Quality and Safety 30(7): 355–365.

Pelletier, F. 2004. Wireless tech allies with low-power gear. EE Times, August 16, 2004. Available online at: *http://www.eetimes.com/article/showArticle.jhtml?articleId=26806906*.

Pennazio, M., R. Santucci, E. Rondonotti, C. Abbiati, G. Beccari, F.P. Rossini, and R. De Franchis. 2004. Outcome of patients with obscure gastrointestinal bleeding after capsule endoscopy: report of 100 consecutive cases. Gastroenterology 126(3): 643–653.

Perlin, J.B., R.M. Kolodner, and R.H. Roswell. 2004. The Veterans Health Administration: quality, value, accountability, and information as transforming strategies for patient-centered care. American Journal of Managed Care 10(11 Pt 2): 828–836.

Pestotnik, S.L., D.C. Classen, R.S. Evans, and J.P. Burke. 1996. Implementing antibiotic practice guidelines through computer-assisted decision support: clinical and financial outcomes. Annals of Internal Medicine 124(10): 884–890.

PITAC (President's Information Technology Advisory Committee). 2004. Revolutionizing Health Care through Information Technology. Arlington, Va.: National Coordination Office for Information Technology Research and Development.

Rae, A., P. Ramanan, D. Jackson, and J. Flanz. 2003. Critical Feature Analysis of a Radiotherapy Machine. Pp. 231–234 in Computer Safety, Reliability, and Security: Proceedings of the 22nd International Conference (SAFECOMP 2003), Edinburgh, U.K., September 23–26, 2003. New York: Springer-Verlag.

Robinson, J.C. 2001. Theory and practice in the design of physician payment incentives. Milbank Quarterly 79(2): 149–177.

Rogers, W.A., A.L. Mykityshyn, R.H. Campbell, and A.D. Fisk. 2001. Analysis of a "simple" medical device. Ergonomics in Design 9(1): 6–14.

Rosenthal, M.B., R. Fernandopulle, H.R. Song, and B. Landon. 2004. Paying for quality: providers' incentives for quality improvement. Health Affairs 23(2): 127–141.

Sarata, A. 2002. Adverse Drug Events, Medication Errors, and CPOE: A Case Study. Prepared for the Committee on Engineering and the Health Care System. Washington, D.C.: National Academy of Engineering.

Sarter, N.B., D.D. Woods, and C.E. Billings. 1997. Automation Surprises. Pp. 1926–1943 in Handbook of Human Factors/Ergonomics, 2nd ed., edited by G. Salvendy. New York: John Wiley and Sons.

Serruya, M.D., N.G. Hatsopoulos, L. Paninski, M.R. Fellows, and J.P. Donoghue. 2002. Instant neural control of a movement signal. Nature 416(6877): 141–142.

Shojania, K.G., D. Yokoe, R. Platt, J. Fiskio, N. Ma'luf, and D.W. Bates. 1998. Reducing vancomycin use utilizing a computer guideline: results of a randomized controlled trial. Journal of the American Medical Informatics Association 5(6): 554–562.

SNL (Sandia National Laboratories). 1996. Strategies for the Future: The Role of Technology in Reducing Health Care Costs. Albuquerque, N.M.: Sandia National Laboratories.

Spelman, F.A. 1999. The past, present, and future of cochlear prostheses. IEEE Engineering in Medicine and Biology Magazine 18(3): 27–33.

Stangel, K., S. Kolnsberg, D. Hammerschmidt, B.J. Hosticka, H.K. Trieu, and W. Mokwa. 2001. A programmable intraocular CMOS pressure sensor system implant. IEEE Journal of Solid-State Circuits 36(7): 1094–1100.

Taylor, D.M., S.I.H. Tillery, and A.B. Schwartz. 2002. Direct cortical control of 3-D neuroprosthetic devices. Science 296(5574): 1829–1832.

Teich, J.M., P.R. Merchia, J.L. Schmiz, G.J. Kuperman, C.D. Spurr, and D.W. Bates. 2000. Effects of computerized physician order entry on prescribing practices. Archives of Internal Medicine 160(18): 2741–2747.

Thompson, T.G., and D.J. Brailer. 2004. The Decade of Health Information Technology: Delivering Consumer-centric and Information-Rich Health Care: Framework for Strategic Action. Washington, D.C.: U.S. Department of Health and Human Services.

Triplett, J.E., ed. 1999. Measuring the Prices of Medical Treatments. Washington, D.C.: Brookings Institution Press.

Triplett, J.E., ed. 2001. Measuring Health Output: The Draft Eurostat Handbook on Price and Volume Measures in National Accounts. Presentation at the Eurostat-CBS Seminar, Voorburg, Netherlands, March 2001.

VHA (Veterans Health Administration). 2005a. Health Community IT Sharing. Available online at: *http://www1.va.gov/vhaitsharing/page.cfm?pg=7.*

VHA. 2005b. What is VistA? Available online at: *http://www.vistasoftware.org/vista/.*

Walker, J., E. Pan, D. Johnston, J. Adler-Milstein, D.W. Bates, and B. Middleton. 2005. The value of health care information exchange and interoperability. Health Affairs Web Exclusive (Jan. 19): W5-10–W5-18.

Wang, S.J., B. Middleton, L.A. Prosser, C.G. Bardon, C.D. Spurr, P.J. Carchidi, A.F. Kittler, R.C. Goldszer, D.G. Fairchild, A.J. Sussman, G.J. Kuperman, and D.W. Bates. 2003. A cost-benefit analysis of electronic medical records in primary care. American Journal of Medicine 114(5): 397–403.

Wears, R.L., and M. Berg. 2005. Computer technology and clinical work still waiting for Godot. Journal of the American Medical Association 293(10): 1261–1263.

Weingarten, S.R., J.M. Henning, E. Badamgarav, K. Knight, V. Hasselblad, A. Gano Jr, and J.J. Ofman. 2002. Interventions used in disease management programmes for patients with chronic illness—which ones work? Meta-analysis of published reports. British Medical Journal 325: 925–942.

Whitten, P., G. Doolittle, M. Mackert, and T. Rush. 2003. Telehospice: end-of-life care over the lines. Nursing Management. 34(11): 36–39.

Winograd, T., and D.D. Woods. 1997. Challenges for Human-Centered Design. In Human-Centered Systems: Information, Interactivity, and Intelligence, edited by J. Flanagan, T. Huang, P. Jones, and S. Kasif. Washington, D.C.: National Science Foundation.

Wise, K.D. 1996. Microelectromechanical Systems: Interfacing Electronics to a Non-Electronic World. Pp. 11–18 in International Electron Devices Meeting Technical Digest, 1996. New York: IEEE.

Wise, K.D. 2002. Wireless Implantable MicroSystems: Coming Breakthroughs in Health Care. Pp. 106–109 in Symposium on VLSI Circuits Digest of Technical Papers, 2002. New York: IEEE.

Wise, K.D., D.J. Anderson, J.F. Hetke, D.R. Kipke, and K. Najafi. 2004. Wireless Implantable Microsystems: Electronic Interfaces to the Nervous System. Proceedings of the IEEE 92(1): 76–97.

Woods, D.D. 2000. Behind Human Error: Human Factors Research to Improve Patient Safety. Washington, D.C.: American Psychological Association.

Yasnoff, W.A., B.L. Humphreys, J.M. Overhage, D.E. Detmer, P.F. Brennan, R.W. Morris, B. Middleton, D.W. Bates, and J.P. Fanning. 2004. A consensus action agenda for achieving the National Health Information Infrastructure. Journal of the American Medical Informatics Association 11(4): 332–338.

Ziaie, B., J.A.V. Arx, M.R. Dokmeci, and K. Najafi. 1996. A hermetic glass-silicon micropackage with high-density on-chip feedthroughs for sensors and actuators. IEEE Journal of Microelectromechanical Systems 5(3): 166–179.

5

A Strategy to Accelerate Change

Many of the problems besetting the health care system are widely recognized, and a growing consensus has emerged that new approaches must be tried to solve them. Health care is commonly described as a system but, as this report shows, it was not created as a system and is not managed as a system. For the most part, management of the highly fragmented health care enterprise does not take into account interdependencies among patients, care teams, organizations, and the political-economic environment. Instead, individual units focus primarily on improving their unit performance with little regard for the impact on others.

A primary purpose of this report is to show that a broad portfolio of systems-engineering tools, information/communications technologies, and associated organizational and business processes are immediately available, or can be readily adapted, to improve health care delivery. Indeed, Chapters 3 and 4 have documented many examples at the patient, care-team, organizational, and environmental levels that demonstrate, albeit on a limited scale, the potential of these tools, technologies, and complementary knowledge to improve health care delivery dramatically. The successful use of many of these tools and technologies by the Veterans Health Administration (VHA), Kaiser-Permanente, Mayo Clinic, Institute for Healthcare Improvement (IHI) collaboratives, and other care providers demonstrates that both the productivity of the system and the quality of its processes can be improved simultaneously. In the committee's view, this may be the only sustainable pathway toward safer, more effective, more patient-centered care.

EDUCATIONAL BARRIERS TO CHANGE

Beyond the islands of progress mentioned above is a vast sea that remains virtually untouched by the portfolio of systems tools, information/communications technologies, organizational/managerial innovations, and cultural changes that have helped transform the quality and productivity of many other industries (both manufacturing and services) in recent decades. As described at length in Chapters 3 and 4, the combined economic, policy-related, technical, cultural, and organizational barriers to the widespread diffusion and implementation of these complementary tools, technologies, and knowledge in health care are formidable. In addition, the health care system faces significant educational barriers.

Currently, very few health care professionals or administrators are equipped to think analytically about health care delivery as a system. As a result, very few of them appreciate the relevance, let alone the potential benefits, of systems-engineering tools. And of these, only a fraction are equipped to work with systems engineers to adapt and apply these tools to meet the challenges in health care delivery. In addition, although most care professionals and administrators now appreciate the relevance of information/communications technologies to improving the quality and efficiency of health care delivery, very few of them are equipped to use these technologies systematically.

There are many reasons for the "systems-education" challenge, some of them related to changes in the structure of medical education early in the twentieth century and the rapid growth of biomedical research in the latter half of the century. In the early twentieth century, medical education underwent a revolutionary change with the development of entrance requirements for medical students, the adoption of a four-year curriculum, and the inclusion of laboratory and clinical experience in medical training. Training sites included academic medical centers, community hospitals, and affiliated facilities.

In the mid-twentieth century, large increases in funding from federal and private sources stimulated basic and clinical research, resulting in advances in knowledge of the biological basis for disease, diagnosis, and treatment. The specialized nature of this knowledge led to the creation of specialties and subspecialties among physicians, and the majority of physicians became specialists in one area or another of medicine (Ludmerer, 1999; Starr, 1992). Graduate medical education—internships, residencies, and fellowships—now supplement medical school education, providing practical training in clinical practice in medical specialties and subspecialties. Specialty boards were created to oversee this training, and eventually the control and regulation of training was transferred from academic medical centers to these specialty boards (Ludmerer, 1999).

Subsequently, new methods of disease prevention, diagnosis, and treatment were developed and tested through clinical research, thus bringing laboratory results to the bedside. Clinical epidemiology provided a scientifically rigorous evidentiary foundation for clinical practice, which has been widely adopted by medical specialties and has led to the notion of "evidence-based medicine." Changes in medical education reflected and reinforced the specialization in fields of medical research and practice, and graduate education of health professionals is now characterized by deep knowledge in narrow fields; a focus on individual patient care, with the primary emphasis on diagnosis and treatment and a lesser emphasis on disease prevention; little appreciation for populations/or public health; and almost no emphasis on the structure and processes of health care delivery. No substantive perspective on the entire system of health care or training in the uses and implications of systems tools and information/communications technologies for managing and improving the system is included in medical education.

Students of engineering and management are much more likely than their counterparts in health fields to be trained in systems thinking and the uses and implications of systems-engineering tools and information/communications systems for the management and optimization of production and delivery systems. Nevertheless, students at most U.S. engineering and business schools are not likely to find courses that address the operational challenges to the quality and productivity of health care delivery.

One major contributing factor to the absence of health care delivery challenges in engineering curricula has been the long-standing lack of demand for engineers in the health care delivery sector. In contrast to engineering careers in device and pharmaceutical companies and other for-profit industries, engineering careers in medical care institutions are nearly nonexistent. In addition, there is a pervasive under-appreciation by engineering faculty, researchers, and practitioners of the magnitude, complexity, and importance of the operational challenges and opportunities facing the nation's health care system combined with a reluctance to meddle in the "art" of highly respected health care professionals.

A PLATFORM FOR INTERDISCIPLINARY RESEARCH, EDUCATION, AND OUTREACH

In the preceding chapters, the committee has recommended a number of actions by industry, government, academia, and the health and engineering professions to begin to break down barriers to the use of systems-engineering tools, information/communications technologies, and business and managerial knowledge. Recommendations have included calls for public- and private-sector investments in research and development, demonstration projects, new approaches to reimbursement, expanded outreach and dissemination efforts by public- and private-sector health care quality improvement organizations, actions to advance the development of health care data, software, and network standards and other components of a National Health Information Infrastructure, and steps to harness the power of wireless integrated microsystems. The committee believes that action on these recommendations will accelerate the development, adaptation, implementation, and diffusion of systems-engineering tools and information/communications technologies in health care delivery. However, breaking down barriers and improving the overall health care system will also require bold, intentional, far-reaching changes in the education of researchers, educators, and practitioners in health care, engineering, and management through interdisciplinary research.

First, the academic research and educational engineering enterprise must be more closely linked to "real-world" needs in the public and private sectors to help bridge disciplinary research-to-application gaps in health care delivery. Some steps have already been taken in this direction. The NSF-sponsored Engineering Research Centers (ERCs) Program—which started in the 1980s and currently supports 22 centers—brings together industrial and academic researchers and graduate students on university campuses to conduct cross-disciplinary research focused on a single topical area and, in the process, encourages multidisciplinary interactions among faculty and students (NAE, 1983) (see Box 5-1).[1] In addition, guidelines for the ERCs explicitly call for strengthening connections between research and the creation of new curricular material (NAE, 1983). ERCs have had a significant impact on both research and academic programs in the institutions where they are located.

NSF and other agencies have also established other university-based interdisciplinary research centers involving engineering (e.g., NSF science and technology centers and materials research science and engineering centers; U.S.

---

[1]These include the Center for the Engineering of Living Tissues at Georgia Institute of Technology and the Emory School of Medicine; the Engineering Research Center for Computer-Integrated Surgical Systems and Technology at Johns Hopkins University; the Engineering Biomaterials Engineering Research Center at the University of Washington; the ERC in Bioengineering Educational Technologies at Vanderbilt University; the Biotechnology Process Engineering Center at Massachusetts Institute of Technology; the Engineering Research Center for Wireless Integrated Microsystems at the University of Michigan; and the Engineering Research Center for Biomimetic Microelectronic Systems at the University of Southern California (NSF, 2004a).

BOX 5-1
Engineering Research Centers Sponsored by the National Science Foundation

In December 1983, NAE was asked by the National Science Foundation (NSF) to provide advice on developing engineering research centers (ERCs), which the NSF described as "on-campus centers that would house cross-disciplinary experimental research activities." In addition to conducting research, the principal purposes of the ERCs are: (1) to provide a means of bringing together people in academia and industry[1] to improve the education of engineers; and (2) to expose a significant number of engineering students to the nature and problems of cross-disciplinary research on engineering systems.

In its report to NSF, *Guidelines for Engineering Research Centers,* NAE emphasized four themes: "(1) the relationship with industry must be real and must be perceived by both sides, the faculty and students of the Centers and the engineers and management of the participating companies, as mutually beneficial and as dealing with problems which are industrially important and intellectually demanding; (2) the Centers are experimental, will take time to grow, and will inevitably require altering protocols and programs; (3) to have an impact, the program must be a significant one, meaning that it is better to have fewer Centers with sufficient funding rather than many with inadequate funding; and (4) the Centers must complement and not supplant, either in size or numbers, the [National Science] Foundation's grants to individual investigators."

---

[1]The reader should substitute "the health care delivery system" for "industry."
Source: NAE, 1983.

Department of Energy materials research centers; U.S. Department of Transportation [DOT] university transportation centers; and university-based nanotechnology research centers sponsored by NSF, National Aeronautics and Space Administration, and DOD) (DOE, 2004; DOT, 2004; NNI, 2004; NSF, 2004a). As the results of interdisciplinary research are translated into classroom materials (e.g., new textbooks and courses) by participating faculty, these centers are directly affecting the way scientists and engineers are educated.

Two important lessons have been learned from these multidisciplinary engineering activities. First, they have contributed both to solving important research problems and to broadening the education of students. Each center, focused on a multidisciplinary area (e.g., tissue engineering, earthquake engineering, or surgical technology), necessarily addresses systems problems. Second, these centers have identified research topics that might not have been undertaken by researchers in a single discipline, which has led to the development of new curricular offerings and materials (NSF, 2004b).

Another instructive, large-scale, multidisciplinary research effort is the NIH-sponsored human genome project. In 1990, NIH embarked on a 13-year, multicenter project to map the human genome. The completion of the map laid the foundation for a wave of multidisciplinary systems research exploring the applications of this new knowledge base to medical practice. The translation of genome research into useful products and services has required a significant expansion of multidisciplinary research, including the establishment of multidisciplinary research centers where physicists, chemists, bioengineers, and mathematicians join forces to undertake the step-by-step progression from gene sequencing to the determination of protein function and the development of applications in screening, diagnostics, and treatment (Collins et al., 2003). These interdisciplinary centers have also demonstrated that multidisciplinary research and education can break down disciplinary barriers between the life sciences and their complements in the physical sciences and engineering (Harvard University, 2004a; MIT, 2004).

These new opportunities for multidisciplinary systems research in engineering and the biological sciences have demonstrated the potential for the development of analogous capabilities to address the challenges of health care delivery based on engineering sciences. The committee believes that a similar approach could build sustainable interdisciplinary bridges between the fields of engineering, health care, and management and begin to address the major challenges facing the health care delivery system. An environment in which professionals from all three fields engage in basic and applied research and translate the results of their research and advances both into the practice arena and the classroom, where students from the three disciplines interact, could be a powerful catalyst for cultural change.

The following recommendations are based on the logic, lessons, and momentum of these recent large-scale, multidisciplinary, research/education/technology-transfer initiatives focused on systems challenges in engineering and biomedical sciences.

Recommendation 5-1a. The federal government, in partnership with the private sector, universities, federal laboratories, and state governments, should establish multidisciplinary centers at institutions of higher learning throughout the country capable of bringing together researchers, practitioners, educators, and students from appropriate fields of engineering, health sciences, management, social and behavioral sciences, and other disciplines to address the quality and productivity challenges facing the nation's health care delivery system. To ensure that the centers have a nationwide impact, they should be geographically distributed. The committee estimates that 30 to 50 centers would be necessary to achieve these goals.

Recommendation 5-1b. These multidisciplinary research centers should have a three-fold mission: (1) to conduct basic and applied research on the systems challenges to health care delivery and on the development and use of systems-engineering tools, information/communications technologies, and complementary knowledge from other fields to address them; (2) to demonstrate and diffuse the use of these tools, technologies, and knowledge throughout the health care delivery system (technology transfer); and (3) to educate and train a large cadre of current and future health care, engineering, and management professionals and researchers in the science, practices, and challenges of systems engineering for health care delivery.

Interdisciplinary research centers could be configured in any number of ways. For example, schools of engineering, health science, and business administration at a single university might be allied with an academic medical center or other health care facility, or a combination of units from two or more academic institutions might work in collaboration with one or more health care facilities, or units from one or more academic institutions and health care facility might join with units from one or more federal laboratories. Whatever their configuration, it is essential that health care facilities (e.g., academic medical centers, regional health centers) be intimately involved, because they will provide a locus where innovations in systems design and operation can be tested, evaluated, and/or implemented.

Multidisciplinary centers would not only blend research and practice, they would also provide a means of demonstrating the value and promoting the use of existing systems tools to the larger community of practicing health care providers. Because each center will choose its focus area based on its inherent strengths, it will be important for the combination of centers to include the full spectrum of health care service providers, patient-advocate organizations, federal and state governments, health care provider organizations, private-sector insurers, technology vendors, medical service companies, university-based researchers and educators, federal laboratories, professional associations, and others. Only through close interactions of researchers, tools, technology developers, end users, and ultimate beneficiaries will the barriers to their widespread use be overcome.

One would expect the research and demonstrations conducted at these centers to inform, complement, and build on ongoing public- and private-sector efforts to promote the use and diffusion of systems engineering and information/communications technologies, such as IHI multiprovider innovation and diffusion collaboratives; the National Health Information Network initiative of the Office of the National Coordinator for Health Information Technology, the Joint Commission on the Accreditation of Healthcare Organizations and the VHA promotion of the use of failure/risk analysis tools; the VHA eHealth Initiative; the Centers for Disease Control (CDC) Centers of Excellence in Public Health Informatics; and the Leapfrog Group's campaign to promote the use of EHRs and CPOE systems (CDC, 2005; IHI, 2005; JCAHO, 2002; McDonough et al., 2004; Milstein in this volume; Thompson and Brailer, 2004; VHA, 2005).

A number of university-based multidisciplinary research centers explored the intersection of engineering and health care delivery during the 1970s and 1980s, but, according to some observers, their impact was significantly muted by the gap between their research results and the capacity of health care providers and organizations to implement them (see Box 5-2). The integration of research and education will be essential for sustained progress. Therefore, as in the NSF ERCs, faculty participating in these centers should be strongly encouraged to develop new curricular materials based on their research (NSF, 2004b). Research faculty could also provide materials for continuing education for health professionals, engineers, and managers involved or interested in becoming involved in the operational management and improvement of health care delivery systems.

The committee estimates that 30 to 50 geographically dispersed centers may be needed to involve and affect a significant number of current and emerging professionals in health care, engineering, and management. This estimate was arrived at in committee discussions on (1) the magnitude of effort at individual institutions of higher learning necessary to attract the attention/interest of faculty and students in relevant fields; (2) the number and geographic reach of the centers necessary to engage a critical mass of individuals and institutional players, including state governments, in the effort; and (3) the relative size of other initiatives (e.g., NSF's Engineering Research Centers Program; NIH's General Clinical Research Centers Network). The centers may vary in size, depending on their area(s) of focus, but core support of roughly $3.25 million annually for an average center would fund the work of eight faculty researchers, 24 graduate students, six support staff, and one senior administrator/center director and provide roughly $500,000 of working capital. An annual core funding level of $100 to $160 million would be anticipated for 30 to 50 centers.

Multiple government agencies (e.g., NIH, NSF, Agency for Healthcare Research and Quality, CDC, VA, and the Defense Advanced Research Projects Agency) would have a stake in the research, technology transfer, and educational missions of the proposed research centers, and these agencies

---

BOX 5-2
Forerunner Research Centers in Systems Engineering and Health Care

From 1970 to 1985, a number of interdisciplinary research centers were established at several academic centers (e.g., Georgia Institute of Technology, University of Missouri-Columbia, University of Pittsburgh, and University of Wisconsin, Madison) to explore the intersection of engineering and health care delivery. Faculty from business schools, engineering schools, medical schools, and nursing schools participated in research in industrial engineering, operations research, quality control, ergonomics, and statistics. At one time, there were more than a half dozen health care multidisciplinary research centers, but by the end of 1985, most of them had been closed down due to a lack of grant money and support from the health care industry. The centers at Georgia Institute of Technology and the University of Wisconsin still exist but are now associated with industrial engineering and have connections with medical schools at Emory University and the University of Wisconsin, respectively (Georgia Institute of Technology, 2005; University of Wisconsin-Madison, 2005).

The scope of research in the network of multidisciplinary centers proposed in this report would go far beyond the modest projects at these forerunner centers. The new centers would be configured not only to carry on research, but also to maintain a parallel focus on demonstration and diffusion of engineering techniques. Application, education, and diffusion would be advanced in living laboratories where engineering, health care, and management professionals and other researchers would work together to identify ways to overcome barriers to the application of currently available tools and to develop new tools.

---

should provide their core financial support. The continuity of funding will be critical for the centers to achieve their full potential. Experience has shown that periodic competitive reviews (for example, every five years) can provide evidence of progress and opportunities for renewing funding. In addition to core funding, center-based researchers and research teams would be expected to compete for additional public- and private-sector funding from health care provider organizations, private foundations, companies, and state governments for research, development, and/or demonstration projects of particular interest to them. An annual meeting of key researchers would ensure that important engineering/health care delivery issues were not overlooked.

Recommendation 5-2. Because funding for the multidisciplinary centers will come from a variety of federal agencies, a lead agency should be identified to bring together representatives of public- and private-sector stakeholders to ensure that funding for the centers is stable and adequate and to develop a strategy for overcoming regulatory, reimbursement-related, and other barriers to the widespread application of systems engineering and information/communications technologies in health care delivery.

The committee believes strongly that the establishment of a national network of multidisciplinary centers focused on improving the quality and productivity of U.S. health care delivery will be critical to achieving and sustaining the critical mass of research, education, and outreach that will be necessary to realize IOM's vision of a transformed twenty-first century health care system. At the same time, the committee believes that support for these new multidisciplinary

centers should not crowd out public- and private-sector funding for research by individual investigators on systems-engineering tools and information/communications technologies for health care. A mix of funding for interdisciplinary centers and individual researchers will ensure that a wide range of individuals from many parts of the research community are engaged in a common effort to improve health care delivery.

Accelerating Cultural Change through Formal and Continuing Education

Making systems-engineering tools, information technologies, and complementary social-science, cognitive-science, and business/management knowledge available and training individuals to use them will require commitment and cooperation among professionals in engineering and health care and changes in the cultures of health professionals and engineering professionals. The committee believes that these long-term cultural changes must begin in the formative years of professional education. Individuals in both professions must have opportunities to participate in learning and research environments in which they can contribute to a new approach to health care delivery.

The recommended interdisciplinary centers are not intended to produce health care professionals who can individually apply systems-engineering tools or engineers who can practice health care delivery. They are intended to provide an environment in which engineers and health professionals can work together and share experiences, thus breaking down disciplinary and linguistic barriers and building mutual trust and a shared understanding of the problems facing health care and the systems-engineering tools and information/communications technologies that can contribute to improving operations.

Recognizing and exploiting the potential contributions of systems engineering to health care delivery will be an enormous challenge for educators of health professionals. The current view of professional excellence accepted by health care providers will have to be expanded to encompass population health and the structure, processes, and systems of health care delivery. Physicians, nurses, and other health professionals will need new skills to work effectively with engineering and management professionals to change the design, implementation, and understanding of structures and processes of health care to ensure that care is safe, effective, timely, efficient, patient-centered, and equitable.

Thus, the training of health professionals will have to be changed. The curriculum will have to include systems-engineering concepts and skills, both directly in specifically focused courses and indirectly as part of other courses and units of study and practice. This will require that faculty with expertise in health care delivery be identified or recruited and educational and research links be established between clinical professions and schools of engineering and management.

This paradigm shift will require new strategies. The health professions have already taken some steps in this direction with the establishment of core competencies, including systems-based practice and practice-based learning and improvement, which have already attracted the attention of every training program and every trainee (Brennan et al., 2004; IOM, 2003; Leach, 2002). If these competencies are extended to requirements for relicensing, they will certainly be incorporated into clinical practice over time (Brennan et al., 2004; IOM, 2003; Leach, 2002; Lynch et al., 2004). Another encouraging sign is the VHA's adoption of formal courses in quality improvement and systems theory (VA, 2004).

New training strategies for interdisciplinary education should include health professional trainees in many aspects of health care working together and learning about each other's disciplines, perspectives, traditions, goals, objectives, tools, and techniques. This would give each clinician an opportunity to see the health care system in a broader context, to work as part of a team, to identify potential problems, and to be better prepared to contribute to system improvements.

Clearly, adding requirements to already crowded health professional curricula poses serious challenges. In medicine, the expansion of core competencies and a new emphasis on the clinician-patient relationship in teaching and testing have already led to a reexamination of the medical school curriculum (Brennan et al., 2004; IOM, 2003; Leach, 2002; Lewin et al., 2001). Core competencies in information technologies have also been identified in nursing at four levels of practice (Staggers et al., 2001).

Dramatic improvements in the efficiency and quality of health care delivery will only be possible with skilled engineers and health care management teams that understand and can implement the types of methods, tools, and technologies described in this report. To ensure that enough engineering and management professionals with these skills are available, curricula in schools of engineering, management, and public health will have to be expanded to encompass problems, concepts, and topics in health care delivery. These changes will have to be incorporated into formal classroom education, applied training, and continuing education for both professions. Thus, new models of education and training will have to be designed, implemented, and evaluated.

In addition to the development of supporting curricula and other resource materials, engineering educators face the challenge of cultivating demand for health care delivery-trained engineering graduates in an industry that has traditionally hired very few engineers and currently has no clearly defined career tracks for engineers. The lack of awareness of career opportunities in the health care industry for managers trained in the quantitative disciplines and tools described in this report may be the most significant reason so few MBAs enter the health care industry.[2] To attract more MBAs and other graduates to health care and to ensure a supply of leaders in health care improvement will require a significant effort to increase the visibility of the health care industry in MBA-related curricula.

The translation of interdisciplinary research results into instructional materials by faculty participants in the multidisciplinary research centers would impact the graduate, undergraduate, and continuing education of students and practitioners in all participating disciplines. In the meantime, however, the committee recommends the accelerated, intense training and development of select health care, engineering, and management professionals who understand the systems challenges facing health care delivery and the value of, and perhaps the application of, the tools and technologies to address them.

Recommendation 5-3. Health care providers and educators should ensure that current and future health care professionals have a basic understanding of how systems-engineering tools and information/communications technologies work and their potential benefits. Educators of health professionals should develop curricular materials and programs to train graduate students and practicing professionals in systems approaches to health care delivery and the use of systems tools and information/communications technologies. Accrediting

---

[2]One might think that the difference between the number of business graduates entering the health care sector and the number entering the financial services sector is attributable to different compensation levels. However, employment statistics from selected business schools show that initial salary levels for health care placements are often close to the initial salaries in financial services (Harvard University, 2004b; Northwestern University, 2004; University of California-Berkeley, 2004; University of Pennsylvania, 2004).

organizations, such as the Liaison Committee on Medical Education and Accreditation Council for Graduate Medical Education, could also require that medical schools and teaching hospitals provide training in the use of systems tools and information/communications technologies. Specialty boards could include training as a requirement for recertification.

Recommendation 5-4. Introducing health care issues into the engineering curriculum will require the cooperation of a broad spectrum of engineering educators. Deans of engineering schools and professional societies should take steps to ensure that the relevance of, and opportunities for, engineering to improve health care are integrated into engineering education at the undergraduate, graduate, and continuing education levels. Engineering educators should involve representatives of the health care delivery sector in the development of cases studies and other instructional materials and career tracks for engineers in the health care sector.

Recommendation 5-5. The typical MBA curriculum requires that students have fundamental skills in the principal functions of an organization—accounting, finance, economics, marketing, operations, information systems, organizational behavior, and strategy. Examples from health care should be used to illustrate fundamentals in each of these areas. Researchers in operations are encouraged to explore applications of systems tools for health care delivery. Quantitative techniques, such as financial engineering, data mining, and game theory, could significantly improve the financial, marketing, and strategic functions of health care organizations, and incorporating examples from health care into the core MBA curriculum would increase the visibility of health care as a career opportunity. Business and related schools should also be encouraged to develop elective courses and executive education courses focused on various aspects of health care delivery. Finally, students should be provided with information about careers in the health care industry.

Recommendation 5-6. Federal mission agencies and private-sector foundations should support the establishment of fellowship programs to educate and train present and future leaders and scholars in health care, engineering, and management in health systems engineering and management. New fellowship programs should build on existing programs, such as the Veterans Administration National Quality Scholars Program (which supports the development of physician/scholars in health care quality improvement), and the Robert Wood Johnson Foundation Health Policy Research and Clinical Scholars Programs (which targets newly minted M.D.s and social science Ph.D.s to ensure their involvement in health policy research). The new programs should include all relevant fields of engineering and the full spectrum of health professionals.

The goal of these recommendations is to make available and encourage the use of engineering tools and information/communications technologies in the health care community and to move toward meeting the six goals of the vision stated by IOM. Meeting the combined objectives of increasing research, demonstrating feasibilities, and diffusing successful demonstrations will require the commitment of many organizations.

CALL TO ACTION

As important as good analytical tools and information/communications systems are, they will not ultimately transform the system unless all members of the health care provider community actively participate and support their introduction and use. Communicating the overall system and subsystem goals to individuals and groups at all levels will be a crucial task for the management of health care organizations. Empowering individuals who do the day-to-day work in health care to make changes will require that everyone understand the overall goals and objectives of the system and subsystem in which they work. Participants must be energized and empowered to make continuous improvements in all processes, and encouraging and recognizing individuals for their contributions to the "continuous improvement" of operations must be a principal operating goal for management.

The committee recognizes the immensity of the task ahead and offers a word of encouragement to all members of the engineering and health care provider communities. Overhauling the health care delivery system will not come quickly, and achieving the long-term goal of improving the health care system will require the ingenuity and commitment of leaders in the health care community, as well as practitioners in all clinical areas. But if we take up the call now to change the system, we can perhaps avoid crises, reduce costs, reduce the number of uninsured, and make affordable, high-quality care available to all Americans.

REFERENCES

Brennan, T.A., R.I. Horwitz, J.D. Duffy, C.K. Cassel, L.D. Goode, and R.S. Lipner. 2004. The role of physician specialty board certification status in the quality movement. Journal of the American Medical Association 292(9): 1038–1043.
CDC (Centers for Disease Control and Prevention). 2005. Request for Applications: Centers of Excellence in Public Health Informatics (RFA-CD-05-109). Available online at: *http://grants.nih.gov/grants/guide/rfa-files/RFA-CD-05-109.html.*
Collins, F.S., M. Morgan, and A. Patrinos. 2003. The human genome project: lessons from large-scale biology. Science 300(5617): 286–290.
DOE (U.S. Department of Energy). 2004. Office of Basic Energy Sciences: BES Scientific User Facilities. Available online at: *http://www.sc.doe.gov/bes/BESfacilities.htm.*
DOT (U.S. Department of Transportation). 2004. University Transportation Centers (UTC) Program. Available online at: *http://utc.dot.gov/.*

Georgia Institute of Technology. 2005. Center for Operations Research in Medicine Homepage. Available online at: *http://www.isye.gatech.edu/~evakylee/medicalor/*.

Harvard University. 2004a. Department of Systems Biology, Harvard Medical School. Available online at: *http://sysbio.med.harvard.edu/*.

Harvard University. 2004b. 2004 Employment Statistics by Industry. Harvard Business School. Available online at: *http://www.hbs.edu/career_services/step5/cd2004-industry.html*.

IHI (Institute for Healthcare Improvement). 2005. Ideas in Action: How health care organizations are connecting the dots between concept and positive change. 2005 Progress Report. Boston, Mass: IHI. Available online at: *http://www.ihi.org/NR/rdonlyres/4CE48D26-2303-4FCD-9BF5-174EA039E725/0/ProgRep020505.pdf*.

IOM (Institute of Medicine). 2003. Health Professions Education: A Bridge to Quality, edited by A.C. Greiner and E. Knebel. Washington, D.C.: National Academies Press.

JCAHO (Joint Commission on the Accreditation of Healthcare Organizations). 2002. Failure Mode and Effects Analysis in Health Care: Proactive Risk Reduction. Oakbrook Terrace, Ill.: JCAHO.

Leach, D.C. 2002. Building and assessing competence: the potential for evidence-based graduate medical education. Quality Management in Health Care 11(1): 39–44.

Lewin, S.A., Z.C. Skea, V. Entwistle, M. Zwarenstein, and J. Dick. 2001. Interventions for providers to promote a patient-centered approach in clinical consultations. The Cochrane Database of Systematic Reviews, No. 4. Article CD003267. Available online at: *http://www.cochrane.org*.

Ludmerer, K.M. 1999. Time to Heal: American Medical Education from the Turn of the Century to the Era of Managed Care. New York: Oxford University Press.

Lynch, D.C., S.R. Swing, S.D. Horowitz, K. Holt, and J.V. Messer. 2004. Assessing practice-based learning and improvement. Teaching and Learning in Medicine 16(1): 85–92.

McDonough, J.E., R. Solomon, and L. Petosa. 2004. Quality Improvement and Proactive Hazard Analysis Models: Deciphering a New Tower of Babel. Attachment F. Pp. 471–508 in Patient Safety: Achieving a New Standard of Care. Washington, D.C.: National Academies Press.

MIT (Massachusetts Institute of Technology). 2004. Computational and Systems Biology at MIT. Available online at: *http://csbi.mit.edu/*.

NAE (National Academy of Engineering). 1983. Guidelines for Engineering Research Centers. Washington, D.C.: National Academy Press.

Northwestern University. 2004. 2003 Employment Report. Kellogg School. Available online at: *http://www.kellogg.northwestern.edu/career/employer/placement/2003/index.htm*.

NNI (National Nanotechnology Initiative). 2004. NNI Centers, Networks and Facilities. Available online at: *http://nano.gov/html/centers/nnicenters.html*.

NSF (National Science Foundation). 2004a. National Science Foundation Engineering Research Center Fact Sheets. Available online at: *http://www.erc-assoc.org/factsheets/start.htm*.

NSF. 2004b. ERC Achievements Showcase. Available online at: *http://www.erc-assoc.org/showcase/education_and_outreach.htm*.

Staggers, N., C.A. Gassert, and C. Curran. 2001. Informatics competencies for nurses at four levels of practice. Journal of Nursing Education 40(7): 303–316.

Starr P. 1992. The Social Transformation of American Medicine. New York: Basic Books.

Thompson, T. G., and D.J. Brailer. 2004. The Decade of Health Information Technology: Delivering Consumer-centric and Information-Rich Health Care: Framework for Strategic Action. Washington, D.C.: U.S. Department of Health and Human Services.

University of California-Berkeley. 2004. MBA Class of 2004, Full Time Employment Report. Haas School of Business. Available online at: *http://www.haas.berkeley.edu/careercenter/03_04Stats.html*.

University of Pennsylvania. 2004. MBA Career Management: 2004 Career Report. Wharton School of Business. Available online at: *http://mycareer.wharton.upenn.edu/mbacareers/report/index.cfm*.

University of Wisconsin-Madison. 2005. Center for Health Systems Research and Analysis Homepage. Available online at: *http://www.chsra.wisc.edu/*.

VA (Veterans Administration). 2004. VA National Quality Scholars Fellowship Program Fact Sheet. Available online at: *http://www.va.gov/oaa/SF_NQSF_Fact.asp*.

VHA (Veterans Health Administration). 2005. Health Community IT Sharing. Available online at: *http://www1.va.gov/vhaitsharing/page.cfm?pg=7*.

PART II

WORKSHOP PRESENTATIONS

Framing the
Health Care Challenge

Crossing the Quality Chasm

Janet Corrigan
Institute of Medicine

The Quality of Care in America Project was started about three years ago. The final report, *Crossing the Quality Chasm*, is a comprehensive review of the overall quality of the health care system, including an assessment of its safety and effectiveness and recommendations for a comprehensive strategy for improvement (IOM, 2001).

The first step in the project was a review of the literature by RAND. About 70 RAND studies have documented serious deficiencies and large gaps between the care people should receive and the care they actually do receive. Deficiencies were observed in all health care settings, in all age groups, and in all geographic areas. In other words, the problems are systemic and permeate the health care industry; problems are just as prevalent in traditional indemnity, or less managed, settings as in managed care settings.

Two factors influence how we approach this problem. The first is the expanding knowledge base, which has clearly overwhelmed physicians and made it all but impossible for an individual physician to provide high quality care on his or her own. A tremendous number of publications now report the results of randomized controlled trials, and the number of new drugs and medical devices and the amount of information flowing into the marketplace has increased exponentially.

The second major factor is the need to care for people with chronic conditions. A very limited number of chronic conditions, 15 or 20, account for the bulk of health care problems. If we targeted those conditions, we could make tremendous progress and affect a sizable proportion of the health care delivery system, as well as of the general population.

The models that are most useful in caring for the chronically ill are very different from our current delivery system models. Providing high-quality care to chronically ill individuals requires well designed care processes focused on information that meets the self-management needs of patients and their families. Patients with chronic illnesses require multidisciplinary care from teams of physicians, nurses, social workers, aides, and others. Team care is essential for high quality care.

Our current health care delivery system, which is organized around professionals and types of institutions, grew out of a need to provide primarily acute care rather than chronic care. This is one kind of chasm we have to cross. The health care delivery system must be reorganized to meet the real needs of patients.

Few clinical programs have the infrastructure to provide a full complement of services to chronically ill patients. Some institutions have well defined programs for particular chronic conditions, but few institutions or systems provide high quality care for the full range of chronic conditions. In addition, we have a problem in "scaling up"—exemplary programs are not replicated throughout the industry.

The lack of standardized performance measures has made it difficult if not impossible to make cross-institutional comparisons. For example, we have no standardized performance or outcome measures that enable us to identify which providers deliver exemplary care for diabetes. This creates two problems. First, we do not know where the best performers are. Second, the best performers are not rewarded for their excellent work. We need much better systems for managing knowledge and for using information technology to help people make decisions, and we need unfettered, timely access to clinical information.

Today, physician groups often operate as "silos" (i.e., in isolation) without benefit of the kind of information, infrastructure, and support they need to provide high quality care. On the one hand, we can no longer deliver health care through a collection of silos. On the other hand, we do not have the organizational support that can, for example, pull together the latest knowledge and make it readily available to providers and patients. If one looks on the Web, one finds 42,000 sites on lupus and 75,000 sites on breast cancer. Individual patients and individual professionals are overloaded with huge amounts of undigestible, disorganized information.

The Committee on Quality of Health Care in America recommended that the redesign process be initiated by focusing on priority areas. Specifically, the Agency for Healthcare Research and Quality should identify 15 priority areas and define them clearly so that everyone involved can work toward the same goals. The committee also recommended that Congress establish a $1 billion innovation fund to seed improvement projects and that purchasers, health care organizations, and professional groups begin to develop action plans immediately for each priority area. The goal should be a 50-percent improvement in quality and safety in the next five years.

Meaningful innovation in the health care delivery system will require some significant changes in the overall health system environment. The *Chasm* report describes changes in four key areas: (1) the use of information technology; (2) payment policies; (3) the development of best practices, decision support tools, and an accountability system; and (4) professional education and training (IOM, 2001).

We have many examples of how information technology can improve quality. For instance, we know that computerized order entry by physicians can reduce adverse drug events by 50 to 60 percent—an enormous improvement in safety. Reminder systems for physicians or patients and their families have been found to be effective in getting people the right services at the right time. The Institute of Medicine is working on a strategic plan for an information technology initiative that should be ready soon.

Second, current payment policies are complex, contradictory, and often work against improving quality. For example, current payment systems do not reward investments in information technology. Unlike investments in medical technology, investments in information technology do not directly generate billable services under Medicare or third-party-payer, fee-for-service systems. Hence, providers may realize a faster return on investments in a new surgical suite than they will on investments in an automated order entry system. Unfortunately, errors in clinical care contribute to rising health care expenditures because patients injured as a result of errors typically require more services and readmissions.

The problem is compounded because the marketplace typically cannot discern differences in quality. Because we do not have good comparative data for measuring quality and performance in medical care and patient outcomes, health care organizations, medical groups, and hospital systems that have better outcomes do no better in the marketplace than providers with poorer outcomes. We must move very aggressively to address these payment concerns before they stifle the adoption of information technologies critical to improving the safety and quality of care.

Third, we need to translate the evidence base into best practices that can be implemented in care delivery and then communicate this information to health care professionals and patients. In addition, we must develop and implement decision-support tools to assist clinicians and patients in

using the clinical knowledge base effectively. Last but not least, the *Chasm* report calls for "transparency"—an accountability system that emphasizes the release of comparative data.

Fourth, we must make major changes in the medical education system. Currently, many providers are trained in environments that are not "wired." Students are not exposed to technology and decision-support systems, evidence-based practices are not emphasized, and learning is not focused on multidisciplinary teams. In other words, we are not training individuals to practice or acquire the kinds of skills they will need to be effective in the health care delivery system we are attempting to create. Changing the medical education system will require the active participation of professional associations, educational leaders, and professional licensing and certification groups.

FIVE-PART AGENDA FOR CHANGE

The committee put forward an agenda for changing the U.S. health care system:

- Commit to a shared agenda for improvement in six areas: safety, effectiveness, patient-centeredness, timeliness, efficiency, and fairness.
- Adopt "10 rules" (see below) to guide the redesign of care processes.
- Implement more effective organizational supports.
- Focus initial efforts on priority areas.
- Create an environment that fosters and rewards improvement.

TEN RULES FOR REDESIGNING AND IMPROVING CARE

Private and public purchasers, health care organizations, clinicians, and patients should work together to redesign health care processes in accordance with the following rules.

1. **Care should be based on continuous healing relationships.** Patients should receive care whenever they need it and in many forms, not just through face-to-face visits. The health care system should be responsive at all times (24 hours a day, every day), and access to care should be provided over the Internet, by telephone, and by other means in addition to face-to-face visits.

2. **Care should be customized based on the patient's needs and values.** The system of care should be designed to meet the most common needs but should have the flexibility to respond to an individual patient's choices and preferences.

3. **The patient should be in control.** Patients should be

given necessary information and the opportunity to exercise as much control as they choose over health care decisions that affect them. The health system should be able to accommodate differences in patient preferences and should encourage shared decision making.

4. **The system should encourage shared knowledge and the free flow of information.** Patients should have unfettered access to their own medical information and to clinical information. Clinicians and patients should communicate effectively and share information.

5. **Decision making should be evidence-based.** Patients should receive care based on the best available scientific knowledge. Care should not vary illogically from clinician to clinician or from place to place.

6. **Safety should be a property of the system.** Patients should be safe from injury caused by the care system. Reducing risk and ensuring safety will require systems that help prevent and mitigate errors.

7. **The system should be transparent.** The health care system should make information available to patients and their families that allows them to make informed decisions when selecting a health plan, a hospital, or a clinical practice or when choosing among alternative treatments. Patients should be informed of the system's performance on safety, evidence-based practice, and patient satisfaction.

8. **The system should anticipate patients' needs.** The health system should be proactive in anticipating a patient's needs, rather than simply reacting to events.

9. **The system should constantly strive to decrease waste.** The health system should not waste resources or patients' time.

10. **The system should encourage cooperation among clinicians.** Clinicians and institutions should actively collaborate and communicate with each other to ensure that patients receive appropriate care.

REFERENCE

IOM (Institute of Medicine). 2001. Crossing the Quality Chasm: A New Health System for the 21st Century. Washington, D.C.: National Academy Press.

Bridging the Quality Chasm

David Lawrence
Kaiser Foundation Health Plan

This presentation focuses on the management of scientific and technological breakthroughs as they are made available to the health care delivery system—specifically on whether health care has kept pace with innovation by moving them into practice safely and responsibly. There is a substantial amount of overuse, misuse, and underuse of available science and technologies in the health care system—regardless of geography, type of payment, or when and where physicians were trained. To address this problem, the Institute of Medicine (IOM) undertook two studies, *To Err Is Human*, published in 2000, which focused on safety issues, and *Crossing the Quality Chasm*, published in 2001, which focused on quality issues. Both reports highlight the symptoms of a broken system. Both reports concluded that there is a mismatch between the rate and quantity of scientific and technological innovations and the ability of the health care system to use them safely and responsibly.

Wide variations in quality were documented as far back as 1975 in a small-area variation analysis by John Wennberg, M.D., and then in a variety of other studies across the country in the last 30 years (O'Connor et al., 1999; Wennberg, 1999). Recent safety studies, primarily but not exclusively studies by Lucien Leape and his colleagues at Harvard, identified a variety of medical errors that result in morbidity and mortality caused not because of physician malfeasance but because of system errors (Brennan et al., 1991; Leape et al., 2002; Thomas et al., 2000). The number of hospital deaths from these errors range from 30,000 to 80,000 per year. At this point, we have no understanding and little documentation of the number of errors in the ambulatory setting. Some early estimates in the United Kingdom and the United States have been published (Bubin, 1999; Fischer et al., 1997; Weingart et al., 2000). The total number of deaths attributable to errors in the health care system we think could be as high as 150,000 or even 200,000 per year.

Another measure was published by Barbara Starfield in an article in *Journal of the American Medical Association* in 2000. Dr. Starfield looked at the whole question of system-related deaths for all reasons, including errors. She concluded that 200,000 to 250,000 deaths per year were attributable to system-related causes, of which error is the most notable (Starfield, 2000). Starfield also made interesting comparisons between our system and others in terms of a variety of health outcomes. She concluded, as have many others, that although we spend an enormous amount on health care and lead the world in scientific innovation and technology, the results in terms of improved health do not match the level of investment.

There are also other symptoms of poor quality in the health care system. One of them has to do with responsiveness. In the Picker Institute studies of patient assessments of their health care experiences, about three-quarters of those surveyed indicated that their experiences with the health care system had led them to conclude that it was a "nightmare" to navigate (Picker Institute, 2000). They identified duplication, lack of communication, conflicting points of view about what should be done, and lack of understanding about what the science suggested. In short, the system is fragmented, fractured, and not patient-centric.

Finally, there is the cost of poor quality care, which has interesting implications for innovation. Between $.30 and $.40 of every dollar spent on health care is spent on the costs of poor quality. This extraordinary number represents slightly more than a half-trillion dollars a year. A vast amount of money is wasted on overuse, underuse, misuse, duplication, system failures, unnecessary repetition, poor communication, and inefficiency.

In this respect, the experience of General Electric Company and others in more tightly managed and highly organized manufacturing systems may be instructive. Companies often find substantial opportunities for improvement in the cost performance of the system by using quality-improvement tools. The health care system does not even come close to a well organized, systematically designed system like a production or manufacturing system.

Our experience in Kaiser Permanente suggests that these numbers are not exaggerations. When we look for ways to improve the organization and delivery of care, we often find that substantial improvements can be made in the underlying cost performance of the organization. In fact, the premise on which we compete is that we can drive costs down by improving quality.

There are five major problems with the health care system. The first is that most of the scientific and technological breakthroughs that have occurred since World War II have not simplified the task of taking care of patients. In fact, they have made it more complex. Here are some examples:

- As we entered the 1950s, there were about 10 to 12 categories of health care professionals in the United States. Today, there are more than 220 categories of health care professionals.
- Right after World War II, there were about six to eight—depending on how you counted them—specialties in medicine. Today, there are more than a hundred.
- In 1970, there were approximately 100 published randomized control trials (RCTs) in the American medical literature. In 1999 alone, almost 10,000 RCTs were published. Half of RCTs published in the United States have appeared in the last five years.

Science and technology have certainly contributed to growing complexity in medicine—increasing the number of people involved, increasing the number of categories of people involved, raising expectations about what can be done to treat people, and increasing the amount of science and technology that must be managed. Largely as a result of advances in science and technology, the medical care system is far more complex today in terms of the number of institutions and types of health care practitioners than it was in 1950.

Second, the health care system, or nonsystem, has grown enormously over the last 50 years but has failed to keep the patient and the patient's family at the center of the enterprise. It is small wonder that people identify the system as a nightmare to navigate. It is not a patient-centered system.

How could the complexity of a system be significantly decreased? First, we could create a highly sophisticated production-design or manufacturing-design process to handle the complexity. Then an investment could be made in an information technology infrastructure. Next, we could create flow systems to manage the support activities required to carry out these processes, retain people, and set new standards of quality.

In medicine, we have done very little of this. Physicians are still trained on the principle of individual, professional autonomy, even though, in reality, they do not work in autonomous situations at all. Production design is a foreign word. In fact, it is considered almost sacrilegious to talk about production design in medicine. To many practitioners medicine is a religion, not a science. Therefore, the tools of production design have not been applied in the units where patients get care.

The third issue is that it is extraordinarily difficult to scale up medical care delivery. There are few examples of integrated care across ambulatory, inpatient, hospice, and home settings. Only a few systems enable us to capture capital and reinvest capital in the delivery system infrastructure. With 80 percent of physicians practicing in groups of fewer than 10, medicine remains largely a single interaction between a patient and a doctor. In reality, although the patient-doctor interaction remains absolutely essential, the enterprise itself now involves a much more complex set of interactions.

Except for the Veterans Health Administration, Kaiser Permanente, which has 10,000 physicians, is the largest health care delivery system. The next largest may be the Mayo Clinic. Most others are small, regional players on the delivery system side. Until there are more scaled-up enterprises, it will be difficult to collect and reinvest enough capital to build and support the production capability essential to the delivery of the science and technology that innovators are creating for us.

Fourth, our public policy environment is structured to inhibit the reshaping of the medical care delivery system. For example, in Wisconsin there are 27 licensed categories of health care professionals, each with its own board of practice. Medicine should be about removing boundaries so that people can flow seamlessly among a variety of practitioners, based on what the technology requires and what the patient needs. Yet regulatory and license-based silos create barriers between professionals. These barriers must be broken down to create teams and to deliver integrated care. This can be done, but only with great effort. The licensing system is designed to protect the interests of particular professional groups in medicine, not to further the delivery of integrated care.

On the reimbursement side, the fee-for-service system is designed to reward individual acts by individual clinicians. Our current reimbursement system does not support integrated delivery capabilities. *Crossing the Quality Chasm* called for experimenting with a variety of reimbursement approaches to determine which ones would stimulate the creation of integrated delivery capabilities—prepayment, perhaps, or capitation or other approaches. The fact remains that the classic fee-for-service system is a barrier to the development of collaborative medicine.

The final issue identified in *Crossing the Quality Chasm* is that information technology is not being used in the delivery system the way one would expect for such an information-rich industry. It is estimated that less than 2 percent of total revenues in health care is being invested in information technology infrastructure. Much more is being invested on the health insurance side, but investment on the delivery system side is much lower than in other industries or in the medical technologies industry. Finding capital, either by aggregating organizations to generate capital or by other means, is a major issue. As the system stands, we cannot make innovations in health care delivery that match the complexity of the science. A physician trying to keep up with 10,000 RCTs in a year cannot practice evidence-based medicine without an information technology decision-support system. It is simply beyond the capacity of the individual to keep up.

Now let's turn to opportunities for innovation, using the problem areas as the focal points. The first priority for innovation is to improve the ways patients can connect with the medical care delivery system. Innovations in monitoring, diagnosis, and treatment technologies will enable patients to self-manage, or at least communicate on a regular, ongoing basis, with the health care system. It makes no sense to continue to invest heavily in the bricks and mortar of classic delivery systems when there are other vehicles for taking care of patients in a far more responsive, patient-centric way. So giving patients the tools and creating bridges between the patient and the delivery system is one focus for innovation.

For example, one of the many promising innovations is the ability to test whether Coumadin is operating at therapeutic levels; this can be done by the patient using a hand-held testing device. A device for testing blood sugar is another. These and many other devices will substantially improve the connection between the patient and the system and put more capability in the hands of the patient. These innovations will also decrease our dependence on brick and mortar solutions for the delivery system.

The second major area for innovation is translating the tools used in the manufacturing and production of goods and services into a language that applies to health care. I would argue that the delivery of medical care today is the most complex production challenge on the planet. Think about what is involved in running a hospital with about 250 beds— a wide array of diagnoses, a multitude of judgments being made by teams of professionals interacting with patients, and all of the support production that makes this happen hour after hour, 24 hours a day, seven days a week. This is an extraordinarily complex production challenge.

The third area of innovation involves organizational design or scaling. It has proven to be extremely difficult to create sufficient scale systemwide to produce the necessary capital, systems, and training capabilities. Scaling up has been done successfully in certain health care settings, for example, hospitals, nursing homes, laboratories, and pharmacies, but it has proven to be extremely difficult to create any kind of organizational scale for building integrated delivery capabilities.

Last, innovation could come through interventions at the national policy level in regulation, reimbursement, and, possibly, the financing of the information technology infrastructure in medicine. Given the current organization of the health care system, the financing of the information technology infrastructure may exceed the capacity of the private marketplace. Perhaps we will have to create the medical equivalent of the Superfund for environmental cleanup to build the information technology infrastructure for the health care delivery system. This infrastructure involves more than electronic medical records, which simply capture and move information to support decision making. A robust infrastructure would incorporate analytic tools that would enable epidemiological studies of disease. Without this infrastructure, it is extremely difficult to test whether or not microproduction units are working well and whether we are getting anywhere with the larger organizational challenges facing us.

In closing, the message of *Crossing the Quality Chasm* should be taken to heart. The mismatch between the pace and scope of innovation in medical science and technology and innovation in the delivery system has created a chasm, which is aggravated by shifting demographics and the shifting of the disease burden from acute to chronic care. The complexity that both add to the task of taking care of patients has not been matched by equivalent sophistication in the delivery system.

REFERENCES

Brennan, T.A., L.L. Leape, N.M. Laird, L. Hebert, A.R. Localio, A.G. Lawthers, J.P. Newhouse, P.C. Weiler, and H.H. Hiatt. 1991. Incidence of adverse events and negligence in hospitalized patients. Results of the Harvard Medical Practice Study I. New England Journal of Medicine 324(3): 370–376.

Bubin, C. 1999. Mistakes happen: improved processes mean fewer mistakes. Ambulatory Outreach (Fall): 23–26.

Fischer, G.F., A.P. Munro, and E.B. Goldman. 1997. Adverse events in primary care identified from a risk-management database. Journal of Family Practice 45(1): 40–46.

IOM (Institute of Medicine). 2000. To Err Is Human: Building a Safer Health System, L.T. Kohn, J.M. Corrigan, and M.S. Donaldson, eds. Washington, D.C.: National Academy Press.

IOM. 2001. Crossing the Quality Chasm: A New Health System for the 21st Century. Washington, D.C.: National Academy Press.

Leape, L.L., D.M. Berwick, and D.W. Bates. 2002. What practices will most improve safety?: evidence-based medicine meets patient safety. Journal of the American Medical Association 288(4): 501–507.

O'Connor, G.T., H.B. Quinton, N.D. Traven, L.I. Ramunno, T.A. Dodds, T.A. Marciniak, and J.E. Wennberg. 1999. Geographic variation in the treatment of acute myocardial infarction: the Cooperative Cardiovascular Project. Journal of the American Medical Association 281(7): 627–633.

Picker Institute. 2000. Eye on Patients. A Report by the Picker Institute for the American Hospital Association. Boston, Mass.: Picker Institute.

Starfield, B. 2000. Is U.S. health care really the best in the world? Journal of the American Medical Association 284(4): 483–485.

Thomas, E.J., D.M. Studdert, H.R. Burstin, E.J. Orav, T. Zeena, E.J. Williams, K.M. Howard, P.C. Weiler, and T.A. Brennan. 2000. Incidence and types of adverse events and negligent care in Utah and Colorado. Medical Care 38(3): 261–271.

Weingart, S.N., R.M. Wilson, R.W. Gibberd, and B. Harrison. 2000. Epidemiology of medical error. British Medical Journal 320(7237): 774–777.

Wennberg, J.E. 1999. Understanding geographic variations in health care delivery. New England Journal of Medicine 340(1): 52–53.

Envisioning the Future

Jeff Goldsmith
Health Futures Incorporated

Our health care system is the largest knowledge-based activity in the world. It is one-third larger than the gross domestic product (GDP) of China and four times the size of Africa's entire economy. The research and development portion of the health care system alone—this year about $50 billion between spending by the National Institutes of Health, venture capital firms, equity markets, and pharmaceutical companies—is as big as the GDP of many Latin American countries. And yet, although we are generating new knowledge at a staggering pace, we are also staggeringly inefficient in assimilating that knowledge and applying it to the delivery of health care services. Even though our health care system is being constantly enriched by new knowledge, we are still using nineteenth-century architectures and sociological constructs for this information.

UNRAVELING THE GENOME AND EXTENDING THE HUMAN LIFE SPAN

The business and mission of the health care system will change with two radical scientific advances. The first is the unraveling of the human genome. There was a tremendous wave of expectation that the mere mapping of the genome would revolutionize medicine and create powerful new tools for intervening definitively in disease processes. My nonscientist's belief is that the results won't be felt until we've done a couple of generations of really hard work. Eventually, genetic information will produce powerful tools for affecting our health, but it is going to take a while.

The second advance is tinkering with the human life span. At the beginning of the twentieth century, a typical American lived to be 47; by the end of the century, average life expectancy was about 80. Most of the increase was the result of eliminating premature causes of death—such as infant mortality and childhood diseases. In the past, most human biologists believed that there would never be much more improvement because the maximum life span of human beings is hardwired into our genome or into the processes by which cells reproduce.

In 1998, discoveries in the processes of cell biology led to the hope that we were close to understanding one of the mechanisms that limit the viability of our cells and tissues and, therefore, the life span of our organ systems. Many gerontologists became convinced that if we could understand the hardwired limits on the capacity of our cells and tissues to reproduce and begin attacking some of them—declining hormone levels, oxidation, etc.—we could dramatically extend the life span of human beings. There is now serious discussion of people living to be 140 or 150 years old.

The stem cell, the Holy Grail of human biology, is the subject of an enormous political debate in Washington, because the principal source of stem cells is discarded embryos from *in vitro* fertilization. Buried in the software of a stem cell is the recipe for each tissue type in your body, as well as the assembly instructions for the organ systems that those tissues ultimately form. A lot of people believe that, once we master the instruction sets buried in the stem cells, we will be able to create, on demand, tissues from our own cells that can be used to repair damage to our organ systems from strokes, spinal cord injuries, and other causes. In combination with growth factors that our bodies produce naturally to encourage cells to grow, we will have the power to replace damaged tissues and, eventually, whole organ systems.

As our understanding of human genetics improves, our paradigm of vaccination will also change. Right now we think of a vaccination as something given to children to protect them against infectious diseases. Soon, however, we will be vaccinating people against chronic diseases, such as breast cancer, asthma, and, perhaps, arthritis. We will be able to vaccinate people any time during the course of the development of the disease. Not everyone will be given the same vaccine, however, because the tools of genetic prediction will enable us to distinguish between risks of disease for each individual all the way down to the level of nucleotide sequences. Instead of building blockbuster drugs to knock out diseases in whole populations of people, the pharmaceutical system will produce highly specific, genetically tailored responses to an individual's genetic risk. Many of these advances in genetics will not be the result of "wet work" (i.e., laboratory research) but of computer modeling and the manipulation of massive computer databases using high-performance computing.

COMPUTERIZED PATIENT RECORDS AND DECISION-SUPPORT SYSTEMS

The Gartner Group, which studies health care systems, has envisioned a computerized five-generation patient record:

- Generation 1 is a passive repository of clinical data based on information gathered manually and on paper.
- Generation 2 is the repository of clinical data plus an electronic version of the paper chart. On this level, passive alerts about drug interactions would be possible. Crude rules built into Generation 2 systems would suggest that doctors reconsider decisions if a deviation from standard practice were observed.
- Generation 3 combines the repository of clinical data, the electronic version of the paper chart, and orders entered by the physician. A Generation 3 record would be able to track patients across inpatient ambulatory settings and provide a full array of passive care alerts. If the patient's status changes, the system would send the doctor a "do you want to do X?" type of message, thus providing an undergirding for making clinical decisions.
- Generation 4 would make the leap from a passive system that mimics a record-keeping system to what might be called "groupware" for clinical decision making. Embedded in the system would be care pathways, work flows, and data on the outcomes of certain courses of action for a particular patient with a particular condition. Creating a Generation 4 record will be very expensive. It will require information based on thousands of hours of structured discussions by physicians regarding what they do and then review of emerging scientific literature on clinical effectiveness and to support clinical decisions. At this level, the patient's chart would become a living document that guides the care process; the system would become a full partner in the care process.
- Generation 5 would be an "intelligent" system capable of self-modification that has acquired knowledge of the context of the patient and of the cognitive style and work flow requirements of the physician or clinical team. With a Generation 5 system, physicians would have complete access to the information they need to make better decisions. Thus, the system would become a trusted source of new knowledge that could help physicians make decisions. The system would create enough options and possibilities for physicians to continue learning, thus encouraging the physician's development, as well as improving patient care.

INTERACTIONS BETWEEN PATIENTS AND THE HEALTH CARE SYSTEM

Changes in the clinical operating system will improve interactions between doctors and patients, who will not have to be in the same room, or even in the same time frame. Enterprise software will provide a patient's personal health record with information from the person's entire clinical history. Patients and caregivers will have a "dashboard" that enables them to control their interactions with the rest of the health care system. Thus, patients will be able to acquire knowledge not only from their doctors but also from the system about managing their own health problems. Once patients understand that this is possible, they will insist on being treated in institutions that have these capabilities.

Patients will hire care managers, particularly for the elderly in a household. Care managers will use Web-based tools to navigate knowledge domains to help make better decisions and get better results. For instance, we will have a search engine that will enable us to ask the questions we really want answered. For example, we could ask where the three most promising clinical trials for drugs that affect lupus are being done and for a link so we can find out about participating in a trial.

SUMMARY

Advances in medicine in the last 25 or 30 years—tools from electrical engineering, miniaturization, and less invasive surgery—have moved our understanding and our interventions closer to the origins of disease. In the nineteenth century, the health care system was focused on acute care—intervening in the late stages of disease and salvaging people from life-threatening events. In the twenty-first century, the health care system will focus on predicting a patient's risk for disease based on genetic screening and powerful clinical chemistry. The system will not only have therapeutic tools but will also have tools to change behavior and disease-management software to modify risk factors and, ideally, eliminate the risk before it progresses into an illness in the first place.

An array of powerful new tools will make our medical care system more humane and more responsive to our needs. But to liberate caregivers and patients from our current cumbersome processes that don't work very well and cost a staggering, even unconscionable, amount of money, we will have to do a tremendous amount of work to renovate the institutions and cultures of medical care.

Improving Health and Health Care

Lewis G. Sandy
Robert Wood Johnson Foundation

Private foundations like the Robert Wood Johnson Foundation are like venture capitalists for ideas. Today, I'm going to talk about our priorities and strategies for improving the health care system and health care. I will reflect on the challenges we face in implementing our agenda, outline strategic directions, and suggest how engineering and medicine can be linked.

I want to make three points. First, I believe the major problem in health care is not a lack of tools, although we have heard about new tools that could and probably should be developed. The major problem is the way we use existing tools. Second, in thinking about using engineering principles, theory, and knowledge, we must think about health, not just health care. We must think beyond the health care delivery system to using technology to actually improve the health of people. We must think beyond the organization and financing of our current health care system. Third, bringing engineering and medicine together is not predominantly a technical problem; it is a cultural problem.

The Robert Wood Johnson Foundation is one of the largest foundations in the country and the largest foundation devoted to improving health and health care for Americans. We have about $8 billion in assets and award $400 million annually in grants. We use a variety of methods to achieve our goals—such as supporting research projects, demonstrations, training, communications, and workshops. Our work is organized around three goals: (1) ensuring that all Americans have access to care; (2) improving care for people with chronic health conditions; and (3) helping the country deal with substance abuse. General improvement is part of our mission, but the specifics are embodied in our goals. We encourage the health care system to do the right things. In some cases, we support innovations. In addition, we promote the diffusion and adoption of existing best practices.

For example, a program called Improving Chronic Illness Care run by the Group Health Cooperative of Puget Sound focuses on improving care for people with chronic illnesses.

Our health care delivery system generally focuses on acute care; the system is geared toward treating infectious diseases and acute traumas. There is a mismatch, however, between that model and the prevalence of disease, predominantly chronic illnesses that require a different model of care with different elements.

A chronic care model of health care delivery includes linkages between the health system and the community, as well as support for self-care and self-management. A health care delivery system organized for chronic care must provide decision-support tools for providers *and* for patients and families. It must also have a supporting information infrastructure; in addition, the health care delivery team must be redesigned and retrained. The foundation has provided $32 million to support projects, research, and demonstrations and provide technical assistance to promote a health care system configured to treat chronic illnesses.

A program called Smoke Free Families focuses on the dissemination of best practices. The goal of the program is to eliminate, or at least reduce, smoking by pregnant women, one of the most important, modifiable risk factors for premature births. Everyone recognizes that prenatal smoking is a problem, but the adoption of proven, effective interventions has not been successful. We provide instructions for providers to assess the situation and advise women to quit smoking during prenatal visits.

We try to implement and evaluate new models of health care being developed by researchers and idea entrepreneurs. Once a better technology has been developed and demonstrated, the difficulty is in getting individuals to use it. It is even more difficult to create an incentive structure that encourages the entire delivery system to adopt and diffuse innovations. We have tried to increase consumer demand for higher quality care and have worked through vehicles, such as a purchaser institute that brings together public and private purchasers. We know that consumer demand can change systems of care. Consider the changes in obstetrical care, which has changed from a technological, sterile practice to a more humane, patient-centered, caring, warm experience through birthing centers. These changes are the result of consumer demand for changes in care.

Not enough attention has been paid to improving overall health care. The health care system needs a "Toyota," someone who can do for health care what Toyota did for the auto industry—engineer the product in a fundamentally different way. No health care delivery system yet has been demonstrated to be better in all respects—in technical quality, interpersonal quality, and so on.

The foundation is providing support to the Institute for Health Care Improvement to develop a demonstration program that would lead to a transformational change in health care. The project, called Pursuing Perfection, is focused on analyzing barriers to improving health care. We want to shake up the current system to show that things can be done in a fundamentally different way. We provide grants and technical assistance for the program, and we are creating a learning network and undertaking a communications campaign. Currently, we are visiting 26 sites to choose awardees for 12 planning grants, some on errors in medication, some on access to care and patient flow, and some on nursing, staffing, and human resource management.

The program has generated a great deal of interest, indicating that there is a pent-up demand among providers for a transformational change in health care. In a recent survey, we found that about 30 percent of physicians think improving care is an important problem and that they personally could affect change (IHI, 2001).

Very little production-process thinking is being used in health care. Even those working on improving quality of care are not using applicable engineering tools. We need to open a bridge between medicine and engineering. People in the engineering community know which tools would be helpful for analyzing problems and effecting improvements.

One of the differences between engineering and medicine is that engineers believe in the theoretical possibility of perfection; doctors do not. Even in highly reliable organizations, adverse events happen all the time. We know from the genome project that human beings are riddled with genetic errors. Doctors understand illness and medical care as part of the human condition and the human tragedy.

But we can make changes through process improvement. Medicine is an ancient story about heroes and tragedies that has only been a high-technology scientific enterprise for the past 50 to 75 years. For the first 3,000 or 4,000 years of the history of medicine, it was considered a calling, a profession that dealt with the inexplicable tragedy of the human condition. This long history is built into the socialization of physicians in a fundamental way.

To bridge the culture gap, engineers who work in health care delivery or operations improvement will need cultural training in some aspects of health care. A good resource is *On Doctoring* by Reynolds and Stone (1991), which is given to all entering medical students by our foundation to socialize them into the practice and culture of medicine.

Physicians also need to be educated in what I call the "engineering culture." Some efforts are being made to train physicians in principles of operations and improvement. However, we need to develop a language and concepts for health care practitioners interested in this field. We also need a research agenda, such as the one being developed for medical errors and patient safety. Another critical area for research is human factors engineering. The burden of malpractice suits and litigation can hardly be overestimated, and we need to create safe harbors for reporting on adverse events or near misses. We must also develop a national agenda for improvement.

We must consider health care at the macrosystem level, that is, the health of the population, and not just the health care system. The Web and other technologies can be used to provide consumers with information on healthy living and to promote behavioral change. The major modifiable determinants of health are in the environment in which people live, choices in individual behavior. Think about how we can use technology and engineering principles to influence those choices. In addition, we should be thinking about designing communities that encourage people to walk or otherwise stay physically active because we know that even minimal exercise can have a huge health impact. We can promote behavioral change strategies to help improve people's diets and help them deal with stress. New organizations and new functions outside the traditional health care delivery system can improve people's lives.

REFERENCES

IHI (Institute for Healthcare Improvement). 2001. Pursuing Perfection. Press release May 8, 2001.

Reynolds, R., and J. Stone, eds. 1991. On Doctoring: Stories, Poems, Essays. New York: Simon & Schuster.

Engineering and the Health Care System

Richard J. Coffey
University of Michigan Health System

I've spent almost 40 years in health care, including 10 years in consulting, which has given me the opportunity to see many different institutions. Today, I will lay out a general format for the issues facing our institution and other institutions across the country.

We can divide health care systems into different levels. Table 1 shows a model with five levels. At the individual patient level (Level 1), the treatment of the patient, we encounter the issue of autonomy. Physicians are trained from the very beginning to work autonomously, to make autonomous decisions. When we try to standardize care, some physicians may feel their autonomy is being challenged. This has made it difficult to standardize equipment, supplies, and pharmaceuticals. Leaders of industrial organizations, for example, often have trouble understanding that health care leaders cannot just order physicians to do something. Academic institutions that have tenured physicians may have the

most difficulty resolving this issue. To compound the problem, institutions tend to recruit interns, residents, and physicians with the same attitude toward autonomy. Mayo Clinic tends to recruit people whose cultural orientation is similar to the prevailing orientation at Mayo. Academic institutions tend to recruit strong researchers who are used to having academic autonomy.

The second level is the department/unit level, such as operating rooms and cancer programs. The third level is the individual hospital. The fourth level, multihospital/multiorganizational systems, try to coordinate operations among multiple sites, multiple kinds of functions, and so forth. These systems have developed largely in the last few years. A few years ago, my colleagues and I wrote a book on a fifth level, virtually integrated health systems, collaborations among multiple organizations to improve health (Coffey et al., 1997).

TABLE 1 A Five-Level Model of a Health Care System

Level	Explanation	Examples
Patient	Treatment of individual patient	• Clinical practice • Surgical practice
Department/unit	Specific systems within a program, unit, or department	• Operating rooms • Cancer program
Hospital	Interacting systems within a hospital	• Multiple departments • Multiple settings
Multi-institutional/ multiorganizational systems	Interacting systems among institutions	• Multiple sites • Multiple hospitals • Multiple functions
Virtually integrated health system	Medical care in the larger context of a community and environment	• Integrations among all systems affecting health and health care

To begin with, we should correct a common mistake. Most of the current U.S. health care system is not focused on health. The current system is primarily a medical care system focused on diseases and illnesses. Primarily, we treat people who are already sick. Some organizations, such as health maintenance organizations, are focusing more on prevention and health; but in large part, the system deals with medicine, rather than health.

Table 2 describes the concept of a six-dimensional, virtually integrated health system. The first dimension, social and environmental conditions, includes crime violence, the community situation, the family situation, and many other factors that have a much stronger effect on health than much of what we do. A health care system that ignores the environmental dimension has a very narrow focus.

The second dimension, health-related human conditions, is familiar to many. A classification system is necessary so we can standardize or categorize diseases and treatments (e.g., diagnosis-related groups). The third dimension, foci, describes types of activity. The majority of work done by health care organizations currently involves diagnosis and treatment, but very little protection. Occupational Safety and Health Administration standards, Joint Commission on Accreditation of Healthcare Organizations (JCAHO), and other organizations address protection more directly than the traditional health care system.

Settings is the fourth dimension. Most of our work right now is done in ambulatory and inpatient settings, facilities to which patients come. An example of health care in the community setting is a cooperative program by the University of Michigan Health System (UMHS) and St. Joseph Mercy Health System, in Ann Arbor, Michigan. The purpose of the program is to discourage smoking by eighth graders and to raise their health awareness.

Core/key processes, the fifth dimension, categorizes major processes, such as leadership, planning, and human resources. These categories are very similar to those used by JCAHO and other organizations. The final dimension categorizes resources.

As an example of how these levels apply, consider the taxonomy we use to address heart disease. What are we doing environmentally to affect heart disease? How do we categorize heart disease? What functions are we and/or others providing? Are we focusing on treatment? The methods of treatment for heart disease are changing radically—especially surgery versus the new drug-eluting stents, which could threaten the role of cardiac surgeons. Recently, radiologists have been testing whether CT scanners can diagnose heart disease as well as or better than cardiac catheterization. Because CT scans are noninvasive, this research has many potential implications for the way we coordinate and provide care. These changes will affect who provides care, where the money goes, and who controls it; there are substantial dollar differences between medical and surgical admissions. The settings may also change. As we consider engineering applications, we must remain mindful that the health care system is much broader than just work in a hospital. Most of you know there has been a sharp drop in the length of hospital stays in the last decade. Much of that change has been possible because some care is now provided in other settings. Most large health care organizations have home-care services. Today, even if you are on IV therapy, you may not have to be in a hospital. Many patients can be treated in a less costly environment than a hospital.

Dr. James L. Reinertsen contrasts the ideas of "high science" and "low science" (Reinertsen, 2003). High science asks if population A is different from population B (you try to control for all other variables). High science studies involve comparative research or clinical trials that generate "descriptive statistics." Low science asks how a process will work the next time a patient experiences it, which involves many complex variables. Methods used to answer this question include quality improvement, run and control charts, and modeling. Low science generates "analytic statistics." Most academic medical and engineering publications do not publish "low science" research.

Academic physicians survive not by the quality of patient care, but by whether or not they get tenure. And tenure is based not on the number of patients seen, but on research and publications. Young professors in engineering colleges are judged in similar fashion. If "low science" is considered substandard, not academically acceptable, young academicians are discouraged from pursuing this type of work in health care. When W. Edwards Deming split from the rest of the statisticians, most academic statisticians advocated theoretical "high science." Deming advocated using statistics to predict system performance. I think we should support research in predictive science, and what Reinertsen calls "low science." If we don't, we will be turning our backs on enormous opportunities to improve systems, health care, and health.

Figure 1 illustrates an example of interacting systems in a hospital. This is not intended to be a flow chart, but it shows some of the interactive processes involved in the care of a patient. Patients come into a clinic or emergency department and may move from there to another area—to the operating room, post-anesthesia care unit, intensive care unit, acute care bed, home care, etc. Physician services and consults are also going on, as well as diagnostic tests. Improved engineering could benefit every one of these processes. There are large variations among patients, which we also need to address. But, most important, we must address the large variations in the way we care for patients. Engineering models could help us address these system variations and minimize their impacts. To reduce health costs, most health care institutions are improving their use of resources, including staff, equipment, and facilities. If systems are not efficient and coordinated, this leads to major bottlenecks,

TABLE 2 Taxonomy for a Virtually Integrated Health System

1	2	3	4	5	6
Social and Environmental Conditions	Health-Related Human Conditions	Foci	Settings	Core/Key Processes	Resources
• Environmental pollution • Crime and violence • Community and social support ICD-9 categories) • Family and living situation with health services • Educational and vocational levels • Employment and income levels • Risk factors and behaviors • Other ___	• Diseases and injuries (17 major ICD-9 categories) • Operations (16 major ICD-9 categories) • Health status and contact with health services (8 major ICD-9 categories) • Causes of injury and poisoning (22 major ICD-9 categories) • Maintenance and enhancement of health (classification of social services) • Other ___	• Promotion • Protection • Prevention • Detection • Diagnosis and assessment • Treatment • Habilitation and rehabilitation • Maintenance • Hospice • Support • Advocacy • Education • Research • Enabling • Other ___	• Area-wide • Community • House of worship • School • Work • Mobile • Home, including assisted living • Ambulatory • Partial-day care • Inpatient • Free-standing support • Other ___	• Leadership and governance • Strategic planning • Human resource management and development • Process and quality improvement • Information planning and management • Continuum of care • Client/patient rights and satisfaction • Prevention and education • Management of the environment • Other ___	• Human resources • Facility resources • Equipment resources • Financial resources • Organizations • Information • Other ___

Source: Coffey et al., 1997.

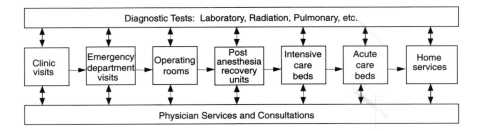

FIGURE 1 Sample of interacting hospital system components.

poor care, delays, lost business, more pain, and so on. This is an illustration of the tremendous opportunities for engineering.

Figure 2 illustrates a breakthrough matrix (Gaucher and Coffey, 2000). Engineering can make major contributions in terms of designing products and processes. We can improve models of customer requirements, interests, and perceptions.

Many kinds of engineering applications (e.g., queuing, operations research, and human factors research) can be applied at all five levels of health care systems (i.e., patient, department, hospital, multi-institutional systems, and virtually integrated health systems). Consider scheduling systems, for example. We have good scheduling systems for individual departments and services, like operating rooms. Where we have failed, as was pointed out in the Institute of Medicine reports, is in "handoffs," the movement of patients from one area of the system to another (IOM, 2000, 2001). At UMHS, for example, we have a good operating room scheduling system, but it isn't linked to staffing of the nursing units or the admitting system. Therefore, we have discrepancies in our schedules. The same is true to some degree in virtually all health care organizations.

Another example of a scheduling problem is the result of our aging population. People often show up in emergency rooms at night with cardiac and other serious problems. These visits lead to increased medical admissions, which often delay the operating room cases the next day and cause huge turmoil in the organization. I believe one of the greatest opportunities for engineering is to improve the coordination of systems throughout a hospital or among multiple institutions.

At the patient system level (Level 1 in Table 1), changes should be planned and implemented in collaboration with physicians, nurses, and other caregivers. Engineers don't deliver care, but they help analyze and model changes, such as comparing the cost effectiveness of different medications. Today, every insurance company and every hospital is doing cost-effectiveness comparisons, but these efforts are not coordinated in any way.

Another frustrating thing is that we do not have a bar coding system throughout the health care industry. Each manufacturer has its own bar code system. Standardized bar codes could improve the quality of care, staffing, speed, and operational effectiveness. Also, we could model and optimize care protocols using decision algorithms and critical pathways. Many protocols have been developed, but few of them are used. I believe this is because individual physicians retain their autonomy rather than deferring to the collective autonomy of a group of physicians to design best-practice protocols. In UMHS, for example, we have a notebook full of critical pathways, but we frequently do not use those protocols.

Don B. Chaffin, professor of industrial and operations engineering at the University of Michigan, is working to improve the handling of patients to reduce back injuries to staff (Chaffin et al., 1999). Although the injury rate for employees in the health care industry is higher than in the construction industry, as an industry, we are not even taking care of our own employees. So there are many opportunities for engineering applications.

At the department level (Level 2 in Table 1), engineering methods (e.g., scheduling systems, inventory control, and staffing models) could improve the quality of care and cost effectiveness. As most of you know, we do not have labor standards in health care. In fact, very few health care managers understand what labor standards are—engineered standards that define a job, measure time, pace-rate the person doing the job, etc. Hospitals don't even have well defined jobs; every nurse does the job differently. Most hospitals don't even have labor standards for nonprofessional staff, such as housekeepers. At U of M, an industrial and operations engineering student group is working on standards for environmental services, establishing a standard for how long it takes to clean a patient room, for example. There is a tremendous opportunity for engineering here, which could also provide fantastic opportunities for engineering students. Every term, 40 to 45 students undertake projects and engineering studies in UMHS. But senior people must oversee the students to make sure they understand cross-departmental, interactive issues.

At the hospital system level (Level 3 in Table 1), a great deal of attention has been given to information technology. Linking scheduling systems among departments or elements

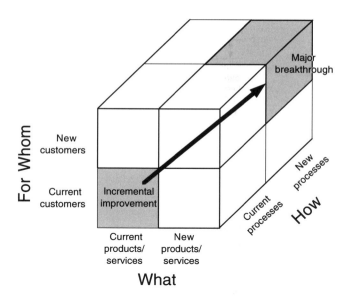

New
customers

For Whom

Current
customers

Incremental
improvement

Major
breakthrough

New
processes

Current
processes

How

Current
products/
services

New
products/
services

What

FIGURE 2 Breakthrough matrix. Source: Gaucher and Coffey, 2000.

offers a great opportunity for engineering applications. Computerized physician order entry systems are being strongly promoted by many organizations, including large employer organizations (e.g., the Leapfrog Group), and there are a few really good systems. For example, Intermountain Health has an excellent system that's been in development for about 30 years. But hospital-wide information systems don't come about quickly, and they are very expensive. At UMHS, we have spent about $30 to $50 million dollars over the last 10 years, and we still don't have an order entry system. We do have an excellent result reporting system, called CareWeb, that includes test results, operating room reports, discharge summaries, clinic notes, and other things—all available at any computer terminal in our system. Now we are spending millions to develop a physician order entry system with built-in logic checks for laboratory results, pharmaceuticals, and other factors. As an industry, we have poor hospital-wide information systems.

The multi-institutional system level (Level 4 in Table 1) addresses issues related to multiple facilities or organizations in a single health care system. For example, how are home-care services linked with hospital discharge planning, and how are both of them linked with ambulatory care clinics? Lack of coordination among departments and organizational units is often a serious problem.

At the virtually integrated health system level (Level 5 in Table 1), the engineering opportunity is to develop processes to enable physicians, hospitals, public health departments, employers, schools, houses of worship, and other organizations to work collaboratively to improve health. I think there are tremendous opportunities here for engineering applications,

but I'm not sure where the political support, leadership, resources, and financial support will come from. Schools, houses of worship, YMCAs, and other organizations may have more effect on changes in behavior than most physicians. Yet few health care systems include schools and other organizations in the foci dimension (see Table 2). Even UMHS, a leader in health planning and delivery, has barely scratched the surface of becoming a virtually integrated health system.

Right now, the health care system in the United States is characterized by fighting over resources and a lack of coordination. Employers, employees, insurance companies, hospitals, doctors, and other stakeholders are fighting with each other rather than trying to coordinate care to improve health. I think each group is so protective of its autonomy that we are not thinking about the broader good for everyone.

In summary, the United States has an aging population, rapidly developing technologies and medical care capabilities, and increasing expectations for care, which are driving our health care costs out of control. Every organization and individual is impacted by these changes. Small employers are perilously close to not being able to afford insurance for their employees. Health care insurance premiums for small employers have been rising by double digits for the past three to five years.

In my opinion, the recognition that we need engineering assistance is greater now than it has been at any time in the past 40 years. At UMHS, the dean of the medical school, many faculty members, and many hospital administrators now recognize that we need models of how UMHS works and engineering tools to help us manage it better. The question is whether, in an environment of very scarce resources, health care leaders are willing to pay for engineering to improve the health care system. In general the answer is no, at least so far. Engineering professionals *must* demonstrate the cost effectiveness of their services, because engineering models and solutions at all five levels of health care systems are vitally important.

REFERENCES

Chaffin, D.B., G.B.J. Andersson, and B.J. Martin. 1991. Occupational Biomechanics. 3rd edition. New York: Wiley-Interscience.

Coffey, R.J., K.M. Fenner, and S.L. Stogis. 1997. Virtually Integrated Health Systems: A Guide to Assessing Organizational Readiness and Strategic Partners. San Francisco: Jossey-Bass.

Gaucher, E., and R.J. Coffey. 2000. Breakthrough Performance: Accelerating the Transformation of Healthcare Organizations. San Francisco: Jossey-Bass.

IOM (Institute of Medicine). 2000. To Err Is Human: Building a Safer Health System, L.T. Kohn, J.M. Corrigan, and M.S. Donaldson, eds. Washington, D.C.: National Academies Press.

IOM. 2001. Crossing the Quality Chasm: A New Health System for the 21st Century. Washington, D.C.: National Academy Press.

Reinertsen, J.L. 2003. Science, Art, and Physician Autonomy. The 22nd Annual Donald P. Shiley Visiting Lectureship, Scripps Research Institute, La Jolla, California, March 23, 2003.

Engineering and the Health Care Organization

Vinod K. Sahney
Henry Ford Health System

Even though as an industry the U.S. health care system spends more than $2 trillion every year, a number of barriers at the organizational level have impeded the performance improvements we are all seeking. Certainly, one should not assume that the leaders who run this industry are incompetent; they invest in whatever is in the best interests of their particular institutions. Because of the environment, the payment systems, and the way things are structured, health care leaders have not invested in engineering approaches that could have a positive impact on quality and productivity.

The Henry Ford Health System is a very large integrated health care system with three major components: hospitals, a medical group, and a health plan with 600,000 enrollees. The system has $2.6 billion dollars in annual revenue, six hospitals, and a medical group with 900 physicians and 16,000 employees in the metropolitan Detroit area.

Changing practices in an environment like Henry Ford or the Mayo Clinic or Kaiser Permanente, where the medical staffs are highly motivated, well paid, and academically oriented, is not the same as changing practices in a community hospital system, where physicians come for part of their time and are independent business people. In a community hospital environment, it can be extremely difficult to change clinical practice. It can be all but impossible to get six orthopedic surgeons to standardize the use of supplies (e.g., to agree on which implant they will use). If they are pressured, they can walk out and go to the hospital across the street. So far, most of the work on quality improvement and engineering solutions is being done in a few leading-edge organizations.

Anyone who thinks the problems of the world can be solved by rational discussion among highly educated people has never attended a faculty meeting. The problem is not intelligence, but self-interest. Every organization that tries to introduce change faces cultural issues that work against the implementation of new solutions. For instance, the Institute for Healthcare Improvement has learned that current best practices are not even implemented consistently by single

institutions, much less by institutions around the country (Sahney, 2003). An institution may implement best practices in its prostate cancer unit, but other groups in the same institution may completely ignore those practices. Problems occur both within institutions and among multiple institutions.

There are four major barriers to improving quality. The first barrier is a lack of metrics for comparison. What do we mean by improving a system's performance? Often, large numbers of patients select one delivery system over another based on their specific needs. For instance, if a patient is getting diabetic care in one system and prostate care in another, comparing quality of health care and productivity becomes a difficult issue. It may be possible to determine that, at a microlevel, a system has improved care for a particular disease. But at a macrolevel, comparison is nearly impossible. It is very hard to evaluate whether any innovations make a difference in cost or productivity.

In the United States, the problem is further complicated because the acute-care sector is highly organized, but the chronic-care system is very disorganized, with large numbers of independent physicians providing care. Another aspect of the metrics problem is the indigent-care sector. Fifty percent of the population within a 10-mile radius of Henry Ford Hospital is either underinsured (Medicaid) or uninsured. The hospital must treat all of these patients for free, which puts an enormous burden on the hospital's services. Before solutions can be proposed for improving organization, it is essential that we agree on the metrics to be used for comparison. As an example of the confusion surrounding rating systems, the ratings issued by *U.S. News and World Report*, AARP, and Solucient are all based on different criteria; as a result, each has rated a different institution as the best in providing care.

The second barrier is a lack of alignment in the reimbursement system. In general, under the fee-for-service system, institutions are paid for procedures and visits but not for improvements in health status. The Advisory Board, a health care industry organization in Washington, D.C., subscribed to by almost all of the major institutions in this country, recently recommended that institutions that want to be successful should focus not on caring for medical patients, but on procedural care (The Advisory Board Company, 2001). In other words, if an institution wants to maximize revenue and profitability, it should keep all of the procedural-based patients and send all of the medical-care patients to the hospital across the street. Here's another problem (or misalignment) in the current system. The reimbursement rate is higher when patients develop complications; this is obviously a perverse incentive. Instead of paying for quality care, the current system pays more generously if patients develop complications.

The third barrier is industry structure. Innovations are made by large hospitals and academic centers, which account for only about 25 percent of total expenditures in health care. A large proportion of care is provided by small community hospitals. For health care to improve nationally, innovations must be implemented in community hospitals. Therefore, improvement protocols should also be tested in these institutions.

A fourth barrier to improvement is that many people, including physicians, think quality health care is synonymous with the use of the latest technology. It is important to understand that there can be enormous gaps between *quality of design* and *quality of conformance*. Take an example from the automotive industry. Ford Motor Company spent millions to develop the Jaguar Lemans racing car, a vehicle that will only be used in races. Ford justified the expenditure by claiming the technology developed would also be used in the manufacture of new cars for consumers (e.g., the Ford Focus). But when the Focus was introduced, it was a mess. It was recalled six times in its first year. The engine compartment would catch on fire, the air bag would catch on fire or deploy spontaneously, the car would stall on the freeway, the front suspension would collapse. Otherwise, it was a good car.

In *The Machine That Changed the World*, the Toyota production system, which is considered the world's best production system, was described in detail (Womack et al., 1990). But when other companies tried to copy that system, they found that they could not convert their production systems without developing the accompanying organizational culture. This is a problem in health care too. American surgeons can do wonderful things; but can they do them every time, consistently? Can quality care be delivered every time? This is a quality-of-conformance issue and not a quality-of-design issue. Making sure every patient gets the same quality of care every time is a serious issue. There are huge gaps here, major problems of conformance in the health care industry.

Across the country, a huge number of projects have been undertaken to improve the experience of patients at the care-delivery level (the microlevel). But at the macrolevel, little has been done to create an organizational environment that will make an overall impact and enable the transfer of knowledge from one microproject to another. In addition, as I mentioned earlier, the current payment system may not generate the will for senior leaders to improve quality. It's not that we can't improve or that we lack ideas—there are plenty of ideas. It's just that we don't have the will to work on improvements.

What would generate the will? If there were enough payment incentives, senior leaders would pay attention to what needs to be done. When clinical service chiefs at major institutions were asked how their senior leaders evaluate them, they all said by financial performance. They said they were never asked about the quality of health care they provide. In the prevailing culture, these questions are simply not asked. The will for improvement is not there.

To change this environment, the first thing we must change is the goals for health care delivery; the goals must be in alignment with population health status goals. To begin with, health care systems must define the populations they serve. If a health care system cannot define the population for which it is responsible, it is extremely difficult to set goals for improving people's health status. If no goals are set, the system cannot be held accountable for failing to meet them.

Next, we should create macro-organizational models to test alternative reimbursement policies for delivery systems. Models that demonstrate the "cost of poor quality" must also be created. A major barrier to investments in quality improvement is the belief on the part of physicians and senior leaders that the investments do not pay back. Models could prove that investing in improvements would actually generate a reasonable rate of return.

Another important step would be to create organizational decision simulators—practical operational tools that would show nurses what to do, if, for instance, the OR or ER is backed up.

And finally, it is important to improve employee and team skills for evidence-based care. It is very difficult to give staff time for training, but it is also important that institutions keep on training care teams. New, cost-effective methods of training must be developed.

In conclusion, major improvements in the health care industry will require not only engineering solutions, but also cultural changes in health care delivery organizations.

REFERENCES

Advisory Board Company. 2001. The New Economics of Care. Washington, D.C.: The Advisory Board Company.
Sahney, V.K. 2003. Generating Management Research on Improving Quality. Accepted for publication in Health Care Management Review.
Womack, J.P., D.T. Jones, and D. Roos. 1990. The Machine That Changed the World. New York: Maxwell MacMillan International.

Equipping the Patient
and the Care Team

Evidence-Based Medicine

Brian Haynes
McMaster University

The idea behind evidence-based health care is the transfer of research results into practice. This means creating operational tools, procedures, and preappraisals of published results to enable practitioners to apply evidence to practice with confidence. But no matter how well we manage evidence or how compelling the evidence is, it has to fit into a framework; it is only one part of the decision process. Machines are not going to control medical care because the evidence has to fit the clinical circumstances of an individual. Best evidence must complement decision making, which must take into account a number of issues, including how severely a disease affects an individual, other diseases competing for the individual's body space, allergies, financial constraints, and so on. Evidence-enhanced health care is perhaps a better term than evidence-based health care. We are not trying to replace the medical care process. We are trying to improve it by providing better access to evidence from research.

What are the barriers to the implementation and acceptance of evidence-based health care? First, our current standards for research claims are very loose, and false messages abound—messages such as "this will help you," "this will be better for you," and so on. These messages come from many sources, and their validity has not always been tested.

Although our resources for synthesizing evidence are generally inadequate, there is one worldwide organization, the Cochrane Collaboration (2002),[1] that attempts to synthesize evidence from research. Because no single study can tell us very much about the value of an innovation, we need the results of several investigations to get a clear picture of an innovation's effectiveness. Therefore, we should invest in synthesis processes to ensure that there is a hard-wired link between evidence and the final picture.

Support for practitioners and patients is also inadequate, which makes it difficult to provide the best evidence when and where it is needed. Consequently, procedures are sometimes done on the very patients who benefit least and are not done on the patients who would benefit most. How can we address the gap between research and practice? First and foremost, the evidence must be clearly understood and assessed so we can develop clinical policies based on the strengths and limitations of the evidence and the settings in which that evidence is going to be applied.

The extraction and synthesis of evidence is one aspect of the process at which we have been successful. Core medical journals put a massive number of published articles through a double filter: (1) the scientific validity of the research; (2) the contribution of the research to practice. An article that meets both criteria may appear in one of the core journals of internal medicine (e.g., *New England Journal of Medicine, Annals of Internal Medicine, Journal of the American Medical Association*, etc.). If one concentrates on these core journals, the number of published articles to be read is somewhat reduced. Nevertheless, a practitioner trying to keep up to date by reading the medical literature hasn't got a chance.

We can now make this mass of information much more tractable by centralizing the evidence-sorting process. The Evidence-Based Medicine Review (EBMR) Service on OVID, for example, provides integrated access to original and reviewed research evidence. Let's say you find a clinical trial on Medline through EBMR and it has been included in a systematic review by the Cochrane Collaboration. You will then be routed right to that review so you can see all of the other studies on the same topic and how they play out when you put them together.

The next step is to develop clinical policies based on

---

[1] The Cochrane Collaboration's mission is "preparing, maintaining and promoting the accessibility of systematic reviews of the effects of healthcare interventions." The collaboration and the online library of databases were developed in response to the call of a British epidemiologist, Archie Cochrane, that information on relevant, randomized, controlled trials be made more widely available.

evidence. This is not simply a matter of taking the evidence as it stands and applying it. Practitioners must first determine how the evidence applies in their own settings. At a few institutions individual practice groups regularly sit down to evaluate evidence systematically, but this is still rare. The Hong Kong Hospital Authority runs about 65 hospitals in the Hong Kong region. Doctors from these hospitals who treat stroke, cancer, and heart disease get together regularly to examine the evidence. They then put together medical bulletins on evidence-based approaches to controversial areas of clinical practice, titled *Evidence*, which they circulate in print form and post on their institution's website (available online at: *<http://www.ha.org.hk/hesd/nsapi/>*).

Now I'd like to comment on the status of continuing professional development. Doctors, and I think most other health professionals, prefer, and are most often offered, continuing professional development in ways that are not very effective—lectures, for example. More effective methods, such as preceptorships, for example, in which a practicing physician returns to an educational institution for a period of supervised training, are expensive and time consuming. In the future, practitioners will have to spend more time using hands-on models. The system will also need ongoing performance reports as feedback so a practitioner's performance can be compared with the performance of his or her colleagues or against quality standards. Many practitioners are resistant to ongoing training, however, because they are reluctant to have anyone oversee their work. In addition, they do not want to spend unpaid time away from their practices, let alone pay for continuing education.

I'll leave you with my wish list:

- Scientists should be looking for treatments that cure. Unfortunately, the people who make money on illnesses will not fund the search for cures, so we must find different financing mechanisms.
- We must develop centralized evidence processing. Despite the volume of research, we can have one central, high-quality, evidence-processing source that examines all of the evidence and evaluates it in terms of certain quality criteria. The next step would be to determine which evidence is relevant to particular practice groups and deliver it to them.
- We must refine computerized decision-support systems and information services. We need a valid code that alerts us to the quality and currency of evidence on the Internet.
- We must develop information-retrieval systems that are both sensitive and precise.
- We must apply human-factors engineering to reduce errors.
- We must develop decision-support systems that integrate clinical data with current, evidence-based, best-practice information and that provide information on when and why it may be appropriate to deviate from best practices.
- We must develop learning systems for busy practitioners that provide them (and the system) with feedback on their performance.

REFERENCE

Cochrane Collaboration. 2002. Online Library of Databases. Available online at: *http://www.cochrane.org/cochrane/cc-broch.htm*.

The Context of Care and the Patient Care Team: The Safety Attitudes Questionnaire

J. Bryan Sexton and Eric J. Thomas
University of Texas Center of Excellence for Patient Safety Research and Practice
and
Peter Pronovost
The Johns Hopkins University School of Medicine

In the words of psychologist John Lauber, a former member of the National Transportation Safety Board, "Human performance doesn't take place in a vacuum, it takes place in an environment engendered and maintained by management, government, and frontline personnel" (Lauber, 1995). Taking the context into consideration is critical for understanding the complexities of human performance. As climate researchers in quality of care, our task is to identify (with methodological rigor) the systems and cultural influences that affect the safe delivery of care.

In the wake of recent reports from the Institute of Medicine and National Health Service, interest in patient safety research has grown substantially (IOM, 1999; Department of Health, 2000). Experience in other safety-critical industries suggests that measuring attitudes toward teamwork and the overall context of work is an important step in improving safety (Maurino et al., 1995; Reason, 1997). In health care, quality of care must also be investigated within the framework of the systems and contextual factors that provide the environments in which errors and adverse events occur (Cook and Woods, 1994; Leape, 1994; Reason, 1995; Vincent et al., 1998). For example, Charles Vincent and his colleagues identify several factors that influence clinical practice: organizational factors (e.g., safety climate and morale), work environment factors (e.g., staffing levels and managerial support), team factors (e.g., teamwork and supervision), and staff factors (e.g., overconfidence and being overly self-assured) (Vincent et al., 1998). These factors are believed to influence the safe delivery of care, but to date, the attitudes of caregivers about these key factors remain largely unexplored (Pronovost et al., 2001; Vella et al., 2000).

Influential organizations in health care agree that caregivers' attitudes about these issues should be examined. Research agencies (Agency for Healthcare Research and Quality, National Patient Safety Foundation, and National Patient Safety Agency), regulators (Joint Commission on Accreditation of Healthcare Organizations [JCAHO]), health maintenance organizations (e.g., Kaiser Permanente), professional organizations (e.g., American Hospital Association), and quality improvement experts (e.g., Institute for Healthcare Improvement) are encouraging the measurement of caregiver attitudes about the context of work. Despite this interest, there is no commonly used metric to measure these attitudes. The lack of a common metric led our research team at the University of Texas Center of Excellence for Patient Safety Research and Practice to develop and validate a tool that can be used across different types of clinical areas, different types of health care providers, and in different national cultures.

THE SAFETY ATTITUDES QUESTIONNAIRE

The Safety Attitudes Questionnaire (SAQ) is a refinement of the Intensive Care Unit Management Attitudes Questionnaire (Sexton et al., 2000; Thomas et al., 2003), which was derived from a questionnaire widely used in commercial aviation, the Flight Management Attitudes Questionnaire (FMAQ) (Helmreich et al., 1993; Merritt, 1996). The SAQ differs from other medical attitudinal surveys (Shortell et al., 1991) in that it maintains continuity with its predecessor (FMAQ), a traditional human factors survey with a 20-year history (Gregorich et al., 1990; Helmreich, 1984). Preserving this continuity allows for comparisons between professions and assists with the search for universal human factors issues. There is a 25 percent overlap in item content between the SAQ and the FMAQ. The new (non-overlapping) SAQ items were generated by focus groups of health care providers, literature review, and roundtable discussions with subject matter experts. More than 100 items were initially generated, but the number was reduced through pilot testing. The SAQ has been adapted for use in intensive care units (ICUs), operating rooms (ORs), general inpatient settings (medical wards, surgical wards), ambulatory clinics, pharmacies, and labor and delivery units. All versions of the SAQ have the same item content, with minor modifications to reflect the clinical area. For example, "In this ICU, it is difficult to discuss mistakes" would be changed to "In the ORs here, it is difficult to discuss mistakes."

The SAQ elicits caregiver attitudes through six-factor analytically derived scales: teamwork climate; job satisfaction; perceptions of management; safety climate; working conditions; and stress recognition. These six scales are based on prior research in the aviation industry and in medicine (Helmreich and Merritt, 1998; Sexton, 2002; Sexton and Klinect, 2001; Sexton et al., 2000; Thomas et al., 2003). The SAQ is a single-page (double-sided) questionnaire with 60 items and demographics information (age, sex, experience, and nationality). The questionnaire takes approximately 10 to 15 minutes to complete. Each of the 60 items is answered using a five-point Likert scale (Disagree Strongly, Disagree Slightly, Neutral, Agree Slightly, Agree Strongly).

To date, we have administered the survey in more than 300 organizations in the United States, the United Kingdom, and New Zealand. Our rule of thumb is that all personnel in a clinical area who influence, or are influenced by, the working environment in that area are invited to participate (e.g., attending/staff physicians, resident physicians, registered nurses, charge nurses, pharmacists, respiratory therapists, technicians, ward clerks, and others). Participation is voluntary, and administration techniques included hand delivery, meetings, and in-house mailings.

The SAQ is a psychometrically valid instrument for assessing the safety-related attitudes and perceptions of front-line health care providers. The SAQ factor structure was replicated in ICUs, ORs, ambulatory clinics, and inpatient settings, as well as three national cultures.

The SAQ results reported here demonstrate the substantial variability in teamwork climate and safety climate across 50 organizations (Figures 1 and 2). Each bar represents the percentage of respondents who reported positive attitudes in each of 50 organizations.

In Figure 1, the right side of the distribution corresponds to organizations with a positive teamwork climate. These organizations are information rich, have good collaboration, effective conflict resolution, and decision making based on input from the team. The left side represents organizations with a negative teamwork climate. These organizations are information poor; the quality of collaboration is abysmal; nurses do not feel comfortable speaking up if they perceive a problem with patient care; conflicts often go unresolved; and decision making does not integrate input from the team. Organizations on the left have problems with turnover and absenteeism, whereas organizations on the right enjoy high levels of retention, good participation, and better working conditions.

In Figure 2, the right side of the distribution shows organizations with a positive safety climate. These organizations have a proactive, rather than reactive, patient-safety posture. Individuals are encouraged to report safety concerns;

medical errors are handled appropriately; rules and guidelines are followed; and it is easy to learn from the mistakes of others.

It is noteworthy that the answers of senior leadership were substantially more positive than the answers of health care providers working at the front line. In fact, senior leadership was four times as positive about teamwork climate as front line personnel and two-and-a-half times as positive about safety climate.

We have established a large archive of SAQ administrations to use as bench marks for comparisons in future research. We hope the SAQ can be used to meet some of the demand for survey assessments of climate and culture in medicine.

The SAQ was designed for organizational diagnoses and interventions relevant to patient safety. Hospitals, federal regulators, quality improvement organizations, and JCAHO could use the SAQ as an economical and efficient means of collecting safety-relevant data proactively, rather than waiting for problems to manifest themselves through adverse and sentinel events. The SAQ can be used to assess strengths and weaknesses in a given organization and to provide a basis for suggesting interventions. Examples of interventions include: briefings, checklists, executive walk-rounds, human factors training, multidisciplinary rounds, and the Comprehensive Unit-Based Safety Program (CUSP).

For example, a poor teamwork climate in the OR may indicate a need for preoperative, multidisciplinary surgical briefings, with participation by anesthetists, surgeons, and nurses. More than 90 percent of OR personnel report that briefings are important for patient safety, but only 23 percent report that briefings are routinely held. On average, surgical briefings require less than two minutes; they cover the plan for contingencies for "this patient, this procedure, this equipment, and this team today," including who is responsible for tasks and what the expectations are. Surgical briefings have been shown to improve nurse retention rates and to have a positive impact on teamwork climate as shown in the higher percentage of respondents reporting that nurse input is well received, that they know the names of the personnel they work with, and that they feel comfortable speaking up if they perceive a problem with patient care.

Poor teamwork climate in the ICU might suggest a need for multidisciplinary rounds (Uhlig et al., 2001), whereas a poor safety climate might suggest a need for executive walk-rounds (Frankel et al., 2003) or CUSP (Pronovost et al., unpublished). CUSP is an eight-step program developed by the Johns Hopkins Hospital Patient Safety Committee and implemented in hospital work units, beginning in ICUs. Improvement teams were identified at each unit; outcome variables included: changes in safety climate from pre-implementation to six months post implementation; and a decrease in medication errors, length of stay, and nursing turnover rates. CUSP was carried out in the Weinberg Intensive Care Unit; a second ICU (the Surgical Intensive

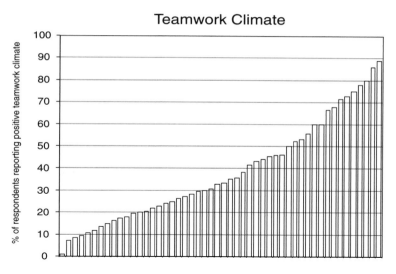

FIGURE 1 Teamwork climate in 50 organizations.

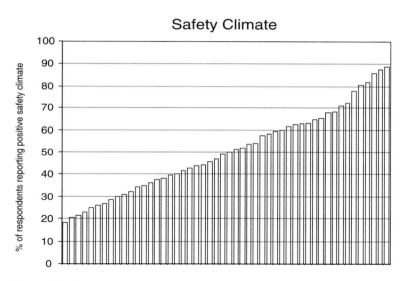

FIGURE 2 Safety climate in 50 organizations.

Care Unit) was used as a control (see Figure 3). The evidence from Johns Hopkins Hospital demonstrates that safety climate can be improved and that these improvements are associated with decreases in medication errors, lower nurse turnover rates, and shorter ICU lengths of stay (Pronovost et al., unpublished).

To date, more than 150,000 copies of the SAQ are in circulation, many being used in longitudinal quality-of-care investigations. As our understanding of health care climates and contextual factors evolves, we are becoming better equipped to improve quality of care. Current research at the University of Texas Center of Excellence for Patient Safety Research and Practice is focused on the relationships between provider attitudes and patient, provider, and organizational outcomes. Some preliminary evidence shows that SAQ factors are related to annual rates of nurse turnover (Roberts, 2002; Sexton, 2002), medication errors, and ICU length of stay (Pronovost et al., unpublished). Additional links to outcomes have been found outside of medicine, where predecessors of the SAQ have been linked to pilot performance (Helmreich, 1984), pilot error management (Sexton and Klinect, 2001), and incident rates among night train conductors in Japan (Itoh et al., 2000). Taken together, these relationships suggest that the SAQ can shed light on important clinical, economical, and administrative issues in medicine and beyond.

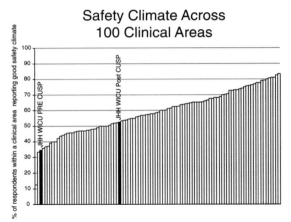

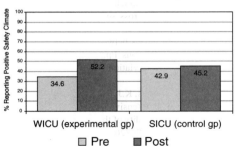

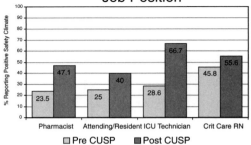

Impact of CUSP on Safety Climate

	WICU (experimental gp)		SICU (control gp)	
	PRE	POST	PRE	POST
% Positive*	34.60	52.20	42.90	45.20
Mean	64.25	71.84	67.98	69.89
Median	62.50	75.00	66.67	70.83
Mode	50.00	83.33	75.00	54.17
SD	19.10	18.18	17.84	18.44

% Positive indicates the percent of respondents answering above neutral on the 5 point scale:
1=Disagree Strongly; 2=Disagree Slightly: 3=Neutral; 4=Agree Slightly; 5=Agree Strongly

FIGURE 3 CUSP results.

REFERENCES

Cook, R.I., and D.D. Woods. 1994. Operating at the Sharp End: The Complexity of Human Error. Pp. 255–310 in Human Error in Medicine, M.S. Bogner, ed. Hillside, N.J.: Lawrence Erlbaum and Associates.

Department of Health. 2000. Organisation with a Memory. London: The Stationary Office, National Health Service.

Frankel, A., E. Graydon-Baker, C. Neppl, T. Simmonds, M. Gustafson, and T.K. Gandhi. 2003. Patient safety leadership walkrounds. Joint Commission Journal on Quality Improvement 29(1): 16–26.

Gregorich, S.E., R.L. Helmreich, and J.A. Wilhelm. 1990. The structure of cockpit management attitudes. Journal of Applied Psychology 75(6): 682–690.

Helmreich, R.L. 1984. Cockpit management attitudes. Human Factors 26(5): 583–589.

Helmreich, R.L., A.C. Merritt, P.J. Sherman, S.E. Gregorich, and E.L. Wiener. 1993. The Flight Management Attitudes Questionnaire (FMAQ). NASA/UT/FAA Technical Report 93-4. Austin, Texas: University of Texas Press.

Helmreich, R.L., and A.C. Merritt. 1998. Culture at Work in Aviation and Medicine: National, Organizational, and Professional Influences. Aldershot, U.K.: Ashgate Publishing.

IOM (Institute of Medicine). 1999. To Err Is Human: Building a Safer Health System, L.T. Kohn, J.M. Corrigan, and M.S. Donaldson, eds. Washington, D.C.: National Academy Press.

Itoh, K., H.B. Andersen, H. Tanaka, and M. Seki. 2000. Attitudinal factors of night train operators and their correlation with accident/incident sta-

tistics. Pp. 87–96 in Proceedings of the 19th European Annual Conference on Human Decision Making and Manual Control, Ispra, Italy, June 26–28, 2000.

Lauber, J. 1995. Putting Professionalism in the Cockpit. CRM Advocate 95.1. Available online at: *http://users2.ev1.net/~neilkrey/crmdevel/resources/crmadvocate/95_1/95_1.htm#2.*

Leape, L.L. 1994. Error in medicine. Journal of the American Medical Association 272(23): 1851–1857.

Maurino, D.E., J. Reason, N. Johnston, and R.B. Lee. 1995. Beyond Aviation Human Factors. Aldershot, U.K.: Ashgate Publishing.

Merritt, A.C. 1996. National Culture and Work Attitudes in Commercial Aviation: A Cross-Cultural Investigation. Unpublished doctoral dissertation, University of Texas at Austin.

Pronovost, P.J., L. Morlock, and T. Dorman. 2001. Creating Safe Systems of ICU Care. Pp. 695–708 in Year Book of Intensive Care and Emergency Medicine, J.L. Vincent, ed. Heidelberg: Springer Verlag.

Pronovost, P.J., B. Weast, C. Holzmueller, B.J. Rosenstein, K.B. Haller, E.R. Feroli, J.B. Sexton, and H.R. Rubin. Unpublished. Evaluating a culture of safety. Submitted to Quality and Safety in Healthcare.

Reason, J.T. 1995. Understanding Adverse Events: Human Factors. Pp. 31–54 in Clinical Risk Management, C.A. Vincent, editor. London: British Medical Journal Publications.

Reason, J.T. 1997. Managing the Risks of Organizational Accidents. Aldershot, U.K.: Ashgate Publishing.

Roberts, P.R. 2002. In Pursuit of a Safety Culture in New Zealand Public Hospitals. Masters Thesis, Victoria University of Wellington, New Zealand.

Sexton, J.B. 2002. A Matter of Life or Death: Social Psychological and Organizational Factors Related to Patient Outcomes in the Intensive Care Unit. Unpublished doctoral dissertation, University of Texas at Austin.

Sexton, B.J., E.J. Thomas, and R.L. Helmreich. 2000. Error, stress, and teamwork in medicine and aviation: cross sectional surveys. British Medical Journal 320(7237): 745–749.

Sexton, J.B., and J.R. Klinect. 2001. The Link between Safety Attitudes and Observed Performance in Flight Operations. Pp. 7–13 in Proceedings of the 11th International Symposium on Aviation Psychology. Columbus, Ohio: Ohio State University Press.

Shortell, S.M., D.M. Rousseau, R.R. Gillies, K.J. Devers, and T.L. Simons. 1991. Organizational assessment in intensive care units (ICUs): construct development, reliability, and validity of the ICU Nurse-Physician Questionnaire. Medical Care 29(8): 709–726.

Thomas, E.J., J.B. Sexton, and R.L. Helmreich. 2003. Discrepant attitudes about teamwork among critical care nurses and physicians. Critical Care Medicine 31(3): 956–959.

Uhlig, P.N., C.K. Haan, A.K. Nason, P.L. Niemann, A. Camelio, and J. Brown. 2001. Improving Patient Care by the Application of Theory and Practice from the Aviation Safety Community. Pp. 1–9 in Proceedings of the 11th International Symposium on Aviation Psychology. Columbus, Ohio: Ohio State University Press.

Vella, K., C. Goldfrad, K. Rowan, J. Bion, and N. Black. 2000. Use of consensus development to establish national research priorities in critical care. British Medical Journal 320(7240): 976–980.

Vincent, C., S. Taylor-Adams, and N. Stanhope. 1998. Framework for analysing risk and safety in clinical medicine. British Medical Journal 316(7138): 1154–1157.

Engineering the Patient and Family into the Patient Care Team

David Gustafson
University of Wisconsin-Madison

The basic message I want to convey is that investing engineering efforts in enabling patients and families to participate more fully in their own care is as important as investing in improving the health care system per se. My focus is on patients and families more than on improving the health delivery system.

In January of this year, my mother died. She had Alzheimer's for about seven years, and when she developed shortness of breath, my sister-in-law took her to the hospital, thinking that she had pneumonia. She may have been right, but within a day that pneumonia, in some way or other, changed to congestive heart failure. The next day she had a heart attack, and on the third day she died. Setting aside the grieving, in a sense, it was fascinating to watch what happened during those three days. I watched a wonderful woman, whose mind had begun to fail but who was still capable of recognizing people and having conversations and who was still physically quite fit, change into a person connected to oxygen tubes, antibiotic IVs, and catheters, surrounded by monitors, hands and body restrained, unable to move, unable to twist, unable to lie on her side. My mother, who never slept on her back, was expected to endure these conditions as part of her "care." All my mother wanted to do was to go home.

It was nice that she died pretty quickly, but she died after more than $20,000 worth of treatment had been given in her last three days. My mom hated health care systems and never went to doctors; she didn't like them, didn't trust them, and didn't think they were very useful. As a result, that $20,000 was a lot more than had ever been spent on her health care during her entire life. And it was spent to see her die in a very unpleasant situation. As a matter of fact, my mom was not unique. In 1997, the Institute of Medicine concluded that "the care of the dying does not even approach the norms of decency" (IOM, 1997). I concluded the same thing from this experience.

One of the fascinating things to me about that experience was that there were so many decisions that could've, should've, maybe would've been made if I and the rest of the family had had access to information and had known what our rights were. Could we have had the tubes removed? All she wanted was to remove the tubes and go home. Did we have the right to do that? Could we have done that? Could we have just taken her home and said, "Look, this is silly. Let's let her die." Would the assisted-living facility have taken her back? How do you manage 24-hour care, if you can find it? Could I have asked her if she wanted to die, and if so what words should I have used to ask her? Should I have called a hospice, and how would I have found a good one? How about a nursing home? I know that nursing homes vary enormously in quality. Which one should I have put her in? How could I have gotten her into the right one, and how could I have ensured that she was getting the right care?

Physicians were not helpful. They are very much "into" curing patients, and I can't blame them. I would be too. But they headed for the hills. In three days, we didn't talk to a single physician! At the same time, the nurses kept telling us they could not answer our questions and that we should talk to the doctors. What we really needed was access to information that we could get on our own. We needed help in making decisions. Techniques like decision analysis might have helped us through this tough time. We couldn't get that help from the health care system.

Tom Ferguson uses a triangle with a waterline dividing the tip of the iceberg of professional care from the rest of health care (Figure 1) (Ferguson, 1987). He argues that the vast majority of health care is self-care, not care from the traditional health care delivery system. Above the waterline is the amount of care delivered by professionals, and below it is the 95 percent of health care that's delivered by individuals and their families. One of the key things that engineering can and should do is find a way to raise the

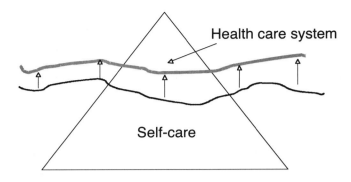

FIGURE 1 Triangle with a waterline dividing the tip of the iceberg (professional care) from the rest of health care. Source: Ferguson, 1987.

waterline, to help the patient and the family provide more care themselves. This will require a multidisciplinary effort that goes beyond industrial engineering to include other disciplines such as biomedical engineering, other professionals, such as psychologists and communications experts, and beyond professionals to include patients and families. If we can raise the waterline, increase the proportion of care delivered by the patient and the family themselves, we will dramatically cut the cost of care and exponentially improve the quality of care.

This goal is not just for the dying, of course. The same kind of problems occur with drug addicts, kids with severe asthma, women with breast cancer, men with prostate cancer, stroke victims, etc. In all of these situations, the family or patients can make a difference, can be involved, can influence outcomes, possibly more dramatically than the health care system itself can. We need to find ways of making that happen, and engineering is uniquely positioned, with the kinds of tools and techniques it offers (and in collaboration with other fields and the patients and family), to do that. I will give you three examples.

One of them is e-health (interactive health communications, consumer informatics). The basic idea is that vehicles, such as computers and the Internet, can make a huge difference in the capability of patients and families to care for themselves. The system I will describe is CHESS (the comprehensive health enhancement support system) (Figure 2), which we developed at the University of Wisconsin in the late 1980s (Gustafson et al., 2002). Since then, it has gone through many evolutions, and it now addresses many topics (e.g., breast cancer, asthma, heart disease, depression, etc.) and offers 17 different services, such as answers to frequently asked questions, an action plan to determine how likely people are to implement changes in your life, and decision analysis to help people better understand their options and their values. Hidden beneath some of these tools, although

patients would never notice, are Bayesian models, multi-attribute utility models, statistical process controls, human-computer interface designs, and several other engineering tools.

Although CHESS has proven to be quite powerful, it has only scratched the surface of what industrial engineering and operations research and other kinds of engineering could do. CHESS does not even take full advantage of statistical process controls as a way of helping patients monitor their own care and helping families monitor the status of their loved ones. We don't use embedded chips to feed information to CHESS about the health status of a patient. And, we have a long way to go for our interface to be extremely easy to use. We could give families of patients approaching the end of life an opportunity to see how pain has changed and how distress has changed. Patients could use that information as a vehicle to communicate with clinicians. We are working on that now.

There are many other ways interactive health communication systems can make a difference in patients' lives. In the last 10 years, we've done a lot of research on CHESS, and the results of our work and other people's work suggest that these kind of tools are extensively used, especially by the elderly and the underserved (Gustafson et al., 1998, 2001). These two groups use them differently from the rest of us, and in fact they are the ones who seem to benefit the most—in terms of improved quality of life and less expensive health care services.

The Internet has great potential. The problem is that not enough of the skills and tools of engineering have been applied. We just completed a study of 300 breast cancer patients: one-third of them got usual care; one-third were given computers with access to the Internet and were trained to use the Internet and given a list of high-quality breast cancer sites; one-third got CHESS (Gustafson et al., 2003). The straight line in Figure 2 (where it says zero) is the impact

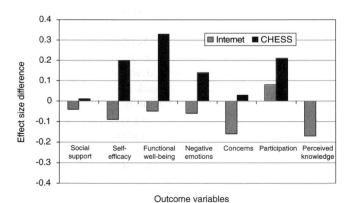

FIGURE 2 The comprehensive enhancement support system (CHESS). Source: Gustafson et al., 2002.

of having usual care; this was our control group. Notice how many things are below the line; those are Internet results.

The results of this study are preliminary but make some important points. First, if you give people access to the Internet, teach them how to use it, and give them high-quality Internet sites, they become, if anything, more confused, more worried, and more depressed. If the results continue to hold, this suggests that, although the Internet has tremendous potential, that potential won't be reached until we can also take full advantage of decision analysis, statistical process control, and other kinds of industrial engineering and operations research tools and integrate them into interactive delivery systems.

I think engineering will be the key to making the Internet a truly useful health intervention. Moreover, this will be the result not only of engineering tools, but also of engineering insight. For instance, decision analysis offers not only tools, such as utility models, but also an understanding of how people make decisions and an understanding of how to communicate uncertainty effectively. These are critical issues in sharing information with patients and families. Other issues relate to the way information is displayed—the appropriate combination of audio, video, and text, for instance. Engineering, such as cost analyses, can help us determine the cost effectiveness of interventions. We also need to address the design and relative roles of PCs, PDAs, cell phones, and monitoring chips embedded in the body.

We ought to convene a panel of experts to address the following problem. Suppose we are caring for people (e.g., with severe asthma), and there is only one rule: no health care professionals can be involved, no doctors, nurses, or any other health care provider—just the patient and family. Let's design a system that's completely technologically based, recognizing, of course, that this could, and should, never happen. Then let's back off the assumption of involving no health professionals, but only involve them when it is absolutely essential to do so. What would that system look like? What tools, techniques, and resources would we need? I think if we took that kind of approach, we would get an idea of the potential of engineering to make a difference that we couldn't make otherwise.

My point is that the National Academy of Engineering and Institute of Medicine should engage in blue-sky work where we assume that we *can* do without the health care system as we know it, and then back into the current health care system only when it's absolutely necessary. Our job should not be to improve the existing system but to develop systems to help patients and families play a more central role in their own care. We can't afford the system we have, and the sooner we get away from the idea of improving it and on to the idea of replacing it, the more likely our work is to make a substantial difference.

In addition, we should not limit ourselves to the acute health care delivery system. There are many other problem areas. I am the national program director for a Robert Wood Johnson Foundation program called Paths to Recovery, which aims to improve access to and retention in substance abuse treatment. When I first got into this area, I didn't know anything about heroin or other addictive drugs. So I took on a persona and got myself admitted for heroin addiction. Everybody knew I was a fake, that I'd never seen heroin in my life; I still don't know what it looks like. But I adopted a persona, and I walked in and said I wanted to get help. And they said, "OK, we need to collect some information from you." They spent two hours collecting information from me, and then they said, "Yes, you need to be admitted, but we don't have a bed. Call back once a week, and tell us if you're still interested." Now heroin addiction is a chronic disease, where timing means everything. A heroin addict can desperately want help one hour and the next hour can give up and desperately look for the next packet of heroin. But they told me to call back. When I called back, I got an answering machine, "leave a message," first week. "Leave a message," second week. "Leave a message," the third week, fourth week, fifth week, sixth week, "leave a message." The loneliness and hopelessness that I felt (even though I don't have the problem) was incredible.

Then I went to my "staffing" where they decide how to treat me, to find out how the process worked. Several professionals were at this meeting talking about what to do with me and other potential patients. Remember this was after I had been interviewed for over two hours to collect data on my condition. The staffing team (which did not include the person who had interviewed me) had one small paragraph of information about me, and that is what they based their decision on. All of the other information collected from me was paperwork compliance, simply satisfying a regulatory body. The inefficiencies and duplications of effort and waste in that system were terrible! I had to travel on a bus route for over an hour to reach the location where my interview took place. Would it have been possible to develop a computer system to interview me that could have saved staff time and allowed me to be interviewed at any public library? Would it be possible to develop an Internet-based system to help the family help heroin addicts? This organization did not have a bed for me, but another one might have. Would it be possible to have an inventory system that could have placed me in an open bed immediately? Did I really need to be placed in an inpatient facility? Could outpatient care have been at least partially effective while I was waiting for a bed? Would it be possible to develop a computer-based protocol that could have made these decisions immediately without my waiting for seven weeks to get an opportunity for treatment? There are so many opportunities beyond the traditional physical health system in areas such as substance abuse and mental health, areas where engineering can make a huge difference.

We also need to ask how engineering can contribute to the diffusion of innovation or the implementation of change. Often changes in the health care field simply disappear, and the system regresses back to its previous condition. One of the things we've got to figure out is how to make changes that stick. That's going to take a lot of work. One way might be to use decision analytic models to predict and explain whether changes will be made and sustained. The problems are much too complex for us to try to solve them alone. We must work with communications scientists, organizational development scientists, psychologists, educators, economists, and others. It's going to take all of us working together to solve them.

Finally, I think we should be trying to put ourselves out of business. Our tools are so powerful. They have so much potential. But too often, we focus on developing more sophisticated tools rather than on asking how we can spread the application of the tools we have. We engineers ought to assume that with the kinds of information technology out there today, we can design systems that will allow a patient or family to do their own simulations and optimization. There's no reason we can't make the technology we have so easy to use and so automated that the assumptions are protected and the data collection mechanisms are developed. Our tools could then be used by the average citizen. We ought to be engaged in developing technologies that automate our field so that everyone can be an industrial engineer. By trying to put ourselves out of business, engineering will find a future that is more dynamic and useful than we can even imagine.

REFERENCES

Ferguson, T. 1995. Consumer health informatics. Healthcare Forum Journal 38(1): 28–33.

Gustafson, D.H., F. McTavish, R. Hawkins, S. Pingree, N. Arora, J. Mendenhall, and G.E. Simmons. 1998. Computer support for elderly women with breast cancer: results of a population-based intervention (letter). Journal of the American Medical Association 280(15): 1305.

Gustafson, D.H., R. Hawkins, S. Pingree, F. McTavish, N.K. Arora, J. Mendenhall, D.F. Cella, R.C. Serlin, F.M. Apantaku, J. Stewart, and A. Salner. 2001. Effect of computer support on younger women with breast cancer. Journal of General Internal Medicine 16(5): 435–445.

Gustafson, D.H, R. Hawkins, E. Boberg, F. McTavish, B. Owns, M. Wise, H. Berhe, and S. Pingree. 2002. CHESS: 10 years of research and development in consumer health informatics for broad populations, including the underserved. International Journal of Medical Informatics 65(3): 169–177.

Gustafson, D.H., R. Hawkins, S. Pingree, F. McTavish, W. Chen, K. Volrathongchai, W. Stengle, and J. Stewart. 2003. The Internet as Source of Health Information and Support: Less than Meets the Eye? The Center for Health Systems Research and Analysis, University of Wisconsin, Madison.

IOM (Institute of Medicine). 1997. Approaching Death: Improving Care at the End of Life, M.J. Field and C.K. Cassel, eds. Washington, D.C.: National Academy Press.

Connecting Patients, Providers, and Payers

John D. Halamka
CareGroup Health System
and
Harvard Medical School

Harvard has moved all of its clinical, financial, and administrative applications to the Web. The changeover began in 1998, when all clinical information was put online. Now one can have complete, ubiquitous, transparent, seamless access to all aspects of the clinical care process. The technologies are robust and secure, and all work flow processes take place on the Web. From an engineering standpoint, the change was made by taking all of the legacy systems that already existed for Harvard's patients and employees and wrapping them, using XML Web services, to provide standards-based information exchanges. Today, I will present this new system.

Everything in the system is secure, and everything is audited. When the system is accessed by a provider, the first screen provides access to the nine million patients in the CareGroup master patient index, reflecting 6 hospitals (Beth Israel-Deaconess, Mt. Auburn, New England Baptist, and three community hospitals).

One serious impediment to using computerized medical records is that there is no universal health identifier in the United States. To search for a patient's record, therefore, the Harvard system uses a statistical, probabilistic match based on demographic information. For example, using this model to gather information about a Martha Ford, one can see (Figure 1) that patients with that name have visited the East Campus, the Mt. Auburn Campus, and the West Campus, with

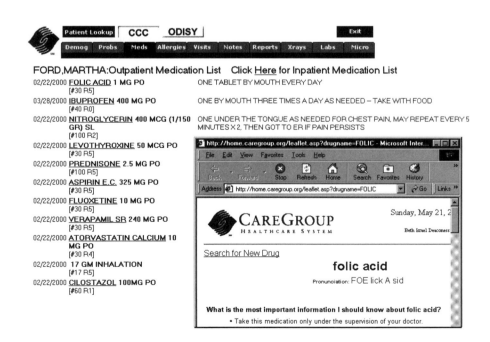

FIGURE 1 Patient record screen.

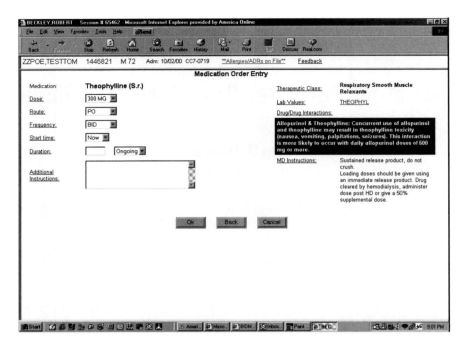

FIGURE 2 Typical flagged drug/drug interaction.

different medical record numbers for each of those visits; but, with consolidated access, it is possible to see that all three Martha Fords are the same person (this patient has given permission for access to her medical records).

Next, one can assemble her entire medical record in real time from all of the places she sought care. Information is stored in very different ways, but, because the legacy systems have been wrapped in a standards-based package, it is possible to click on, for instance, medications, and get a complete look at the medications she is using. That information can be forwarded, for instance, to a drug interaction engine, that could list in order of severity the interactions of all the medications she has taken in the entire continuum of her care. It is possible to look at text data, such as her last echocardiogram, to obtain all of the echo parameters. It is also possible to pull out telemetry data, even data stored in an old, non-standards-based system, convert it to a standards-based display, and deliver it. This is truly a time series, scalable object that can be measured, printed, and manipulated.

All medical record images are also online and are DICOM based. Because Martha's chest x-ray is an object, it can be examined in many ways, and old films can be pulled up for comparison. Moreover, with this system one can also look at laboratory results over time, such as her CBCs trended over time for the last 10 years. This is the organizational context of information ubiquity, pulling together all of the data from wherever it is stored.

Provider order entry is also complete; there is 100 percent compliance throughout the entire organization. To achieve this, many processes had to be changed. Now, no voice or handwritten orders are done anywhere at Beth Israel-Deaconess Medical Center.

Here is an overview of how provider order entry works. Farr 2 is a typical medical ward. From a dashboard of all patients in that ward, one can click on any patient and get the patient record and a snapshot of the patient. All the standard orders that would appear on paper are available on the Web. When orders are entered, the system response includes queries as rules or reminders. One can, for instance, set rules that a flu vaccine has to be given to a patient per the standard protocol. One can then click a button to document that the patient has received the flu vaccine or click a button to order the vaccine. The system offers a quick pick list of all medications the clinician has ordered in the past for the patient, the most common orders, as well as overlays of some pharmacy and therapeutics standard formulary medications.

The physician order entry system has some fail-safe mechanisms. If a clinician orders something that might be bad for the patient—for instance cefazolin for a patient allergic to penicillin—the system notifies the clinician of a potential drug/drug interaction (Figure 2 shows a typical flagged interaction). If the clinician overrides the warning and continues ordering, the system queries the order. Let's say the clinician thinks the allergy history is questionable and wants to monitor the patient. The system then immediately fires off another set of care pathways or rules that advise about the drug. Based on the newest information about the patient's size and test results, it calculates the recommended dose of the drug, the dose frequency, and suggests body parameters that a clinician may want to follow while administering this drug. Thus, this system helps reduce adverse drug events.

If the clinician orders a different drug that may be restricted, an ID fellow may have to approve it. This is a form of consult. The system presents a built-in work flow: click on the button and the system pages the ID fellow via the Web to get approval for the drug. By the way, disapproval happens less than 10 percent of the time. The clinician may choose to default to the standard dose and standard route, which also requires only one click.

The system covers all aspects of ordering care plans and processes and contains standard order-sets for diseases, such as congestive heart failure and asthma. The system has also proven to be very helpful in the emergency room, where it has resulted in a 30-minute decrease in patients' length of stay. At the same time, customer and provider satisfaction has gone up a lot—before implementation, 60 percent rated the ER experience as excellent; after implementation, 85 percent rated it as excellent.

The system also gives the care team the organizational context to enable patients to take part in their care. Here is an example. In 1999, Harvard created a patient site, working with people in the patient-centered movement, that allows patients to have ubiquitous access to their own medical records, with secure, encrypted, doctor–patient e-mail and convenient transactions, such as appointment scheduling, referrals, and prescription renewal.

The patient site begins at patientsite.caregroup.org. (A typical screen shot is shown in Figure 3). For an overview, you just click on the "Take a Tour" button. This is how it works. A patient enters the system. The patient has a unique portal with access to messages of the day from the doctor; links to providers and websites; and life events such as

appointments, a flu vaccine, or a colonoscopy. The patient can send secure—not standard—e-mails to doctors at any time. The patient sites are backed up with behind-the-scenes triage rules so that the medical staff can observe patient transactions and route messages appropriately, for instance, to a doctor, the appointments desk, or a nurse practitioner. The information on the transactions goes into the permanent medical record, where it is retained for 30 years. All of this happens in a secure, audited way. Patients can see the same medical records their doctors see, with certain limitations; patients can access information about their medications, visits, reports, x-rays, allergies, and problems, but cannot access laboratory reports, microbiology, or DICOM imagery. That happens across all institutions and outpatient facilities. CT, MRI, pathology, and psychology results are delayed for 14 days, to ensure, for example, that patients do not first read about a cancer diagnosis online; bad news does not transmit well electronically. The idea is to get information to patients as soon as possible without compromising the doctor–patient relationship.

One question about such a system is "cyberchondria." It's midnight, say, and a patient decides to type in a complete 27-page medical history, including every brand new symptom, such as sudden chest pains. What is the liability issue? Harvard has not encountered this problem. First of all, the site is full of disclaimers and warnings, and patients are repeatedly told to call 911 in case of emergency. Patients have been extraordinarily reasonable when it comes to interplay with their doctors. They have been using the system correctly, even adding in their over-the-counter medications. For example, a patient came in with refractory hypertension. He was treated with ACE inhibitors, beta blockers, and calcium channel blockers, but nothing helped. At the patient

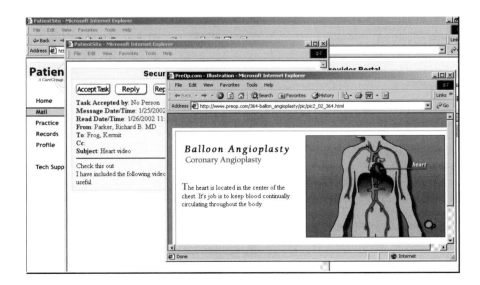

FIGURE 3 Online communication between a patient and doctor.

site, the patient documented that he was taking ephedra five times a day for energy. That was good to know because that is like drinking 40 gallons of coffee a day. Of course, this exacerbated his hypertension.

In another example, a post-liver transplant patient who was feeling depressed took St. John's wort for the depression. One thing St. John's wort does is wrap up the liver's cytochrome P-450 system so immune rejection drugs are processed extraordinarily rapidly, leading to subtherapeutic levels and rejection of the transplant. This problem was picked up entirely because of the shared medical record, amendable by the patient and seen by the care staff.

The patient portal also makes available standard services, such as medication renewal. Patients go to the list of their medications, click on the one that needs renewing, and a prescription renewal request appears, querying dose, quantity, and pharmacy. After review by a doctor, the renewal is autofaxed to the pharmacy. The portal also has an appointments feature. Twenty percent of our doctors allow patients to self-schedule into their calendars. There is also compliance with the Health Insurance Portability and Accountability Act, so that patients can find out who has been looking at their medical records over time.

About 10,000 patients a month use this system, and 2.5 million transactions have been carried out. The average patient sends 1.2 e-mails to the provider every month. Ninety percent of those are triagable to extenders, such as nurse practitioners. Even in a busy practice, the doctor does not see more than five or ten clinical messages a day, which, moreover, usually replace phone calls. The system has become an asynchronous communication medium, allowing doctors to answer e-mails at will instead of having to place phone calls that break up the day. This makes the work flow much more efficient. As long as there is a framework with good engineering principles giving the patient and the doctor shared information and a mechanism for questions and answers, problems with excessive volumes of e-mail do not arise.

To ensure that the system is improving quality and using resources appropriately, the performance of the system is evaluated with metrics. This can be done because all data are warehoused; there are about 40 terabytes of health care data. Metrics based on good data, patient involvement, and control systems give doctors an understanding of how well and how appropriately they are performing. It is also possible to assess performance at the organization level.

The entire enterprise has really helped Harvard, as an organization, meet some of the challenges of the last few years. The Web is an ideal technology for connecting payers, providers, and patients. Creating this system did involve some challenges, which were mostly adaptive and organizational. The important thing about the system is that patients can access their information and participate more often in their own care. Consumer empowerment is a reality that is already redefining the practice of medicine.

New Paradigms for Working and Learning

Richard Bohmer
Harvard Business School

Most of us think of the health care process as the tasks and activities we see performed by doctors and nurses and the technologies and settings they use. However, behind these tasks and technologies are problem-solving activities, predominantly information gathering and decision making, undertaken by members of the patient's caregiving team. These decisions are based on a huge body of medical knowledge developed over centuries. Hence, at its heart the practice of medicine is the application of a general body of medical knowledge to a specific patient for the purpose of resolving the health-related problem for which the patient sought treatment.

Learning (the development and dissemination of the knowledge underlying medical care and medical decisions) plays a pivotal role in this endeavor. Learning is the mechanism by which we advance the practice of medicine and ensure that these advances are widely applied. Learning occurs at many levels in the health care industry. The most prominent levels are the industry level (learning that derives from funded basic research and new technology development) and the individual practitioner level (learning that occurs in medical school and through continuing medical education). At the industry level, learning means the creation of new knowledge; on the individual practitioner level, it refers to the dissemination of existing knowledge. Learning occurs at other levels, too. Patients learn through their experiences of medical problems, and whole organizations learn as they develop experience with particular classes of problems or as they implement new technologies.

One particularly important setting in which learning takes place is inside a delivery organization during the adoption of innovations, such as new services or technologies. Some innovations are, by their nature, nettlesome, difficult to adopt, and significant learning challenges. I call these innovations "interactive," to distinguish them from what I call "component" innovations, which cause relatively little disruption to the processes and systems in which they are used. Consider

a "me-too" drug. For example, we have an existing process of care for treating patients with congestive heart failure, and we simply substitute one drug for another (e.g., we replace ACE inhibitor "A" with ACE inhibitor "B"). The adoption of an interactive innovation occasions a redesign of a process of care, a redistribution of tasks, a change in sequencing—in effect, a disruption of organizational routines.

Interactive innovations are technologies that disrupt *processes*. Medical devices and new information systems are frequently interactive innovations. A new generation of biopharmaceuticals targeted more specifically based on a genetic profile may also disrupt processes of care, organizational routines, and team configurations by requiring members of the care delivery team to work together in new ways. As interactive innovations occasion rearrangements of organizational roles and routines, care delivery teams have to learn to use new technologies, perform new tasks, and develop new relationships and new ways of working together. Hence, organizational learning, as well as learning at the individual practitioner level and the health care industry level, is an important aspect of the adoption of a new technology.

Both organizational and individual learning are correlated with experience. In cardiac surgery, for example, where much of the volume-outcome debate has taken place, this insight has motivated a requirement for mandatory minimum case numbers to credential an individual surgeon or surgical unit. The underlying assumption of the so-called volume-outcome hypothesis is that if you do something often enough, you will become good at it. Practice makes perfect.

When we mandate minimum volumes to ensure competency, we assume that all individuals learn at the same rate and that all institutions learn at the same rate. In effect, we assume that for a given aliquot of experience all surgeons and all institutions will abstract the same amount of learning. This might not be the case, however. Organizational learning is not simply the accumulation of individual learning experiences in one organization. It also requires that teams learn new ways of working together.

We recently undertook a research project to examine the learning rates of 16 surgical units in the adoption of a new surgical procedure for minimally invasive cardiac surgery. With this technique, the surgeon places the patient on femoral bypass and uses long-shafted instruments to operate through a small chest incision (Edmondson et al., 2001). This seemingly simple modification to a well understood operation involves a substantial change in the traditional activities of each member of the surgical team and in the way team members interact with each other. The change occurs because the direct visualization of the heart in the conventional open method is replaced with remote monitoring via pressure traces and transesophageal echocardiogram images displayed on various screens in the operating room. The result has been that the new technology—a good example of an interactive innovation—has been difficult for many teams to learn to use, which has slowed its adoption.

The learning rates of the teams in our study varied significantly (a finding that was not predicted by the volume-outcome hypothesis) as did their success in adopting the new technology. Even more intriguing were the factors associated with rapid learning and successful adoption. Type of institution (academic or community) and seniority of the adopting surgeon were not particularly important factors. What mattered was whether the process of adoption of the new technology was managed as a "project." This meant careful selection of the team members and adequate preparations, such as practice sessions before the first case, the selection of simple cases to operate on early, and debriefings after every early case to reflect on what went well and what did not. For successful adoption, these learning activities took place in an environment conducive to team-based learning—a "psychologically safe" environment. Learning as a team is made easier if team members can fail publicly—make an error or be criticized or warned of an impending error by another team member—and not be disadvantaged.

In short, team learning cannot be left to chance. As the example illustrates, although experience is clearly necessary for learning, experience alone is not enough. Learning takes place at both the individual level and the team level, but unlike individuals, teams do not learn naturally. Team learning requires an environment that is deliberately structured and managed to be conducive to learning. The role of team leader and project manager was new to the surgeons in our study. In the context of new technology adoption, they had to be not only clinical decision makers and practitioners but also team leaders and project managers.

We are becoming increasingly aware of the importance of organization in care delivery. Solo practice is giving way to group practice, and care that was once delivered by an individual is now delivered by a team. In addition, the size and complexity of the health care team has increased dramatically in the last century. Many current innovations in health care (e.g., new services, processes, and technologies) are interactive and thus have the potential to disrupt routines and processes. The successful introduction of these innovations into day-to-day care will require that team members learn to work together in new ways. And as we have seen, team learning depends on leadership more than anything else—a very different role for the rank and file physician.

Engineers have already undergone the change from solo professionals practicing their craft to members and leaders of teams of professionals who collaborate to realize difficult goals. An engineer used to be a technologist who functioned in a tightly defined engineering specialty; now engineers are project managers who use their knowledge base to manage multidisciplinary teams to complete complex projects. Health care practitioners are just beginning to undergo a similar transition. So, we can learn a great deal from engineers, not just about modeling—the subject of many of these presentations—but also about leadership and about restructuring the role of professionals.

REFERENCE

Edmondson, A.C., R.M.J. Bohmer, and G.P. Pisano. 2001. Speeding up team learning. Harvard Business Review 79(9): 125–132.

Designing Caregiver- and Patient-Centered Health Care Systems

H. Kent Bowen
Harvard Business School

The engineering discipline, with its proclivity for seeing the world as it really is and then designing systems to make things better, offers a good perspective for addressing the dilemma facing our health care systems. Like many people, I was not aware of the chaos on the front lines of the health care system until my 14-year-old son suddenly became gravely ill. Because of a brain aneurysm, he went from an active, vibrant young man to a paralyzed boy within minutes. My wife and I essentially lived at Massachusetts General Hospital for three weeks while a team of "the best of the best" worked to save his life. During that time, I observed how the actual practice of medicine affects patients, and it became clear to me that the system was not designed to prevent errors and defects. At one point, because important information was not communicated, a grievous mistake (not directly related to the aneurysm) nearly cost my son his leg. Even though the medical team corrected the error, after I caught it, I wondered how such a mistake could have occurred in the first place. After much thought, I came to the conclusion that the nurses, physicians, and technicians were not at fault. Our *ad hoc* system for delivering health care conspires against the best intentions of care providers, making it extremely difficult for them to provide patient-centered, defect-free care.

Many industries have revolutionized their approaches to deliver products and services that are more customer centered, high quality, and cost effective. The automotive industry, for example, has made dramatic improvements to avoid both design and production failures. Toyota, in particular, has an operating system that delivers award-winning quality year after year. Toyota's system is designed to bring problems to light, resolve them, and improve the system to ensure that the problems are not repeated and that the organization learns. Toyota's approach helps frontline workers (as well as all others) be successful, as defined by the customer's (or patient's) needs. The goal is "defect-free operations" and learning (Spear and Bowen, 1999).

Based on examples from industry, a young colleague of mine, Professor Steven Spear, developed a case study to determine the applicability of systems-thinking to health care. He engaged a former medical administrator and surgeon, Dr. John Kenagy, to work with leaders of a small community hospital in the Boston area. Like most people in the medical profession, the dedicated hospital staff wanted to provide the best care. He initially focused on a system for the administration of medications using the Toyota production system (TPS) as a model for defect-free operations. First, he taught Dr. Kenagy to look at the hospital through the TPS lens. Early on, he discovered that not only does the medical staff itself not fully understand its system for providing care, but also that the staff was not equipped with the tools, processes, or organizational structure to solve problems (Spear, 2001; Spear and Kenagy, 2000a,b).

Anita Tucker, a doctoral student at the time (now an assistant professor at the Wharton School, University of Pennsylvania), expanded the initial findings with studies of nursing care in 20 additional hospitals. Her studies revealed that nurses' care of patients was constantly interrupted because of system failures (Tucker, 2003). Nurses are trained to evaluate and diagnose patients and administer a care plan based on a physician's recommendation. Over the course of a shift, however, nurses spent only 33 to 50 percent of their time caring for patients. The rest of the time, they were searching for information, equipment, or materials or correcting mistakes. Thus, they spent most of their time compensating for the faulty system, becoming frustrated and cynical of management's work design and rules.

The current design of most hospital work systems is disrespectful to both patients and frontline caregivers, as evidenced by the high turnover of nurses and the complaints of patients. Think about the service you receive at the best commercial establishments and compare that with the service you receive when you are admitted to a hospital. One reason for the difference is the constant and conflicting demands on hospital service personnel and caregivers. For example, a typical nurse, in a single hour, works in eight different physical locations, makes 22 location changes among those eight places, has conversations with 15 partners on 25 different topics, while taking care of five patients in three rooms (Spear and Kenagy, 2000a). If one of the patients requires critical care, which means following strict care guidelines, it is nearly impossible for the nurse to follow the care plan. The critical-care routines are constantly interrupted because of wrong medications, faulty equipment, poor information, or requests to assist colleagues.

Observations of the flow of information necessary to patient care revealed other problems. Information that originates at the patient (e.g., the patient's insurance provider, family history, medications, medical history, symptoms, etc.) flows along many pathways to physicians, nurses, and pharmacies. In spite of large investments in information technology, getting the correct information to the people who need it when they need it is very problematic. Any of the pathways over which critical information flows can be blocked, and there is a high probability that this will happen on a daily basis. If the medication-administration pathway breaks down, for example, the medication will not be administered in the right dose at the right time under the right conditions. The medication error rate has been shown to be in the parts-per-hundred range (Bates et al., 1995). The most frequent failures occur between shifts.

Most hospitals do not have defect-free standards for exchanges of information. Anita Tucker identified the best hospitals from her pool of 20 for more detailed analysis of this problem. Her study showed that even at facilities renowned for the high quality of their nursing care, the work of a frontline caregiver is filled with interruptions and poor information flow. When she asked why health care workers "live this way," she concluded that most of them actually expect the work system to be defective. Because problems often cross organizational boundaries or are so complex a single person cannot hope to eliminate the root cause, they expect to have to "work around" problems (Tucker et al., 2002).

In hospital after hospital, because no resources have been allocated for solving problems, health care workers confront the same problems every day. At this point, the health care system is incapable of fixing itself. This is a significant contrast to a Toyota factory where improvements are made continuously in the course of accomplishing daily work, crossing organizational boundaries if necessary, sending problems to the appropriate management level (Spear and Schmidhofer, 2005).

We did find some medical facilities that have designed systems to reduce defects, improve the work systems of frontline caregivers, and improve the patient experience. For example, we studied an eye surgery clinic in Boston with 18 top ophthalmic surgeons (Miguel and Bowen, 1997). One of the surgeons, Dr. Barry Shingleton, was three times as productive as other surgeons in terms of time spent performing similar surgeries. When Dr. Shingleton was designing his diagnostic and surgical procedures, he had turned to the business literature for guidance. His service model is centered on the patient experience, from the first encounter through post-surgical follow-ups. In addition, he collects outcomes data much more rigorously than his colleagues as feedback for improving procedures and processes. He developed his own patient scheduling algorithm to improve service and efficiency, and he schedules simpler procedures earlier in the day to minimize disruptions and delays. He also eliminated unnecessary variabilities during surgery by standardizing procedures. For example, to reduce changeover time between surgeries, he maintains contact with the anesthesiologist prepping the next patient; in this way, he has been able to reduce the time between the administration of the drug and the beginning of surgery by as much as 50 percent. More important, as a result of his efficiency, his patients experience less surgical trauma, which speeds the healing process.

In a more recent study, we looked at Intermountain Health Care, where doctors, under the leadership of Dr. Brent James, have applied the entire quality-management concept to the hospital's functions (Bohmer et al., 2002). The study was focused on two intensive care units (ICUs) located next to each other in LDS Hospital in Salt Lake City (Tucker et al., in progress). We found that, even though the hospital had developed an overarching quality system, frontline care was administered differently in the two units. In addition to some structural differences, the medical directors of each ICU had different design models for operating their units. In one ICU, problem solving was more prevalent, especially root-cause elimination (much like Toyota's TPS). This ICU also stressed patient-centered care: the number of admitting physicians was small; interns spent more time on the rotation; a nurse manager was available to assist in problem solving and problem prevention; and the unit developed and used more medical protocols. In the second ICU, the quality of care was also very high, but operations were more physician centered: because there was a different set of patients, there were more admitting physicians; by design, interns spent less time on this rotation; no nurse manager was available for problem solving; the unit had fewer protocols and did not generate any of its own. To further learning at LDS, the two ICU medical directors have now exchanged positions, which should provide a wonderful natural test of how much the differences relate to design choices and how much they relate to differences in the patient mix, structure, etc.

A recent study at the Pittsburgh Regional Health Initiative demonstrates what can be achieved with a systematic approach to redesigning work systems. In one study, the goal was to eliminate central-line-associated bloodstream infections using techniques like those practiced at Toyota. By implementing simple but elegant tools and devices, transmissions of infection were reduced dramatically. In 2003, Allegheny General Hospital's MICU and CCC (Cardiac Critical Care) Units had 37 patients who suffered central-line-associated bloodstream infections, 19 of whom died. In 2004, there were six infected patients, one of whom died (Shannon et al., in progress).

Solutions to the health care problem are being offered from many directions. Our own suggestions are based on the perspectives of the patient and frontline caregiver. We can summarize what we learned through direct observation of how frontline caregivers do their work:

- Most hospitals have evolved complex work systems that conspire against defect-free health care.
- Caregivers have come up with "work arounds" and other ineffective approaches to solving problems. Frontline workers spend a significant fraction of their time doing nonvalue-added work caused by fundamental failures in the design of work systems.
- The delivery of patient-centered care by nurses and other frontline caregivers is limited under current work systems designs.
- Systems approaches perfected by industrial corporations (e.g., Toyota's TPS) appear to provide useful models for improving health care work systems.

The challenge for engineers and managers outside the health care system is to bring the lessons learned in other settings to clinics and hospitals.

REFERENCES

Bates, D.W., D.L. Boyle, M.B. Vander Vliet, J. Schneider, and L. Leape. 1995. Relationship between medication errors and adverse drug events. Journal of General Internal Medicine 10(4): 199–205.

Bohmer, R., A.C. Edmondson, and L.R. Feldman. 2002. Intermountain Health Care. HBS Case No. 603-066. Cambridge, Mass.: Harvard Business School Publishing.

Miguel, M.F., and H.K. Bowen. 1997. Ophthalmic Consultants of Boston and Dr. Bradford J. Shingleton. HBS Case No. 697-080. Cambridge, Mass.: Harvard Business School Publishing.

Shannon, R.P., et al. In progress. Eliminating Central Line Infections in Two Intensive Care Units: Results of Real-time Investigation of Individual Problems. Harvard Business School Working Paper. Cambridge, Mass.: Harvard Business School Publishing.

Spear, S. 2001. Deaconess-Glover Hospital (C). HBS Case No. 602-028. Cambridge, Mass.: Harvard Business School Publishing.

Spear, S.J., and H.K. Bowen. 1999. Decoding the DNA of the Toyota Production System. HBS Case No. 99509. Harvard Business Review (September-October): 96–106.

Spear, S., and J. Kenagy. 2000a. Deaconess-Glover Hospital (A). HBS Case No. 601-022. Cambridge, Mass.: Harvard Business School Publishing.

Spear, S., and J. Kenagy. 2000b. Deaconess-Glover Hospital (B). HBS Case No. 601-023. Cambridge, Mass.: Harvard Business School Publishing.

Spear, S.J., and M. Schmidhofer. 2005. Ambiguity and workarounds as contributors to medical error. Annals of Internal Medicine 142(8): 627–630.

Tucker, A.L. 2003. Organizational Learning from Operational Failures. Unpublished dissertation, Harvard University, Cambridge, Massachusetts.

Tucker, A., H.K. Bowen, and B.C. LaPierre. In progress. Quality Improvement in Intensive Care at LDS Hospital. HBS Case No. 604-071. Cambridge, Mass.: Harvard Business School Publishing.

Tucker, A.L., A.C. Edmondson, and S.J. Spear. 2002. When problem solving prevents organizational learning. Journal of Organizational Change Management 15(2): 122–137.

Engineering Tools
and Procedures
for Meeting the Challenges

Systems Engineering: Opportunities for Health Care

Jennifer K. Ryan
Purdue University

Systems engineering involves the design, implementation, and control of interacting components or subsystems. A system consists of interacting, interrelated, or interdependent elements that form a complex whole, a set of interacting objects or people that behaves in ways individuals acting alone would not. The overall goal of systems engineering is to produce a system that meets the needs of all users or participants within the constraints that govern the system's operation. The objectives can generally be divided into two broad categories: service and cost. Service can be measured by a variety of criteria, such as availability, reliability, quality, and so on. Cost is usually measured by how much costs can be reduced or at least controlled.

A final objective of systems engineering is to gain a better understanding of system behavior and the problems associated with it. Models enable us to study the impact of alternative ways of running the system—alternative designs or controls and different configurations and management approaches. In short, systems engineering models enable us to experiment with systems in ways we cannot experiment with real systems.

Systems engineers generally prefer to work with analytical or mathematical models rather than with conceptual models because they are generally better defined, have more clearly defined assumptions, and are easier to communicate, manipulate, and analyze. We begin with a graphical representation of the system, which often includes a diagram showing the flow of information and resources. We then create a mathematical description that includes objectives, interrelationships, and constraints. The components of the mathematical model can be divided into four categories: (1) decision variables, which represent our options; (2) parameters or givens, which are the inputs to the decision-making process; (3) the objective function, which is the goal, the function to be optimized; and (4) the constraints, which are the rules that govern operation of the system.

When dealing with large complex systems, we often deconstruct it into smaller subsystems that interact with one another to create a whole. The decision-making structure provides natural breaks in the system. We model and analyze the subsystems and then connect them in a way that recaptures the most important interdependencies between them.

Systems engineering requires a variety of quantitative and qualitative tools for analyzing and interpreting system models. We use tools from psychology, computer science, operations research, management and economics, and mathematics. The quantitative tools include optimization methods, control theory, stochastic modeling and simulation, statistics, utility theory, decision analysis, and economics. Mathematical techniques have the capability of solving large-scale, complex problems optimally using computerized algorithms.

Mathematical models clarify the overall structure of a system and reveal important relationships. They enable us to analyze the system even when data are sparse. Models, combined with analyses, reveal the most critical parameters and enable us to analyze the system as a whole. Sensitivity analysis involves testing out trade-offs. Before we can convert a model solution to an implementable solution, we must test and validate the model to ensure that it actually predicts the behavior of the system.

A logistics system can be defined as a network of suppliers, manufacturing centers, warehouses, distribution centers, retail outlets, and end consumers. The system includes raw materials, work in process, inventory, finished products, all of the materials in the system, all of the information that flows within the system, and all of the resources in the system (e.g., people, equipment, etc.). Logistics-systems engineering can be defined as the planning, implementation, and control of the system to ensure the efficient, cost-effective flow and storage of all materials and information from point of origin to point of consumption for the purpose of meeting customer requirements. Our goal is to ensure that the right amount of materials or resources is in the right place at the right time at minimum cost.

We deliberately leave the definition of service (i.e., meeting customer requirements) somewhat vague so we can define the needs and requirements of different customers in different ways. Logistics-systems engineering involves the difficult problem of simultaneously improving customer service and quality, improving timeliness, reducing operating expenses, and, if possible, minimizing capital investment. We are also interested in answering strategic questions, such as where we can expand capacity or what types of collaboration with customers or suppliers would be most beneficial.

Systems engineering problems have some common characteristics. They tend to be interdisciplinary, involving both technical and nontechnical fields. They require multiple, high-level, or strategic metrics or performance measures, often measurements of nonquantitative factors (e.g., customer satisfaction). They involve many participants with different value systems and many decision makers; therefore, we have to find optimal solutions that meet conflicting criteria. The systems and issues tend to be hierarchical and complex, but the systems also evolve and change over time; they generally involve significant uncertainties. Much of the current research in logistics is driven by the needs of public and private organizations, such as health care systems, that operate in environments characterized by intense competition, constant change, and a strong focus on customer needs.

Health care delivery systems, for example, consist of a variety of health care organizations, caregivers, and patients. State and federal governments are involved, as well as a variety of other organizations. These complex systems also involve a large number of interconnections between the components and the system—multihospital systems and provider networks with linkages between hospitals, physician groups, insurers, and others. There are also many decision makers who often have conflicting criteria, and there are complex interactions between participants. The effective organization and management of a health care delivery system requires careful management of resources to ensure that the necessary staff and equipment are in the right place at the right time. The problem is complicated by uncertainties and system complexity.

Some aspects of the health care delivery system, such as government intervention, the level of uncertainty, and the nature of the demand, appear to be unique to health care. But similar problems can be found in other industries, such as the telecommunications and electricity industries, which also have to factor in government intervention. The nature of the uncertainties may be different, but they have similar effects on the system. Both the telecommunications and electricity industries have used logistics models to their advantage.

Systems engineering models can provide structured, quantitative methods of studying alternative control policies and system designs for almost any industry. The methods can be used to help coordinate information systems, operations, and capital investment; develop control policies; predict and evaluate outcomes; and evaluate the benefits and costs of a given program or system design.

The elements included in the model depend on the question or problem to be solved. For the output of the model to be useful, it must mimic the expected behavior of the real system. To control the behavior of one part of the system, the incentives driving that aspect of the system must be built into the model.

A good deal of literature is now available on research in this area. Operations research tools and systems engineering tools have been used to address a wide variety of problems, from the operation of a hospital to higher levels of complexity, such as incentives, efficiency, and payment schemes. Quantitative models can provide important input for making decisions that involve complex societal, ethical, and economic issues.

Supply-Chain Management and Health Care Delivery: Pursuing a System-Level Understanding

Reha Uzsoy
Purdue University

In recent years, effective supply-chain management has emerged as a significant competitive advantage for companies in very different industries (e.g., Chopra and Meindl, 2000). Several leading companies, such as WalMart and Dell Computer, are differentiated from their rivals more by the way they manage their supply chains than by the particular products or services they provide. A supply chain can be defined as the physical and informational resources required to deliver a good or service to the final consumer. In the broadest sense, a supply chain includes all activities related to manufacturing, the extraction of raw materials, processing, storing and warehousing, and transportation. Hence, for large multinational companies that manufacture complex products, such as automobiles, machines, or personal computers, supply chains are highly complex socioeconomic systems.

The ability of successful firms to make the effective management of supply chains a source of competitive advantage suggests that there may be useful knowledge that can provide a point of departure for the development of a similar level of understanding of certain aspects of health care delivery systems. Similar to the supply chains in manufacturing and other industries, the health care delivery system is so large and complex that it has become impossible for any individual, or even any single organization, to understand all of the details of its operations. Like industrial supply chains, the health care "supply chain" consists of multiple independent agents, such as insurance companies, hospitals, doctors, employers, and regulatory agencies, whose economic structures, and hence objectives, differ and in many cases conflict with each other. Both supply and demand for services are uncertain in different ways, making it very difficult to match supply to demand. This task is complicated because demand for services is determined by both available technology (i.e., available treatments) and financial considerations, such as whether or not certain treatments are covered by insurance. Decisions made by one party often affect

the options available to other parties, as well as the costs of these options, in ways that are not well understood. However, almost all of these complicating factors are also present, to one degree or another, in industrial supply chains; the progress made in understanding these systems in the last several decades is a cause for hope that some insights and modeling tools developed in the industrial domain can be applied to at least some aspects of health care delivery systems.

In general, a centralized approach to controlling the entire system is clearly out of the question, although centralized decision models may be useful for coordinating the operations of segments of the larger system controlled by a single decision-making body. Designing decentralized models of operation that render the operation of the overall system as effective as possible is the main challenge for both health care delivery and industrial supply chains.

In the following section, I shall briefly discuss how the study of industrial systems has evolved from individual unit processes to considerations of complex interactions among many different components of an industrial supply chain. I shall then describe some examples of modeling approaches that have been applied to supply chains and close with some comments on how these tools might be adapted for the health care delivery environment.

FROM UNIT PROCESSES TO SUPPLY CHAINS

If we examine how industrial operations, particularly manufacturing operations, have evolved since the beginning of the nineteenth century, we can see that many efforts were motivated by a desire to understand and optimize individual unit processes (see, for example, Chandler, 1980). These efforts led to many innovations, among them the development of improved machine tools and fixtures, a significantly better understanding of the chemistry of processes (e.g., steelmaking), and through the work of the early industrial engineers, such as Frederick Taylor and Frank and Lillian Gilbreth, the optimization of interactions between workers and their environment.

As the understanding of unit processes developed, engineers began to consider larger and larger groupings of unit processes, trying to understand interactions between them and optimize the performance of entire systems, sometimes to the detriment of individual components. Hence, from considering individual unit processes, we progressed to considering departments of factories that perform similar operations, entire manufacturing processes from raw materials to finished products, and eventually, the operations of entire firms, as well as their suppliers and customers. It has often been observed that most significant new opportunities, both for cost reduction and the generation of new products and services, have been based on an understanding of interactions between different subsystems, or different agents, operating in the supply chain.

Among today's leading companies, examples abound. Many automotive companies, for instance, have developed joint ventures with transportation firms; the objective is to optimize the interface between the production and distribution functions and facilitate the just-in-time operation of automakers' final assembly plants. Software companies that provide supply-chain planning software for multilocation companies is another strong indicator of the advantages companies perceive will accrue to them by the effective management of the various elements of their supply chains. The strong trend in industry to outsource noncritical functions has increased the need for companies to effectively manage and clearly understand their relationships with other companies. As a final example, we can point to the collaborative forecasting, planning, and replenishment initiative in the retail sector; retailers work closely with major suppliers to develop demand forecasts for products through information-sharing and joint planning processes.

Clearly, the basic process of improving a system by a detailed understanding of the most fundamental unit processes, in other words the "atomic" elements of the system, and steadily extending that knowledge to interactions among larger and larger groupings of these elements is directly applicable to health care delivery systems. The individual unit processes in this case include the processing of a patient in an emergency room, the process by which a medical insurance claim is approved, and the scheduling of hospital operating rooms to optimize their performance. The need for a better understanding of how the operations of individual elements affect each other is apparent; these interactions can be quite complex because of long time lags between cause and effect. For example, the decision by a regulatory agency to disallow a certain kind of preventive procedure for infants may result in the emergence of an unexpectedly large number of children with special needs in the elementary school system several years later. The same kinds of problems are present to some degree in industrial supply chains, and a significant body of knowledge has been developed over the years to address them.

Based on the history of industrial enterprises, we know that the development of today's enterprises required substantial organizational innovations, such as capital budgeting to allocate scarce capital between competing activities, cost accounting to develop an understanding of factors contributing to product costs, and the development of multidivisional corporations with complex structures of management incentives and coordination mechanisms. An important development in recent years has been the recognition of the need for a cross-functional view of supply-chain operations. All aspects of a firm's operation, from the design of a product to the specific timing of marketing promotions, have a direct effect on the operation of the supply chain. Therefore, different functional specialties must actively collaborate to develop solutions to optimize the performance of the overall system. Similarly, in health care delivery a number of different constituencies, such as doctors, government agencies, insurance providers, and patient groups, are all involved in the operation of the health care delivery supply chain.

KNOWLEDGE OF SUPPLY-CHAIN MANAGEMENT

In the domain of industrial supply chains, it is probably safe to say that we have developed a fairly good understanding of the operation and economics of individual unit processes, including functions such as transportation, distribution, warehousing, and information processing. In particular, we have developed a substantial understanding of the often complex dynamics of capacity-constrained systems subject to variability in both demand and process (Hopp and Spearman, 2000). However, in general we are only beginning to learn how to integrate the solutions to these individual elements to reach a reasonable understanding of the operation of the overall supply chain.

Integrated planning models based on linear and integer programming have been applied to the segments of the supply chain controlled by a single company for at least four decades (e.g., Johnson and Montgomery, 1974). Although these models have been successful in many instances, they have not been effective in addressing the needs of a supply chain that involves many different companies with potentially conflicting objectives. In recent years, considerable efforts have been made to use some of the tools of economics, such as contracts, as a mechanism for coordinating the operation of complex supply chains (Tayur et al., 1998). However, these models are generally subject to long-run, steady-state assumptions that can be carefully evaluated relative to market conditions.

Conventional Monte Carlo simulation techniques (Law and Kelton, 1991) have proven extremely effective for systems in which the operational dynamics can be described at a high level of detail, such as segments of manufacturing processes or hospital operations. The difficulty with these models is that for large-scale systems the level of detail required to unequivocally model system behavior accurately becomes prohibitive in terms of both data collection and computation time. Systems dynamics models used to model large systems work by establishing input-output relationships for their components and simulating their operation through time using techniques based on the techniques used for the numerical solution of differential equations (Sterman, 2000). Although these techniques are capable of modeling large, complex systems, they usually do so by specifying aggregate input-output relationships for large subsystems, which must be validated and whose parameters must be estimated carefully. Nevertheless, these models can capture many critical aspects of supply-chain behavior, such as the "bullwhip effect," in which variability in orders is amplified as it passes down the supply chain from the consumer towards the producers of raw materials (Forrester, 1962).

RESEARCH NEEDS AND FUTURE DIRECTIONS

At the risk of overgeneralizing, it appears that most of the tools required for analysis of the individual unit processes in health care delivery, such as efficiency of hospital facilities, have been developed in the engineering literature and have, in fact, been applied intermittently to a variety of systems over the last several decades (e.g., Pierskalla and Brailer, 1994). However, if our experience with industrial supply chains is any guide, only limited improvements in health care delivery can be obtained by these means. Repeated experience has shown that far greater improvements can be obtained by a thorough understanding of the interactions between different elements of the system and restructuring them in a way that leaves all parties better off. This brings the modeling issues squarely into the region where current supply-chain research is weakest (the effective coordination of socioeconomic systems consisting of multiple, independent agents); but this is also the area that is developing most rapidly. The development of novel models at the intersection of conventional engineering and economics promises to provide a wide range of challenging research problems for many years to come.

To support this agenda, the most pressing research need is for techniques that can be used to model systems at the aggregate level, where one can accept some level of approximation to obtain computationally tractable models that achieve the correct qualitative behavior and provide useful insights into interactions between systems. This means that the aggregate models must capture the often nonlinear relationships between critical variables correctly, which has not always been the case in supply-chain modeling. The literature on systems dynamics may be a good starting point for this initiative, but it must be complemented by a variety of other techniques, such as economic models of competition and collaboration and agent-based techniques for modeling complex systems.

It is important to bear in mind that the purpose of these models is far more likely to be descriptive than prescriptive, that is, models are far more likely to be used, and arguably far more useful, to inform debate between the various parties involved in health care delivery than to deliver decisions to be executed. Hence, the development of large-scale computational simulations of different scenarios with different actors and interaction protocols between the actors appears to offer interesting research challenges. These tools would be extremely beneficial to decision makers in health care delivery.

REFERENCES

Chandler, A.D. 1980. The Visible Hand: The Managerial Revolution in American Business. Cambridge, Mass.: Belknap Press.

Chopra, S., and P. Meindl. 2000. Supply Chain Management: Strategy, Planning and Operations. Englewood Cliffs, N.J.: Prentice-Hall.

Forrester, J.W. 1962. Industrial Dynamics. Cambridge, Mass.: MIT Press.

Hopp, W., and M.L. Spearman. 2000. Factory Physics. 2nd Edition. New York: McGraw-Hill/Irwin.

Johnson, L.A., and D.C. Montgomery. 1974. Operations Research in Production Planning, Scheduling and Inventory Control. New York: John Wiley & Sons.

Law, A., and W.D. Kelton. 1991. Simulation Modeling and Analysis, 2nd edition. New York: McGraw-Hill.

Pierskalla, W.P., and D.J. Brailer. 1994. Applications of Operations Research in Health Care Delivery. Vol. 6, pp. 469–505 in Handbooks in OR & MS, S.M. Pollock, M.H. Rothkopf, and A. Barnett, eds. Amsterdam, The Netherlands: Elsevier Science.

Sterman, J.D. 2000. Business Dynamics: Systems Thinking and Modeling for a Complex World. New York: McGraw-Hill.

Tayur, S., M. Magazine, and R. Ganesham, eds. 1998. Quantitative Models for Supply Chain Management. Amsterdam, The Netherlands: Kluwer Academic Publishers.

The Human Factor in Health Care Systems Design

Kim J. Vicente
University of Toronto

The simplest way to think about the discipline of engineering is that engineers design things that are useful to society and satisfy important needs based on what we know about the physical world. When a bridge fails, we do not usually blame the bridge. We look to its design, trying to find a mismatch between what we know about the physical world and the outcome.

We should apply this same logic to people. But when a system is poorly designed, we often blame the person using it rather than the flaws in the system. For example, when we design a mechanical lathe, we must place the mechanical controls in a way that respects what we know about human bodies. But sometimes, if a lathe is poorly designed, we blame the user rather than the design.

Although we know a great deal about teamwork and about human behavior at the organizational and political levels, that knowledge is not always taken into account by designers of health care systems and devices. Clearly, improvements could be made, and not just in terms of safety. The lack of respect for human nature in the design of health care systems causes injuries and deaths, but it also costs money.

Contrast that to the field of aviation. Despite September 11, 2001 was not a bad year for aviation safety. The average number of deadly crashes for the previous decade was 48 per year. In 2001, however, there were only 34 deadly crashes—worldwide, not just in the United States. That's the lowest number since 1946 when there were far fewer flights.

One reason for the improvement is that aviation engineers pay attention to the human factor. A familiar example is the rather high rate of crashes in a certain type of aircraft that occurred because pilots tended to raise the landing gear as the plane was landing, causing the airplane to scrape along the runway. When Al Chapanis, an aviation engineer, studied the problem, he found that the controls for the landing gear and the wing flaps were right next to each other and that they looked and felt identical. He realized that pilots could easily grab the wrong control, but he also realized that he could not redesign the whole cockpit. He came up with an idea, now called shape coding. He did not move the controls, but he altered the feel of the landing gear control. The controls are still right next to each other, but the change eliminated the errors. It was as simple as that.

Can we apply the same type of thinking to health care systems? Patient-controlled analgesic devices, which allow patients to self-administer analgesics (usually morphine), are a case in point. A number of parameters are programmed into these devices by the nurse, the most important being drug concentration. These devices rely strictly on the programming and cannot independently verify either the concentration or even the type of analgesic in the syringe. Therefore, errors in programming can mean underdoses or overdoses; and errors have enduring effects, that is, the problem lasts until the programming is corrected.

For the particular device that we studied, programming errors were associated with five to eight *reported* patient deaths. Adverse drug events and adverse events in general in medicine are severely underreported—roughly only 1.2 to 7.7 percent are reported (Vicente et al., 2003). In other words, adverse events may be 13 to 83 times higher than the reported rate. We calculated that programming errors had lethal results for this particular device at least 65 times, and perhaps as many as 667 times, over a 12-year period. To put these numbers in context, the manufacturer reports that the device was used safely over 22 million times.

We then examined the existing design using traditional human-factor principles to see if there was room for improvement. We also talked to nurses, the users of this device. One serious problem we found was that the layout of the buttons on the interface was confusing and counterintuitive. So we came up with a new design by resegmenting the buttons and changing some of the labels. The new design offered the same functionality but changed the mode of interaction between the programmer and the pump. The system now provided more feedback and gave the user an overview of the programming sequence. The redesigned device told the programmer the drug concentration, what was coming up next, how to program the mode, and then showed the settings. In essence, the new programming sequence was much less convoluted.

We tested the redesigned interface in a laboratory setting with professional nurses who had more than five years of experience programming the commercial device. With the commercially available design, there were eight programming errors for drug concentration, three of which were undetected. With the new interface, there were no errors in drug concentration. They were eliminated.

Given the epidemiological data, the change was obviously important for safety reasons. But it was also important in terms of cultural attitudes. If the problem had originated with the person programming the device, then changing the interface should have made no difference in the error rate. In fact, changing the design did eliminate the errors. Therefore, we concluded that the problem was not with the people, or, at least, not only with people.

Surprisingly, we had a great deal of difficulty getting this research published. One journal refused it because the editor took for granted that what we had scientifically demonstrated was not true. We went through some pretty hard times, both in terms of getting the work published and dealing with the response from the public. One reviewer even suggested that a lawyer look at the research because of potential legal action by the manufacturer. We had chosen the particular device because it was relatively new, but soon after our research was completed, the media began to report some deaths as a result of errors in programming the device.

This example shows three important points. First, we know how to design technology that works for people because we know a lot about people at many levels—physical, psychological, team, organizational, and political. We do not always make the most of this knowledge when we design health care devices, but lack of understanding is not the problem. Second, not making the most of that knowledge results in a tremendous loss to society. Tens of thousands, perhaps even hundreds of thousands, of people are injured or die every year unnecessarily. Finally—the most difficult lesson— change is important and necessary, but there is a great deal of resistance that must be overcome before we can make progress.

REFERENCE

Vicente, K.J., K. Kada-Bekhaled, G. Hillel, A. Cassano, and B.A. Orser. 2003. Programming errors contribute to death from patient-controlled analgesia: case report and estimate of probability. Canadian Journal of Anesthesia 50(4): 328–332.

Changing Health Care Delivery Enterprises

Seth Bonder
The Bonder Group

The health care delivery (HCD) system in the United States is in crisis. Access is limited, costs are high and increasing at an unacceptable rate, and concerns are growing about the quality of service. Many, including the Institute of Medicine, believe the system should be changed significantly in two ways: (1) HCD enterprises should be reengineered to make them more productive, efficient, and effective; and (2) substantially more effort should be devoted to a strategy of prevention and management of chronic diseases instead of the current heavy reliance on the treatment of diseases. Although operations research can make substantial contributions to both areas, the focus of this paper is on: (1) reengineering HCD enterprises, particularly areas in which operations research can provide valuable support to senior health care managers; and (2) enterprise-level HCD simulation models to determine the reengi-neering initiatives with the biggest payoffs *before implementation.*

HCD enterprises are very large, complex operational systems comprised of large numbers of people and machine elements. Tens of thousands of people are involved as providers, patients, support staff, and managers organized into specialties, departments, laboratories, and other organizations that are considered independent service units ("stovepipes"). Machines include durable medical equipment, information technologies, communications equipment, expendable supplies, rehabilitation equipment, and so on. These elements are affected by many clinical and administrative processes (e.g., arrivals, testing, diagnosis, treatment, scheduling, purchasing, billing, recruiting , etc.), most of which are probabilistic (i.e., uncertain) and change significantly over time.

Perhaps most important, these processes involve large numbers of *interactions* within units, among units, and across processes. Decisions by enterprise managers regarding one unit may have second, third, and fourth order effects, which may be more significant than the first order effect. HCD enterprises are driven by endogenous and exogenous human decisions made by providers, patients, insurers, administrators, politicians, government employees, and others. Demand and supply issues have complex feedback effects. A great many resources are required for the development and operation of an HCD enterprise. For example, the University of Michigan's budget for its HCD enterprise is more than $1 billion; the Henry Ford Health System's budget is $2.5 billion, and these are relatively small HCD enterprises. Billions of dollars have been spent on cost containment initiatives over the past 15 years by the Agency for Healthcare Research and Quality (formerly the Agency for Health Care Policy and Research), the U.S. Department of Defense, the Veterans Administration, National Institutes of Health, foundations, universities, and others to reengineer the HCD system. Nevertheless, costs continue to rise at double-digit rates.

We need better ways of analyzing systems of this magnitude. The operations research community has been involved with HCD enterprises for more than 40 years working on a wide range of problems, such as inventory for perishables; management of intensive care units; laboratory and radiology scheduling; relieving congestion in outpatient clinics; nurse staffing, scheduling, and assignments; and layouts for operating and emergency rooms. These efforts have focused on the small, stovepipe units, referred to by Don Berwick as clinical and support "microsystems," and have produced some useful information for unit managers but have not addressed enterprise-level reengineering and planning issues (the so-called "macrosystem"). Macrosystem issues have interactive effects across the enterprise and have large cost, access, and effectiveness impacts. Some of these interrelated issues are listed below:

- the mix of health *services* necessary to support a given population
- the *staff* required (e.g., specialties, numbers, locations) to provide necessary services
- the impacts of changing demands (e.g., aging populations, effects of preventive measures)

- the impacts of new HCD models (e.g., home health care, task performance substitution)
- the effects of centralized radiology services
- the impacts of primary care outreach
- facility capacity for the next 20 years and the best way to provide it
- operational changes to adapt to regulatory changes (e.g., Medicare)

These and other macrosystem issues can be addressed quantitatively using enterprise-level simulation models that represent all of the elements, units, and processes in the enterprise *as well as the interactions among them.* Because analyses of these issues are necessarily prospective, the models must be *structural* rather than *statistical.* Statistical models, which are usually used in economics and the social sciences, use existing system data to develop aggregated statistical relationships between system inputs and outputs (i.e., the model). Statistical models are used primarily retrospectively, that is, for making *inferences* and *evaluations.* In contrast, structural models are usually developed in the engineering and physical sciences by modeling the detailed physics of each process and activity. Structural models are used prospectively, that is, for *predictions* and *planning.* Statistical models are less appropriate to prospective analyses of future systems because the data used to develop statistical models are intrinsically tied to the existing system.

Figure 1 provides an overview of a particular enterprise-level HCD simulation model. The figure shows the elements in the Healthcare Complex Model (HCM), which was developed seven years ago and has been continually updated in a prototyping process by Vector Research Incorporated (now the Altarum Institute). HCM simulates individual patient episodes in a network of facilities for a population of patients. The network of facilities, with its entities and processes, is referred to as a "complex" (synonymous with an

enterprise). Complexes usually have one or two major medical centers (where much of the tertiary care is provided), five to ten hospitals, and many clinics. The model can be adapted to represent specific features of any HCD enterprise.

Inputs to the model include demographics of the population that receives care. A model preprocessor converts the demographics into a stream of patients entering the complex; each patient's condition is described by an International Classification of Diseases, ninth edition (ICD-9) code. Patients can enter the enterprise at a clinic, a hospital, or a medical center. They can be referred physically or via telemedicine consults from clinics to hospitals or to a medical center. Providers of various types are located at each facility in the complex. The *care protocols* represent practice guidelines and patient pathways, define what service patients receive next, where patients receive the service, and the type of personnel who will provide it. The model keeps track of the resources used and estimates costs using related cost models. Each protocol is a tree with many probabilistic branches to simulate that different providers may provide patients having the same condition with different medical services. The care protocols may be tailored for simulations of specific enterprises and facilities. The model represents various ancillary personnel (e.g., nurses, nurse assistants, medical technicians, etc.) and various ancillary resources (e.g., laboratories, pharmacies, beds, CAT scans, MRIs, and durable medical equipment). Finally, the model represents various clinical (e.g., computerized patient record system) and administrative (e.g., billing, scheduling) information technologies and communications systems.

Because the HCM explicitly simulates all of the entities, processes, and activities in the system, any one or combination of them can be changed, and the impact on various output costs and access metrics can be observed. For example, HCM can determine how a change affects the cost of running the enterprise, a hospital, or a particular unit in a

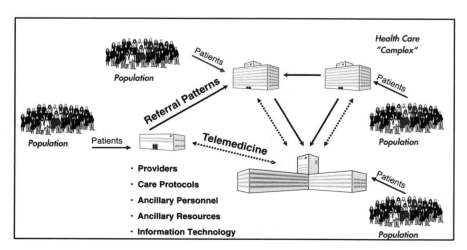

FIGURE 1 Overview of the Healthcare Complex Model.

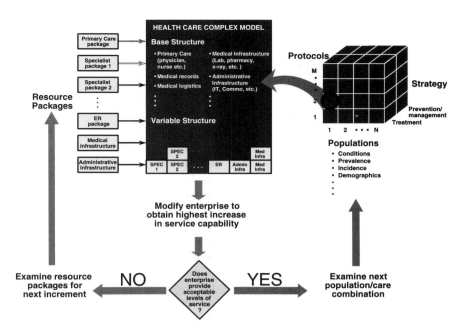

FIGURE 2 Zero-based HCD enterprise design.

hospital. It can calculate the impact on access metrics for the enterprise, a hospital, or a unit in a hospital. Because the model is being enhanced continually via a prototyping process, consideration has been given to simulating false positive and false negative statistical errors and their effects. Although these are not outcomes, they would provide useful quality information about the simulated HCD enterprise.

HCM has reasonable fidelity at this stage in its development. It contains more than 1,200 ICD-9 code conditions (e.g., acute appendicitis, asthma, cellulite, open chest wound, viral hepatitis, low back pain, etc.) and more than 1,500 clinical tasks/procedures (e.g., preoperative anesthesia, computer tomography for staging/radiation, EEG, interpretation of angiogram, administration of antibiotics, etc.). The model simulates 60 different kinds of health care providers, 17 types of ancillary resources (e.g., x-ray, ultrasound, pathology, dialysis unit, etc.), 6 different inpatient beds, and 23 combinations of telemedicine equipment. And its fidelity improves with every study.

The model was tested on one of the smaller regional HCD enterprises in the military health system (MHS). The enterprise has one major medical center, two hospitals, two clinics, and a managed care support contractor that provides additional capacity for the region. Together they handled about 1.6 million outpatient visits in fiscal year 1999. The model was adapted to represent the facilities, workforce, ancillary resources, information technologies, and clinical protocols used by the regional complex. Using population demographics provided by the government, regional operations for the year 1999 were simulated a number of times (because of the probabilistic nature of the protocols) to develop stable average outputs. These were compared to the historical values

from the enterprise's 1999 operations with encouraging results. Total outpatient visits differed by 0.11 percent, same-day surgeries by 1.02 percent, inpatient admissions by 2.99 percent, emergency room visits by 6.04 percent, and average length of stay by 0.94 percent. More detailed comparisons of outpatient visits by individual facility and individual specialty all differed by less than 4 percent. Although this was not a true validation study (which would require implementing model-suggested changes and comparing predicted impacts with actual results after the changes), it did show that simulation models can represent the complex dynamics of health care enterprise operations and can generate useful information and insights for enterprise managers.

HCM has been used in a number of other studies including the geographic distribution of primary care providers for a large, dispersed enterprise; telemedicine needs for a MHS regional complex; centralization of radiologists to service a 20-facility enterprise; and determining return-on-investment for information technologies. HCM is currently being used to determine capacity requirements for an enterprise that would experience increased demand following a bioterrorist attack.

Enterprise-level simulation models like HCM can be used to address a broad range of issues facing enterprise executives. Here is one challenge that could be posed: Given a population of patients, how can operations research determine an efficient set of resources to provide an acceptable level of services to that population. Assuming the HCD enterprise is a shell with no existing medical services, models like HCM can be used to address difficult issues, such as designing a system from scratch to serve a given population (sometimes referred to as "zero-based" design). A schematic drawing of the analysis process is shown in Figure 2. For purposes of this discussion, we assume that an acceptable level of service can be defined in terms of some access/quality metrics, cost of enterprise operations, and cost of the resources.

The resources required to service the specified population depend not only on characteristics of the population (e.g., conditions, prevalence, incidence, etc.), but also on the protocols, as well as the degree to which the enterprise strategy for servicing the population focuses on treatment or prevention/management of medical conditions. The three-dimensional structure shown on the right side of Figure 2 allows the analysis team to select a population, a protocol set, and a mixed treatment/prevention strategy as input to the analysis process. (The protocols are obviously related to the strategy and designed to reflect the strategy.) Figure 2 shows that input (1, 2, T), representing population 1, protocol set 2, and a treatment-focused strategy is used to begin the analysis.

Regardless of the input set, the enterprise will need a "base structure" consisting of a primary care package, medical records, medical logistics, a medical infrastructure package, and other base resources, as shown in the figure. Enterprise operations with the base-level resources, protocol set 2, and strategy T can then be simulated for a period of time to see if it provides an acceptable level of service to the selected population (#1). If the answer is no (as shown by the decision diamond), the analysis can then try adding individual resource packages to see which provides the most improvement in service capability to the population. Resource packages are designed by the user team (e.g., pediatrician/internist/obstetrician/ENT package, which can be substituted for a primary care package; a gastroenterologist/orthopedist package; an oncologist/urologist package; a cardiologist/thoracic surgeon package; an emergency room package; and other resource groupings). Enterprise operations are simulated for each package to determine the improvement in service capability above the base level. The resource package with the most improvement on the margin is added to the enterprise (as shown under the variable structure).

This process is repeated, and resource packages with the most marginal improvement to the enterprise are added until an acceptable level of service is reached. (Mathematical programming techniques would likely make this iterative search process more efficient.) When this process is complete, the sum of the base and variable resources constitute an *efficient*

set of resources that provide an *acceptable level of service* (measured by access/quality and cost metrics) to the *designated population* using the *specified protocols*. The effect of different protocols on the resource requirements, as well as resource requirements for other populations, can be determined in a similar way. This process could be used to design a "versatile" set of resources that would provide a capability to serve multiple populations using different protocols.

Operations research could address some of the important enterprise-level issues but would require cultural changes on the part of enterprise management, as well as the operations research community. Enterprise management would have to encourage centralized planning for enterprise design and resource allocation issues, simultaneously maintaining decentralized operations. Higher order (and usually large) effects of interactions across stovepipes can only be identified at this level. Enterprise management would have to encourage a culture of prospective analyses to identify necessary changes that would be useful and would provide a high return on investment. (Retrospective analysis is an expensive trial-and-error process to learn what doesn't work). Enterprise management would have to establish a "requirements-pull" process for equipment and IT decisions, rather than the existing "technology-push" process, which is based on what is available from industry rather than what is needed. Management would also have to require that processes be reengineered when implementing new technologies (technology changes overlaid on existing processes produce zero value).

The health operations research community would also have to make important cultural changes. It needs to begin addressing enterprise-level issues, which should not remain in the purview of health econometricians who have failed to solve the cost, access, and quality problems that have beleaguered health enterprises and the nation. The operations research community would have to start working with enterprise-level structural models and begin using them for prospective analyses. Health operations research practitioners must become integral partners with senior enterprise managers in their business planning. They should use their 40 years of tactical-level support as an entreé and then demonstrate (and market!) the value of enterprise-level analyses to enterprise managers.

Transforming Current Hospital Design: Engineering Concepts Applied to the Patient Care Team and Hospital Design

Ann Hendrich
Ascension Health National Clinical Excellence Operations Office

Health insurance premiums and the cost of hospital services and care have risen significantly over the past few years. Public and private data recently analyzed by PricewaterhouseCoopers (2003) for the American Hospital Association and the Federation of American Hospitals confirmed that, from 1997 to 2001 spending on hospital care increased by $83.6 billion. Increased volume, the most important reason for this increase, accounted for 55.4 percent; 33.4 percent was attributed to increased use and 21.0 percent to population growth. Since 1996, adjusted admissions increased at least 3 percent every year except 1998, when the increase was 2 percent. Other factors included an aging population; lack of effective care management and patient education; less restrictive benefit plans; and new, more expensive technologies.

Spending on hospital services increased 61 percent over the last 10 years and is still the largest component of rising national expenditures on health care (31.7 percent in 2001). Increased compensation is the most significant driver of the rising cost of goods and services purchased by hospitals. Nearly three-fifths of hospital expense goes to the wages and benefits of caregivers and others. Furthermore, labor costs accounted for 38.8 percent of the increase in spending on hospital care between 1997 and 2001. The study also determined that improved hospital efficiency accounted for $15 billion in savings between 1997 and 2001. These initiatives resulted in shorter hospital stays, less inpatient capacity, higher productivity, and consolidations.

Labor costs (related to the nursing shortage) are anticipated to account for the largest share of the current increase in spending on hospital services. Between 1995 and 2000, hospital wages exceeded increases paid in private industry, and, as a result, financial margins eroded. In addition to wages, hospitals have absorbed other expenses to retain or recruit nurses, such as tuition reimbursement, sign-on bonuses or referrals, loan repayments, and financing of child care centers. This has put great financial pressure on hospitals to be more efficient, which in turn has put significant stress on the workforce. The lack of significant, sustained efforts at improvement, coupled with efforts to reduce labor costs, have led to caregivers spending less time with patients and lower job satisfaction. These statistics suggest that we have an enormous opportunity to improve efficiency, safety, and environmental designs to counteract increases in labor costs and inflation.

My presentation is divided into three sections: (1) a study of how health care workers spend their time; (2) a study of current and future hospital designs, with a focus on the patient room (about 400 new hospitals are currently being built from the ground up, many of them designed the same way they have been designed for 100 years or more raising concerns about their sustainability); and (3) the results of changes in design.

BACKGROUND

In Methodist Hospital, a large time-and-motion video study of patient care processes and the patient care team, with Ann Hendrich as the principal investigator, was done to determine how improvements could be made (Hendrich and Lee, 2003a). Four video cameras were installed in hospital patient units: one in the nursing unit hallway, one on each side of the nursing station, and one in each patient room. (This was an informed Institution Review Board consent study.) The four cameras fed video data into a quad screen for data review and analysis. About 1,000 hours of continuous work were studied in a hospital nursing unit very similar to units in most hospitals in this country. Almost 4,000 events in the patient room and thousands more in the nursing station and the nursing hallway were tracked and "trended" to measure how health care workers spend their time.

We found that in this typical unit a nurse executive budgets for about five-and-one-half to six hours of direct nursing hours per patient day. But patients received less than

10 percent (about 20 to 40 minutes) of direct care in their rooms. Nursing-acuity systems cannot account for the waste and inefficiency we were able to measure in design, distance, transfers, and differences among units. We concluded that the built environment (new or transformed) enabled by technology is a nearly untapped opportunity for improving the cost, quality, and access to hospital care. A main reason nurses are unhappy in their professional roles is that most of their time is spent doing things other than professional nursing. For the most part, their time is not spent with patients on healing, intervention, care, or teaching. It is spent instead on what I call "hunting and gathering"—hunting and gathering paper, supplies, medical records, equipment, trays, carts, linen, and so on. Thus hour by hour, much more time is spent in the nursing unit hallway and the nursing station than in the patients' rooms.

In addition, many patients are moved two to five times during short hospital stays, which adds to waste, inefficiency, and the workload index. Patients are moved from unit to unit for two reasons: (1) the head wall and technology; and (2) nursing skills. Admittedly, these are very important reasons, but if hospitals address these issues, a whole new level of care and efficiency could be provided.

In a separate patient-transport study, patient-placement data (the chance of transfers, waits, and delays) were entered into a simulation model to show actual patient flow (Hendrich and Lee, 2003b). This study affirmed the need for changes in the current hospital design to reduce waste and inefficiency, improve safety, increase meaningful work for caregivers, and align facilities with future needs. The need for flexible, acuity-adaptable rooms for current and future hospital designs is imperative. The need for comprehensive care and progressive-level care will continue to increase with anticipated changes in demographics and technology. The model clearly demonstrated the high cost and inefficiency of running hospitals the way they are run now and the potential improvements of doing things differently. The model suggested that we have a multimillion dollar opportunity to reduce waste for both patients and caregivers.

A NEW DESIGN

Based on the internal and external trends revealed in these studies, a demonstration unit was established at Methodist Hospital, shortly after it was consolidated with University Hospital and Riley Hospital for Children. Additional bed space was needed for the cardiovascular consolidation, but we chose not to replicate the familiar nursing unit design. A coronary critical-care unit was combined with a coronary medical unit into a future-state patient room. The head wall was acuity adaptable, and patients were admitted and discharged from the same room. The unit was called the comprehensive coronary critical care unit (Hendrich et al., 2003).

The simple change in the head wall required minimal investment (approximately $100 dollars per room) to provide the pounds per square inch necessary to handle multiple gases (oxygen and suction) up through a multilevel tower. Other monitoring technologies would cost more and could be added when needed. Private rooms with acuity-adaptable head walls, adequate space for family, and lighting and temperature controlled by the patient could help reduce infection rates and bed placement times. This design offers maximum flexibility for hospitals of the future.

Hospital patient flow also requires a major transformation. The demonstration unit showed the value of not moving patients from unit to unit. When patients are moved, not only do we lose their dentures, but we also make serious clinical errors because of communication gaps. Every time a patient is moved from one nursing unit to another, the patient comes into contact with another 25 or so caregivers.

The new room design balanced privacy with high observation and created a healing environment for the patient. The windows facing the interior hallway were electronically charged. With the flip of a switch located on the wall, the window in front of the decentralized nursing station could become clear or opaque. (The same effect could be provided with an inexpensive blind.) The nurses used an infrared tracking system to reduce hunting and gathering time to find each other on the unit. The phone was modem capable for family or patient use, and blood analysis modules were in each patient room, so routine blood tests could be done quickly, at the point of care, to reduce lead time for physicians and caregivers.

As electronic medical records become more prevalent, hospitals should think about changing how they use the space of a centralized nursing station. This centralized space could become a business/care center for interdisciplinary practice (nurses and physicians), which would in turn make physician office and department practices more efficient. The nursing stations could be decentralized to reduce travel time and workload index and increase direct-care time. Problems relating to cultural change and human factors (nurses are most familiar with centralized stations) can be resolved with concerted effort. The data are clear—decentralized stations reduce the waste and inefficiency of typical work patterns of hospital nurses (see Figures 1 and 2).

When we consolidated the two units (coronary critical-care and the coronary medical unit), we had a definite moment in time for comparison because patients from both units were moved to the new unit on the same day. We were able to compile true pre-baseline data, and, with this case-control comparison, we were able to measure the impact of change on a variety of levels (clinical, cost, satisfaction). The case-mix was unchanged in the new unit. We measured sentinel events, length of stay, cost of care, medication errors, nursing turnover, and patient falls. The decrease in errors and adverse events was a direct result of the changes in design and care model. Patient dissatisfaction decreased greatly and more rapidly in this unit than in any other unit in the hospital. Nursing hours returned to 1997 levels—patient-care time

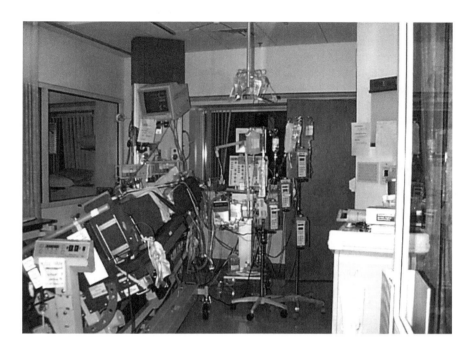

FIGURE 1 Typical critical-care patient room.

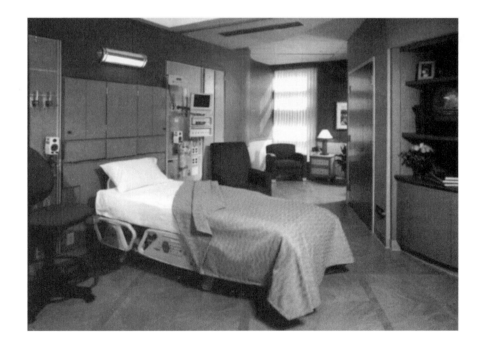

FIGURE 2 Comprehensive cardiac critical care: acuity-adaptable room for single stay.

was increased, not decreased. Direct-care contact was increased, and hunting and gathering time was decreased.

Previously these two units had transported 200 patients a month back and forth between them; the number dropped to fewer than 20. Remember that the average time for a transport is 25 minutes to 48 hours in most acute-care facilities. Theoretically, we had predicted that acuity-adaptable rooms would be more efficient and that there would be less need to move patients; this was demonstrated in the outcome data. Although the total number of beds was reduced by seven, there were dozens more patient days handled on fewer beds. When the data were entered into the simulation model, the results showed millions of dollars in efficiency improvement. This suggests that smaller, more efficient facilities would bring some relief from workforce shortages and growing demand in the future.

At the heart of the hospital capacity and flow problem (or the cause and effect) is the tension between medical and surgical care specialties and critical care. Many patients don't require critical care, but because progressive beds are usually full, they are often assigned to a critical care bed. Emergency departments and operating room recovery areas are often backlogged with patients waiting for the "right" bed. Thus, patients who are between the critical care and medical–surgical care levels ("tweeners") create a bottleneck in hospital flow. Physicians and nurses tend to err on the side of safety and "hold them" until critical care beds become available. This bottleneck phenomenon tells us something about future demands for care and the necessity of migrating the middle section of care to the "next generation" of care delivery (Hendrich and Lee, 2003c).

The built environment, enabled by technology, provides an enormous untapped opportunity for reducing waste and improving care when non-value-added analysis is used to improve caregiver work spaces. The development of new care-delivery models to match new hospital environments will be an imperative for the future. This demonstration unit, which provided a healing, patient-centered design to support the patient and caregivers, improved both clinical and fiscal outcomes.

REFERENCES

Hendrich, A.L., J. Fay, and A.K. Sorrells. 2003. Cardiac comprehensive critical care: the impact of acuity adaptable patient rooms on current patient flow bottlenecks and future care delivery. American Journal of Critical Care. Accepted for publication.

Hendrich, A., and N. Lee. 2003a. A Time and Motion Study of Hospital Health Care Workers: Tribes of Hunters and Gatherers. Manuscript in progress.

Hendrich, A., and N. Lee. 2003b. The Cost of Inter-Unit Hospital Patient Transfers. Manuscript in progress.

Hendrich, A., and N. Lee. 2003c. The Cost of Current Hospital Patient Flow: A Simulation Model. Manuscript in progress.

PricewaterhouseCoopers. 2003. Cost of Caring: Key Drivers of Growth in Spending on Hospital Care. Washington, D.C.: American Hospital Association and Federation of American Hospitals.

Discrete-Event Simulation Modeling of the Content, Processes, and Structures of Health Care

Robert S. Dittus, M.D., M.P.H.
Vanderbilt University and
Veterans Administration Tennessee Valley Healthcare System

The Institute of Medicine (IOM) report, *Crossing the Quality Chasm*, challenged health care providers to deliver care that is safe, timely, effective, equitable, patient-centered, and efficient (IOM, 2001). To meet these challenges, health care providers must redesign, implement, and continually improve current health care systems, including: (1) the content of care (what is being delivered); (2) the processes of care (how care is delivered—the microsystems of care); and (3) the structures of care (how delivery systems are organized and financed—the macrosystems of care). Although biomedical and clinical researchers will continue to identify potentially modifiable risk factors for disease and improve methods for diagnosis and treatment through observational and experimental studies, such advances alone cannot address the IOM challenges.

CONTENT OF CARE

The content of care will be shaped largely by advances in biomedical and clinical research. In colorectal cancer, for example, new chemotherapeutic agents have recently been developed that can prolong life for patients with advanced colorectal cancer (Rothenberg, 2004). In addition, new diagnostic modalities have been developed, such as radiographic "virtual colonoscopy" and a fecal DNA test, to detect early colorectal cancer (Winawer et al., 2003).

Traditional clinical research designs can address the efficacy and effectiveness of treatment and the sensitivity and specificity of diagnostic tests, but cannot easily address many important clinical management questions. Clinical research cannot readily examine the cost-effectiveness of screening colonoscopy at different ages, the most cost-effective time for surveillance colonoscopy among patients who have had a polypectomy, or the combination of age and morbidity at which colorectal cancer screening should be stopped. The myriad of possible solutions to these questions precludes comparing alternatives using traditional research designs and

the size of a clinical study for adequate power would be prohibitive. In addition, the time required to gather study results would be measured in decades because of the slow growth of adenomatous polyps, the precursor of colorectal cancer. However, simulation modeling is a study design that could effectively address these questions (Banks et al., 2004; Law and Kelton, 2000).

PROCESSES OF CARE

Biomedical research can contribute little to improvements in the processes of care. Clinical observational and experimental studies on the processes of care could be helpful, but little work has been done to date in this area. In the past decade, management science methods have been introduced into clinical medicine more formally and extensively than in the past. A set of such methods, often referred to as continuous quality improvement, have been used worldwide to reduce variations in care delivery. Because health care is generally operating far from the efficiency frontier, these reductions in variation are often accompanied by improvements in quality and reductions in cost. However, the "plan-do-study-act" incremental approach to improvement is not always applicable because external forces, such as governmental or professional regulations, may require significant sudden change. Simulation modeling can be used to explore the implications and consequences of alternative processes of care. Simulation modeling can also generate new insights into underlying systems of care and identify new approaches that might not otherwise be apparent.

STRUCTURES OF CARE

The structures of care will also require substantial modifications. For example, financing systems are not designed to align incentives to improve the quality and efficiency of care delivery. Even though care delivery systems have changed over the past decades, they are still based on the same general structures as they were a century ago. For example, the relationships and tasks among health care workers have changed very little. In the past two decades, questions have been raised about the effects of long hours (usually more than 80 hours per week) put in by residents on the quality and safety of care. In response to these concerns, the Accreditation Council for Graduate Medical Education recently established work-hour restrictions for residents. However, it is difficult for residency programs and hospitals to make small, incremental changes to their residency programs. Changes are generally made once a year, and implementing a poor system can affect a program's reputation and subsequent resident recruitment. In this situation, simulation modeling can again be an effective way of examining the potential impact of alternative systems of resident scheduling on both residents and the quality of care.

TWO SIMULATION MODELING PROJECTS

In this paper, I will describe two simulation modeling projects that highlight the benefits of this systems approach to improving health care. Both projects have been previously published. The first project is a disease-based simulation model that examines the content of care for colon cancer; the project also demonstrates how the model can affect the structure of care. The second project is a hospital-based scheduling simulation that examines the structure of care; the results of this simulation led to improvements in both the structure and processes of care.

Disease-Based Simulation Model

Colorectal cancer is currently the second leading cause of death from cancer in the United States (Jemal et al., 2003). There are more than a million deaths per year from colorectal cancer, predominantly among the elderly; mortality rates rise logarithmically with age. There is no cure for unresectable disease, although when discovered at an early stage the disease is curable through resection. Several different screening tests are available for early detection, and studies have shown that screening decreases mortality by 15 to 30 percent and that the removal of adenomatous colorectal polyps (e.g., during colonoscopy) decreases the incidence of cancer by 70 to 90 percent (Winawer et al., 2003). Based on these data, a single screening colonoscopy at an appropriate age might be an appropriate diagnostic and therapeutic strategy. Our objective was to develop a decision model and examine the cost-effectiveness of one-time colonoscopic screening for elderly patients (Ness et al., 2000).

A discrete-event network simulation model was used as the platform. The model included the biology of the disease, risk factors for incidence and prognosis, and the health care system that screens for and treats the disease. Input parameters for the model were described as distributions with characteristics, including distribution shapes, and fit to the data. To measure the cost-effectiveness of alternative screening strategies for colorectal cancer, the outcomes of colorectal cancer had to be described; to measure quality-adjusted life years (QALYs), a standard metric for cost-effectiveness analyses; utilities (as morbidity weights) needed to be measured for each outcome (Gold et al., 1996). Two clinical studies were conducted to create these outcomes, develop a utility instrument, and measure the utilities associated with the outcome states (Ness et al., 1998, 1999). Next, a comprehensive review of the literature (more than 2,500 citations) was conducted. Cost information for diagnosis and treatment were derived from a variety of sources. Once the process was conceptualized and the model formally constructed, verification and validation tests were conducted (Ness et al., 2000).

In constructing the model, an attempt was made to match polyp prevalence data measured through autopsy series and cancer incidence data measured through cancer registries, under the assumption that all adenomas progress to cancer. However, matching the adenoma prevalence rate and the cancer incidence rate required using a dichotomous population of "slow-growing" and "fast-growing" polyps, with mean transition times from adenoma to carcinoma of 52 years and 26 years, respectively. As a result, it was revealed that adenomas progress to cancer at substantially different rates and that some, perhaps many, adenomas regress without treatment. Subsequent data have also suggested that adenomas may regress. As this experience shows, modeling can not only lead to insights into the effectiveness and efficiency of alternative strategies of care, but can also inform the basic biomedical sciences and generate hypotheses regarding the pathophysiology of disease.

The main study results revealed that, among men who had not previously been screened for colorectal cancer (unfortunately, a significant percentage of the population), one-time screening colonoscopy between the ages of 55 and 59 not only reduces the incidence of colorectal cancer, but is also less costly overall than no screening (Ness et al., 2000). In a hypothetical cohort of 100,000 40-year-old men, a screening colonoscopy between the ages of 55 and 59 reduced the overall incidence of colorectal cancer from 5,672 to 2,060 and reduced deaths from colorectal cancer from 2,177 to 654. One-time screening colonoscopy thus was demonstrated in this model to reduce the incidence and mortality of colorectal cancer by approximately 65 to 70 percent. At the same time, the cost of care (colorectal cancer screening, follow-up, and treatment) for these 100,000 men was reduced by 15 percent, from $75 to $63 million. If the screening was done five years earlier, between the ages of 50 and 54, the incidence and mortality were reduced even more, but at a slightly higher cost. The marginal cost per QALY was less than $4,000, which is generally considered a very favorable cost-per-quality ratio. Similar findings were demonstrated for women. The results of this study thus informed changes in the "content" of health care, that is, the specific, recommended care.

A clinical trial to compare the costs and effectiveness of screening different age groups would be prohibitively expensive and take a very long time. A simulation model is feasible and, in addition, can also examine other features of these strategies of care, such as differential risk patterns among subgroups for the formation of adenomas or the speed of transformation from adenoma to cancer. The impact of differential sensitivities and specificities of diagnostic tests and new diagnostic modalities can be examined quickly. The model can also be used to examine the timing of a repeat "surveillance" colonoscopy after a polyp has been identified and removed. The frequency of surveillance colonoscopies can have a significant impact on the effectiveness and costs of a screening strategy. Given the current lack of capacity in this country to meet the need for colonoscopy under current recommendations, any strategy that reduces demand (such as lengthening the interval for surveillance colonoscopy) can be important. The simulation model can also examine the importance of compliance with certain elements of the strategies on the overall effectiveness and cost-effectiveness of care.

Clinical trials, observational studies, and decision analyses, such as the one described above, have since been used to inform Medicare payment policy. Prior to 2001, Medicare did not reimburse for screening colonoscopies. When cost-effectiveness models demonstrated the overall impact and potential cost savings of screening compared to not screening, this policy was changed. With potential reductions of 70 percent in deaths from colorectal cancer and simultaneous reductions in costs, the "structure" of health care was improved significantly, in this case by a financing change.

Workforce-Scheduling Simulation Model

Outside of healthcare, simulation modeling has been most commonly used to address facility design, inventory management, scheduling, and workforce deployment. Simulation modeling has also been used in a variety of settings to examine and design new structures and processes of health care (Klein et al., 1993). The second project described in this paper addressed issues related to workforce scheduling.

As a result of a variety of pressures to improve patient safety and reduce resident fatigue, many residency programs began in the 1980s to review and implement changes in house staff work schedules. The initial focus was on the frequency of in-hospital call and the amount of resident sleep time. In the 1970s, first-year residents in internal medicine in some programs were on call either 5 nights out of 7 or every other night, with the norm being every third night, and the work hours regularly exceeded 100 per week. Over time, the frequency of call has been reduced, and recently, the work week has been limited to 80 hours by professional training regulations. In addition, the number of continuous work

hours and the quantity of work, such as patient volume, have also been regulated. As a result, residency programs have been forced to redesign their resident work hours and, at the same time, hospitals have had to redesign their workforces to make up for the reduction in resident work. Resident work scheduling remains an ongoing problem for academic health centers.

In 1989, simulation modeling was used to examine resident scheduling in a county hospital affiliated with an academic medical center (Dittus et al., 1996). A goal of the project was to show whether a discrete-event simulation model of an internal medicine service constructed from easily obtainable information could make valid predictions of residents' experiences; the major focus was on the amount of sleep residents experienced while on call. A two-stage study was conducted. First, a network simulation model of the internal medicine service of the teaching county hospital was constructed, parameterized, verified, and validated using readily available hospital data and physician surveys. Second, the model was used prospectively to predict the effects of changes in the resident work schedule; the changes were made the year after the model was built.

The setting for the study was a 450-bed municipal teaching hospital with an average daily census of 90 patients on the internal medicine service (78 ward patients and 12 intensive care unit [ICU] patients). Each week, approximately 91 new patients were admitted. The service averaged eight admissions per night, one-third of which went to the ICU. To care for these patients, the medicine service had six teams; each team included a faculty member, a second or third year resident (resident), two first-year residents (interns), a senior student, and several junior medical students. In the baseline call schedule, two of the six teams were on call each night—one ward resident and his or her two interns and senior student, as well as a consulting resident and two interns from another team. Interns were on call every third night and residents every sixth night. Interns averaged 97 hours per week in the hospital.

To model the service, a discrete-event network simulation model was constructed using the INSIGHT simulation language (Roberts, 1983). The model characterized hospital schedules, such as the on-call schedule, the nighttime cross-coverage plan, clinic and conference schedules, and weekday versus weekend work schedules. The model described patient arrivals based on both scheduled and emergency admissions either to the ward or the ICU and characterized 38 house staff activities (residents and interns), including routine patient care, patient-initiated requests for care, and other activities. A decision-priority list established the order in which tasks would be addressed by the house staff following completion of any task. Twenty preemption levels described the prioritization of new tasks added to the work list, which described the interruption of a task prior to completion when a more urgent request was received. Because tasks were time sensitive, their preemption levels could change over time. The baseline model was constructed and validated against observational data not used in the parameterization of the model.

In contrast to other types of decision analyses, a discrete-event network simulation model is flexible enough to accommodate such representations. The model also allowed for complete flexibility in the description of the input parameters. A flexible distribution system was used to characterize and parameterize input data elements by mean, variance, skewness, and kurtosis.

The model was used to inform a change in the call system from four interns on call every third night to three interns on call every fourth night. To test the predictive validity of the model following this change, a second phase of the project, a prospective work-measurement study, was conducted. Senior medical students were assigned to track the house staff and record the time for the beginning and end of each task. In a pilot study, we measured interobserver variability among the medical students, and, after making clarifications, more than 96 percent agreement was established. The predictive validation study was conducted on 18 house staff days and 6 house staff nights during which house staff were followed and their tasks recorded. We then programmed the simulation model to reflect the change in call schedules and replicated the timing and number of admissions to the hospital to reflect the actual workload managed during the observed time periods.

The simulation model was able to make accurate predictions of the observed house staff work and very close predictions of house staff sleep time, the principal objective of the study (Dittus et al., 1996). For example, in the work-measurement study observations, interns spent 32 percent of their time during the day providing ward and ICU care; the model had predicted 31.5 percent. Residents spent 22.6 percent of their time on ward and ICU time; the model had predicted 23.5 percent. The observed measurements were then compared to the model prediction for total house staff sleep time when on call. The measurement study observed that each member of the house staff spent 3 hours and 30 minutes sleeping; the model had predicted 3 hours and 27 minutes. Thus, the model appeared to be a valid representation of the actual work. Once validity was established, the model was used to improve work and care delivery.

One advantage of the model is that it can examine a number of parameters and monitor outcomes. For example, a quality-of-care metric might be based on the percentage of care provided by "tired" house staff members, the percentage of emergency or urgent care delivered by "tired" house staff members, or the average time taken to complete a care request. The model allows for a very flexible definition of "tired" (e.g. the total number of minutes of sleep over a past period of time and/or the total number of minutes of uninterrupted sleep, etc.). In addition, the model could track the percentage of time that an emergency or urgent care request was managed by a member of the patient's true team, and

not a covering member of another team, who wouldn't know the patient as well. The new and old call schedules were compared against these quality metrics using varying definitions of "tired." The results showed that the new call schedule, although designed to reduce house staff fatigue, resulted in significantly less sleep on call because the house staff teams were busier during their nights on call. As a result, the quality metrics deteriorated.

The model also allowed for the examination of potential improvements in the "processes" of care. An examination of the causes of interruptions of sleep time revealed a common demand for starting intravenous lines and drawing blood at various times during the night. The model illustrated that relieving the house staff of these jobs would result in a substantial increase in uninterrupted sleep time. As a consequence, a phlebotomy and intravenous placement team was hired by the hospital, which had an important impact on the quantity and quality of house staff sleep time.

CONCLUSION

As the colorectal cancer and house staff scheduling models demonstrate, discrete-event network simulation modeling can be used to analyze and improve the content, processes, and structures of health care. Continued advances in computational speed and modeling software should make this technology increasingly accessible to health care leaders and managers. The incorporation of such models into the routine planning, examination, and improvement of health care systems holds promise for helping health care become increasingly safe, timely, effective, equitable, efficient and patient-centered.

REFERENCES

Banks, J., J. Carson, B.L. Nelson, and D. Nicol. 2004. Discrete-Event System Simulation. Upper Saddle River, N.J.: Pearson Prentice Hall.
Dittus, R.S., R.L. Klein, D.J. DeBrota, M. Dame, and J.F. Fitzgerald. 1996. Medical resident work schedules: design and evaluation by simulation modeling. Management Science 42(6): 891–906.
Gold, M.R., J.E. Siegel, L.B. Russell, and M.C. Weinstein, eds. 1996. Cost-Effectiveness in Health and Medicine. New York: Oxford University Press.
IOM (Institute of Medicine). 2001. Crossing the Quality Chasm: A New Health System for the 21st Century. Washington, D.C.: National Academy Press.
Jemal, A., T. Murray, A. Samuels, A. Ghafoor, E. Ward, and M.J. Thun. 2003. Cancer statistics, 2003. CA: A Cancer Journal for Clinicians 53(1): 5–26.
Klein, R.L., R.S. Dittus, S.D. Roberts, and J.R. Wilson. 1993. Simulation modeling and health care decision making. Medical Decision Making 13(4): 347–354.
Law, A.M., and W.D. Kelton. 2000. Simulation Modeling and Analysis. Boston, Mass.: McGraw-Hill.
Ness, R.M., A. Holmes, R. Klein, J. Green, and R.S. Dittus. 1998. Outcome states of colorectal cancer: identification and description using patient focus groups. American Journal of Gastroenterology 93(9): 1491–1497.

Ness, R.M., A. Holmes, R. Klein, and R.S. Dittus. 1999. An assessment of patient utilities for outcome states of colorectal cancer. American Journal of Gastroenterology 94(6): 1650–1657.

Ness, R.M., A. Holmes, R. Klein, and R.S. Dittus. 2000. Cost utility of one-time colonoscopic screening for colorectal cancer at various ages. American Journal of Gastroenterology 95(7): 1800–1811.

Roberts, S.D. 1983. Simulation Modeling and Analysis with INSIGHT. Indianapolis, Ind.: Regenstrief Institute.

Rothenberg, M.L. 2004. Current status of second-line therapy for metastatic colorectal cancer. Clinical Colorectal Cancer 4(Supp.1): S16–S21.

Winawer, S., R.H. Fletcher, D. Rex, J. Bond, R. Burt, J.T. Ferrucci, T.G. Ganiats, T. Levin, S.H. Woolf, D. Johnson, L. Kirk, S. Litin, and C. Simmang. 2003. Colorectal cancer screening and surveillance: clinical guidelines and rationale—update based on new evidence. Gastroenterology 124(2): 544–560.

Measuring and Reporting on Health Care Quality

Dana Gelb Safran
New England Medical Center

I will address a crucial question in this talk—what brought us to the point that we mistrust or question our doctors and our insurance companies? The answer is complex. Research has shown that medical practice varies greatly across the country, raising the question of how much of medical practice is really science. Research has also been done on health care spending and cost inflation—but efforts to contain spending have raised concerns about compromising quality. Gradually, the idea of accountability through measurement and reporting is gaining support.

Several definitions of "health" and "health care quality" have been proposed over the years. Back in 1952, Lembeke proposed this definition:

> The best measure of quality is not how well or how frequently a medical care service is given but how closely the result approaches the fundamental objectives of prolonging life, relieving distress, restoring function, and preventing disability.

In 1948, the World Health Organization defined health in the Declaration of Human Rights: "Health is a state of complete physical, social, and mental well-being, not merely the absence of disease and infirmity." We are just beginning to measure health in these terms and to study the impact of medical care on functional health status and well-being.

One of the many difficulties in measuring health care quality is determining how overall health relates to health care spending. Managed care raises the question of where we are on the hypothetical curve that economists propose reflects the relationship of health care to health (Figure 1). Will spending more or providing more care lead to better health? If we are on the ascending part of the curve, then more care or more spending will lead to better health. But if we are on the flat part of the curve, and that is the theory of many managed care organizations, then we can afford to cut back on care without doing harm. This is a fundamental question in health services research, and the answer depends on who you ask.

The most widely used instrument for measuring health in the multidimensional terms outlined by the World Health Organization is the Short Form 36-Item Health Survey (SF-36), which measures eight dimensions of health—physical function, the physical component of role function, bodily pain, general health perceptions, vitality or energy, social function, the emotional component of role function, and mental health. These eight dimensions combined yield two global assessments—one of physical health and one of mental health.

The Health Care Financing Administration and the National Committee on Quality Assurance are using the SF-36 to study the health outcomes of Medicare beneficiaries in Medicare HMOs. This Medicare Health Outcomes Survey is the first to follow data on patients' health longitudinally. The goal is to be able to hold systems accountable for patients' health as defined by the World Health Organization. There has been tremendous resistance to this approach. Many have questioned how doctors can be expected to affect multiple aspects of patient functioning. My answer is that, until they try, they probably can't.

From 1986 to 1992, I had the privilege of participating in the Medical Outcome Study, a large-scale, longitudinal study by leading scientists at New England Medical Center; the study was performed in conjunction with RAND. Two goals of the study were: (1) to determine where we are on the health care curve; and (2) to assess how differences in health care delivery and specialty care are reflected in health outcomes (Tarlov et al., 1989). This study could start a new dialogue about health care and the way patients think about their health.

In the early 1990s, we began measuring and reporting on the performance, or quality, of health care plans. The impetus for the study was a demand for data by large employers

Health

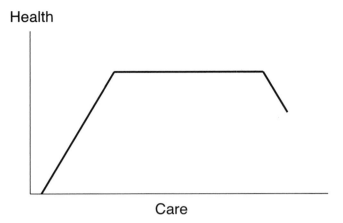

Care

FIGURE 1 The health care curve.

in the United States who needed information about health plans for themselves and their employees. The website for the National Committee for Quality Assurance (*www.ncqa.org*) now provides report cards (by zip code) rating health maintenance organizations (HMOs) in the following categories: Access, Service, Qualified Providers, Staying Healthy, Getting Better, Living with Illness. Each HMO is given an overall rating of Commendable or Excellent.

Unfortunately, this two-dimensional system of information is not very helpful to patients. First, an increasing share of Americans don't have a choice of plans. Second, even those who do have a choice find it difficult to process this much information. Third, the information is not presented in a user-friendly way; it does not allow the user to prioritize the aspects of care or to add dimensions. One of the things we learned from quality measurement on the health plan level is that plans don't vary much in a given market, especially in the provision of care.

However, it is important to note that our analyses and others have demonstrated considerable variability across markets—suggesting that where you live has an important bearing on the quality of care you can expect to receive. But assuming that the public will not use health care quality data to make "relocation" decisions—but rather to make health care decisions, the question remains as to what level of data are most appropriate and most relevant.

The next level of quality measurement that has been attempted, after health plans, is performance at the medical group level. And, indeed, within markets there appears to be considerably more variation among medical groups than among health plans. However, our own analyses reveal that the variability *within* groups is considerably greater than the variability between them. In other words, a medical group's overall performance does not provide an accurate representation of the performance of individual physicians within that group. So knowing how a group performs, on average,

doesn't tell me very much about the quality of care I will receive from an individual physician in that group whom I might select. And for patients, choosing a doctor—not a group—is almost always the relevant choice. There are exceptions in a few select U.S. health care markets, but for the most part, patients choose a specific physician to take care of them, not a group. Indeed, recent studies confirm that the kind of health care quality data that is a priority for U.S. adults is information that will help them choose a doctor (Tumlinson et al., 1997).

So, what do we know about measuring performance at the individual physician level? First, although there is some momentum for measuring physician performance, there is also tremendous resistance. Our research group developed a tool to measure each attribute of primary care based on the definitions of the Institute of Medicine Committee on the Future of Primary Care (IOM, 1996):

> Primary care is the provision of integrated, accessible health care services by clinicians who are accountable for addressing a large majority of personal health care needs, developing a sustained partnership with patients, and practicing in the context of family and community.

We measured access (a defining characteristic of primary care), continuity, and comprehensiveness of care, including knowledge of the patient. We measured two aspects of clinical interaction, the quality of communications and the thoroughness of physical exams. We measured the quality of interpersonal relations and trust, both of which relate to sustained partnerships. We then used these measurements to get an understanding of the organizational and individual characteristics that predict performance in these areas and to determine whether performance is a meaningful predictor of outcomes.

We have studied three outcomes so far: (1) a patient's adherence to a doctor's advice; (2) a patient's voluntary disenrollment from a doctor's practice; and (3) a patient's functional health outcome. We found that two attributes of primary care predict a patient's adherence to the doctor's advice: the patient's trust in the doctor and the patient's feeling that the doctor has "whole-person knowledge" about him or her. Lack of trust and lack of comprehensive knowledge of the patient are strongly correlated with patients voluntarily leaving a doctor's practice. Over a three-year period (from 1996 to 1999), 11 percent of patients who had the most trust in their doctors voluntarily left the practice; 37 percent of patients with the least trust in their doctors voluntarily left. For an individual doctor, that translates to a loss of 400 patients over a three-year period, a lot of patients to replace. We need to find ways to improve the interpersonal dimensions of health care and thus close the gaps in performance in these attributes.

So far, we have not improved on them. Our three-year follow-up study in Massachusetts showed that patients who had stayed with their primary care doctors had noticed an erosion in their relationships with their doctors. Physician satisfaction and physician morale had also declined, especially in terms of professional autonomy, time spent with patients, and time for family and personal life (Murphy et al., 2001; Safran et al., 2001).

We have also attempted to assess the current medical environment, specifically the experiences of clinicians and nonclinicians who work together. We developed an instrument to gauge medical care culture by job classification. First, the data suggest that physicians are dissatisfied, and, if physicians are dissatisfied, the feeling probably cascades to everybody else in the health care setting. When we measured several aspects of the quality of the medical workplace, including job demand, job control, leadership quality, supervisor support, interactions with physicians, interactions with patients, team culture, overall mood, and job benefits, the results were alarming. A survey of residents, for example, showed that they were satisfied with their interactions with other residents but very dissatisfied with their interactions with nurses. In addition, because of the complexity of health care and time constraints on clinicians, patients must rely on teams for their care. Our study showed that both patients and team members were dissatisfied with team care. To engender a true team culture, we will have to change the way physicians and other caregivers are educated.

REFERENCES

IOM (Institute of Medicine). 1996. Primary Care: American's Health in a New Era. Washington, D.C.: National Academy Press.

Lembeke, P.A. 1952. Measuring the quality of medical care through vital statistics based on hospital service areas. Part 1. Comparative study of appendectomy rates. American Journal of Public Health 42: 276–286.

Murphy, J., H. Chang, J.E. Montgomery, W.H. Rogers, and D.G. Safran. 2001. The quality of physician-patient relationships: patients' experiences 1996–1999. Journal of Family Practice 50(2): 123–129.

Safran, D.G., J.E. Montgomery, H. Chang, J. Murphy, and W.H. Rogers. 2001. Switching doctors: predictors of voluntary disenrollment from a primary physician's practice. Journal of Family Practice 50(2): 130–136.

Tarlov, A.R., J.E. Ware, Jr., S. Greenfield, E.C. Nelson, E. Perrin, and M. Zubkoff. 1989. The Medical Outcomes Study: an application of methods for monitoring the results of medical care. Journal of the American Medical Association 262(7): 925–930.

Tumlinson, A., H. Bottigheimer, P. Mahoney, E.M. Stone, and A. Hendricks. 1997. Choosing a health plan: what information will consumers use? Health Affairs 16(3): 229–238.

Archimedes: An Analytical Tool for Improving the Quality and Efficiency of Health Care

David M. Eddy and Leonard Schlessinger
Care Management Institute, Kaiser Permanente
and Kaiser Permanente Southern California

The practice of medicine has become extraordinarily complex, and it promises to become even more complex as the pace of innovation accelerates. Managing that complexity requires good information about the effects of different courses of action on health, logistic, and economic outcomes. The preferred method of obtaining that information is through empirical clinical research. Unfortunately, in medicine the ability to conduct clinical research is severely limited by the high cost of enrolling and following patients, the long follow-up times, the large number of options to be compared, the large number of patients, unwillingness of people to participate (e.g., to be randomized or to follow a specified protocol), and unwillingness of the world to stand still until the research is done. A typical clinical trial comparing just two options requires thousands of patients, costs tens or hundreds of millions of dollars, takes 3 to 15 years, and is likely to be outdated before it is completed.

In other fields, mathematical models have been used to help make decisions and design systems. However, the variability of human biology and behavior, the size and complexity of health care systems, and the wide variety of important questions to be addressed all place special demands on health care models. We have designed a new type of model, called Archimedes, to try to address these special demands. This paper describes the basic structure and scope of the model, the modelling methods, how we can validate the model, and its potential uses.

STRUCTURE AND SCOPE

Archimedes has three main parts. At the core is a model of human physiology that describes the pertinent aspects of anatomy, physiology, pathophysiology, occurrence of signs and symptoms, effects of tests and treatments, and occurrence of health outcomes. The second part consists of care process models; these describe what providers do when a person seeks care or what providers can do to prevent a

person from needing care. The third part, system resources, includes such things as personnel, facilities, equipment, and costs. The full Archimedes model is applied in a specific health care setting defined by specific care processes and specific system resources.

A complete description of all the objects and their attributes, functions and interactions is not possible here. But to give you a sense of the model's scope, I will describe some of the main classes of objects and give examples of their attributes and functions.

Patients. We use the term "patient" to mean anyone who might receive health care from the system, including people when they are well. The attributes of patients can be as detailed as required; they can include age, sex, risk factors, behaviors, education level, type of employment, and insurance coverage. All patients have physiologies, which include all pertinent organs and biological variables. As governed by the equations, patients can get diseases, which can modify the functions of their organs and can cause signs, symptoms, and health outcomes. Patients have perceptions, memories, and behaviors that determine how they respond to signs and symptoms and how they adhere to interventions. Their risk factors, physiologies, and behaviors can respond to interventions, which in turn can affect the occurrence and progression of their diseases. As in reality, each patient is different, and the spectra of physiologies, behaviors, and other characteristics correspond to the spectra seen in reality.

Health Care Providers. All pertinent types of personnel involved directly or indirectly in providing health care are included. Examples are nurses, pharmacists, physicians, telephone operators, and case managers. Within each of these types are the appropriate subtypes to model a particular problem (e.g., physicians $\rightarrow$ surgeons $\rightarrow$ cardiac surgeons $\rightarrow$ pediatric cardiac surgeons). Health care providers have attributes (e.g., ages, skill levels, behaviors), as well as functions (e.g., cardiac surgeons can perform bypasses, but telephone operators can not).

Interventions. Archimedes includes two main types of interventions. "Tests and treatments" encompass *what* care is delivered. This type includes: changes in risk factors and preventive treatments; tests that provide information about the existence, severity, or prognosis of a disease; "curative treatments" that directly affect the progression and outcomes of a disease; and "symptomatic treatments" that affect the symptoms of a disease, without affecting its progression. The other type of intervention, "care processes," determines *how* tests and treatments are delivered. Examples are: use of case managers, creation of a registry to increase compliance with a performance measure, and development of criteria for referrals to specialists. For either type of intervention it is possible to specify the types of providers who can deliver it, the types of facilities or locations where it can be provided, and the types of equipment and supplies it requires. In the model, such things as the use, effectiveness, and cost of an intervention can vary depending on many factors, such as patient characteristics, type of provider, skill of provider, time of day, delivery site, and random factors.

Policies, Protocols, and Regulations. The use and effectiveness of any intervention can be determined by a set of policies and protocols that describe such things as: who delivers it, where it is delivered, the criteria for determining which patients should get it, the sequence of events for implementing it, and the decision rules applied at different steps. Clinical practice guidelines, performance measures, strategic goals, and the "what-to-do" parts of disease management programs are examples of policies that affect tests and treatments. Continuous quality improvement projects, nursing protocols, instructions to telephone operators, and the "how-to-do-it" parts of disease management programs are examples of policies that affect care processes. The accuracy with which any of these is applied can allow for variations and random factors that mimic the variations and randomness of real practice. For example, adherence to a particular guideline can be different for a primary care physician than for a specialist, for a physician who has attended a continuing medical education class within the last 12 months, or for a physician who sees more than 50 patients a year who are candidates for the guideline.

Facilities, Equipments, and Supplies. Archimedes can include all types of facilities, equipment, and supplies that are involved in the management of a disease. Any type of any of these classes can be expanded to any level of detail (e.g., bed → monitored bed → monitored bed in the emergency department).

Logistics and Finances. Archimedes can record the cost, location, time, and any other important circumstance of every event. Thus virtually any type of budget, table of accounts, utilization report, or forecasting report can be calculated.

METHODS

The mathematical foundations of the Archimedes model are described elsewhere (Schlessinger and Eddy, 2002).

Briefly, it is written in differential equations and programmed Smalltalk, an object-oriented language. The most difficult part of the model is the representation of physiology. We conceptualize the physiology of a person as a collection of continuously interacting objects that we call "features." The concept of a feature is very general, but features correspond roughly to anatomic and biological variables. Examples in the current Archimedes model are systolic and diastolic blood pressures, patency of a coronary artery, cardiac output, visual acuity, and amount of protein in the urine. Features can represent real physical phenomena (e.g., the number of milligrams of glucose in a deciliter of plasma), behavioral phenomena (e.g., ability to read an eye chart), or conceptual phenomena (e.g., the "resistance" of liver cells to the effects of insulin).

The model is largely driven by the trajectories of features—their values as continuous functions of time. They register the effects of patient characteristics, interact continuously with each other, determine the occurrence and progression of diseases, trigger the onset and determine the severity of signs and symptoms, are measured by tests, respond to treatments, and cause health outcomes. Specifically, differential equations are used to define the progression of each feature as a function of patient attributes as well as other features. At any given time, the values of features can be measured by tests, subject to both random and systematic errors. Equations define clinical events, such as signs, symptoms, and health outcomes, as functions of the magnitudes and trajectories (e.g., rate of change) of various combinations of features. Diseases, which in reality are human-made labels for constellations of biological variables, are defined in the model in the same way. For example, in the model as in reality, a person is said to have "diabetes" if the fasting plasma glucose exceeds 125 mg/dl or the oral glucose tolerance test exceeds 199. Treatments are included as parameters in the equations for features, being able to change their values, rates of progression, or both. In the model, treatments do this at the level at which their actual mechanisms of action are understood to occur. For example, in the model the drug Metformin affects the equation that determines the amount of glucose produced by the simulated liver cells. Finally, the signs, symptoms, and behaviors caused by changes in features set in motion all the logistic events and use of resources that occur in a health care system.

In general, several dozen features and 10 to 30 equations are necessary to calculate the occurrence of any particular outcome (e.g., the rate of heart attacks in a specified population). The model currently includes the features pertinent to coronary artery disease, congestive heart failure, diabetes, and asthma. Features relating to other diseases are being added continually. Other formulas describe the clinical, logistic, and economic events. These formulas are typical of decision trees, flow charts, and accounting models. All of the formulas can include person-to-person differences, random variations, and uncertainty.

The level of detail of the model is determined by the intended users. We build the physiology part of the model to the level of detail clinicians tell us they consider necessary for their decisions. As a result, the physiology model corresponds roughly to the level of biological detail found in patient charts, general medical textbooks, and the designs of clinical trials. Care processes, logistics, resources, and costs are modelled at an equally high level of detail, as determined by administrators. For example, there are 37 different types of outpatient primary care visits.

BUILDING THE MODEL

Archimedes is built from existing basic research, epidemiological studies, and clinical trials of treatments (Schlessinger and Eddy, 2002). When person-specific data are available, they can be used to derive equations for features as functions of other features. When person-specific data are not available, aggregated data, such as those routinely published for registries, population-based studies, and clinical trials, can be used. In general, the results of any well designed study can be used to build the part of an Archimedes model that addresses biological phenomena, outcomes, and interventions that were investigated in the study.

The data to describe care processes are not routinely collected or published. In practice, we develop our models of care processes through examination of administrative data, existing protocols, interviews, and on-site observations, checked against any available data. Pilot studies can be conducted as needed for processes that are determined through sensitivity analysis to be critical.

VALIDATION

Methods. Ultimately, the value of a model depends on how accurately it can represent reality. The deep level of physiological detail coupled with the care processes in the Archimedes model provide a rigorous way to test this. The validation strategy is to identify an epidemiological study or clinical trial, conduct a "virtual study" or "virtual trial" in the virtual world of the model, and then compare the results. The basic steps are: (1) Have the model "give birth" to a large population of simulated people. Imagine a large city of simulated people with a representative spectrum of characteristics (e.g., age, sex, race/ethnicity, and genetic background) and medical histories. They are all unique, and most will never get the disease to be studied in the trial. (2) Run the model to let them age naturally until they reach the age range of the people who were candidates for the real trial. (3) Identify those who would meet the inclusion criteria for the trial, and select from them a sample that corresponds to the sample size of the real trial. (4) Randomize the simulated participants into groups, as was done in the real trial. (5) Have simulated providers give the patients the treatments

according to the protocols described for the real trial. (6) Run the model for the simulated duration of the trial, with the simulated providers applying whatever follow-up and testing protocols were used in the real trial. (7) Count the outcomes of interest that occurred to the participants in the simulated trial. (8) Compare them to the results observed in the real trial. We use Kaplan Meier curves to make the comparisons because they contain the most information about the outcomes in all of the arms of a trial at all time periods.

All of this is done at whatever level of detail is necessary to simulate what was done in the real trial, using whatever descriptions are available from publications. For example, if "hypertension" is defined as "a finding on at least two of three consecutive measurements obtained one week apart . . . of a mean systolic blood pressure of more than 135 mm Hg or mean diastolic blood pressure of more than 85 mm Hg, or both," that is what we have the simulated physicians do.

Each trial that is simulated in this way provides a sensitive test of the model. For each, the simulated results come from thousands of simulated individuals, each of whom has a simulated liver, heart, pancreas, and other organs. Each liver produces glucose, each coronary artery can develop plaque or thrombus at any point, and each kidney clears urine. The progression of the pathological process is different in every person, just as in reality. The simulations also include simulated physicians following simulated practice patterns or guidelines, with different degrees of compliance . . . on through to the performance of tests, reporting of results, making of errors, giving of treatments, use of facilities and equipment, and generation of costs. All told, each simulation tests scores of equations in every patient and hundreds of other equations that all have to work correctly in concert.

At the end of a simulation, the results of the virtual study should closely match the results of the real study, within the bounds of random variation related to sample size. We say there is a "statistical matching" of results if there is no statistically significant difference between the model's results and the real results.

To help probe different parts of the model and to check its validity for different populations, organ systems, treatments and outcomes, we test the model in this way against a variety of different trials. Each validation exercise uses the same model with the same parameter values; parameters are not set to "fit" one trial and then reset to fit another trial. The trials are chosen by an independent advisory committee, which also reviews the results.

In some cases, some information from a trial is needed to help build some part of the model. When this occurs, the information from the trial is used to help derive only one equation out of the 10 to 30 used to calculate the outcome of interest in the population of interest. Thus a validation exercise involving such a trial not only confirms the equation it helped build, but also provides an independent validation of the other equations. Furthermore, the equation built with help of any particular trial is independently tested by all of the

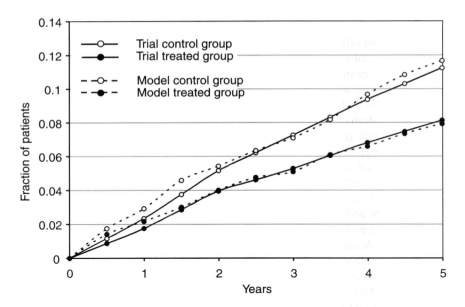

FIGURE 1 Comparison of model and trial of fraction of patients having major coronary events in the Heart Protection Study (2002).

validation exercises involving other trials. Out of the 18 trials used to validate the model thus far, 8 were used to help build the model, 10 were not.

Validation Results. Using these methods, the Archimedes diabetes model has been validated against 17 epidemiological studies and 18 clinical trials thus far. The example shown in Figure 1 compares the model results with the trial results for the Heart Protection Study (2002). This trial randomized about 25,000 high-risk people to receive either a placebo or a cholesterol-lowering drug, Simvastatin. People were defined as being at high risk if they had coronary artery disease, occlusive arterial disease, or diabetes. The primary outcome was the fraction of people who developed heart attacks. No information from this trial was used to help build the model.

Counting the different arms and outcomes of the 18 trials, a total of 74 validation exercises have been conducted to date. (Figure 1 illustrates 2 of the 74.) In 71 of the exercises, the model's results statistically matched the real results. For the three exercises that were not a statistical match, in one case the difference in results was just barely statistically significant (p = 0.04), which is to be expected in 74 exercises. In the other two, the difference was due to the model underestimating the underlying rate of the outcome in the trial population by about 35 percent. (The model estimated the effect of the treatment accurately.) The advisory committee concluded that this discrepancy was most likely due to a risk factor in the trial population that was not described in the publication and therefore could not be included in the model. Considering all 74 exercises, the correlation between the model's results and the real results is r > 0.99. Considering only the 10 trials that were not used to help build the model, the correlation was still r > 0.99.

USES OF AN ARCHIMEDES MODEL

Archimedes is meant to create a virtual world at the level of detail at which real clinical and administrative decisions are made. Once created and validated, the virtual world can be used to explore a wide variety of scenarios and questions, much as a flight simulator can be used to simulate different types of flying conditions and emergencies. Applications include: (1) designing and testing clinical management tools, such as guidelines, performance measures, strategic goals, disease management programs, priorities and continuous quality improvement programs; (2) evaluating and performing cost-effectiveness analyses of clinical and administrative programs; (3) designing and interpreting clinical research, including setting priorities for new trials, planning trials (e.g., sample size, duration, clinical costs), projecting long-term Phase 3 results from short-term Phase 2 results, estimating outcomes in subpopulations, and extending the results of a trial (e.g., predicting 15-year outcomes from 3-year outcomes, predicting outcomes that were not initially measured); (4) estimating outcomes for specific patients who are contemplating different treatment options; and (5) creating a "living library"—a place where the current body of knowledge about a disease is not only organized and stored, but is also integrated in a quantitative way that can be used for the other types of applications just described.

DISCUSSION

Archimedes is distinguished from other models by several features. It is a person-by-person, object-by-object simulation. It covers a broad spectrum, spanning features from biological details to the care processes, logistics, resources, and costs of health care systems. It is written at a deep level of biological, clinical, and administrative detail. It is continuous in time; there are no discrete time steps, and any event can occur at any time. Biological variables that are continuous in reality are represented continuously in the model; there are no clinical "states" or "strata." It includes many diseases simultaneously and interactively in a single integrated physiology, enabling it to address comorbidities, syndromes, and treatments with multiple effects. Finally, it has been validated by simulations of a wide range of clinical trials.

Archimedes is not intended to replace reality. If a question can be answered with a well designed empirical study, that approach is always preferable. Our goal is to provide a trial-validated method that can be used to address problems that can not be feasibly addressed through empirical studies, because of high cost, long follow-up times, large sample size, unwillingness of providers or patients to participate, large number of options, or the rapid pace of technological change. In the way that a flight simulator provides valuable experience, shortens the time needed in real planes, and simulates experiences that are too dangerous or rare to attempt for real (like severe wind shear), the Archimedes diabetes model should be a useful tool for sharpening our understanding of diseases and their management.

The model, which was developed and is owned by Kaiser Permanente, is currently being prepared to be made accessible to individuals and organizations, over the Web, through a friendly interface on a nonprofit basis. The website is expected to be completed by the end of 2005. In the meantime, the authors can be contacted by e-mail about access (eddyaspen@yahoo.com).

REFERENCES

Heart Protection Study Collaborative Group. 2002. MRC/BHF Heart Protection Study of antioxidant vitamin supplementation in 20,536 high-risk individuals: a randomized placebo-controlled trial. Lancet 360(9326): 23–33.

Schlessinger, L., and D.M. Eddy. 2002. Archimedes: a new model for simulating health care systems—the mathematical formulation. Journal of Biomedical Informatics 35(1): 37–50.

Applying Financial Engineering to the Health Services Industry

John M. Mulvey
Princeton University

The primary goal of operations research (OR) is to improve the efficiency of public and private organizations. There have been many significant success stories since the field began during the Second World War. For example, military war planners employ OR methods to assist in the logistics of moving people and equipment to designated locations and time points; the last two wars in Iraq show the critical benefits of efficient logistical planning. In another application, both the airline and telecommunication industries rely on optimization for scheduling and planning purposes. OR methods improve the efficiency of these complex logistical decisions.

The goal of financial engineering is to analyze, manage, and transfer risks efficiently within and across organizations. To achieve this goal, we focus on modeling uncertain elements as stochastic systems of equations. Financial engineering has been used to price options, design structured securities, employ dynamic portfolio theory for investors, and manage asset-liability for institutional and individual investors. In contrast to traditional OR, financial engineers must model risks and create instruments for transferring risks. Financial engineering addresses both tactical and strategic decisions. At the strategic level, we optimize complex organizations (enterprises) in the face of uncertainties.

There are differences, of course, between traditional engineering and service-sector engineering (such as financial engineering). Traditional engineers typically design physical objects, machines, and networks. Financial engineers design financial products and services. Traditional engineers build upon physical reality, whereas financial engineers attempting to solve problems using advanced mathematics build objects that are not physical in nature, such as novel securities. Traditional engineers typically take on professional responsibility; they are personally liable if harm results from a failure. Financial engineers have little personal liability at this time. And finally, perhaps because of personal liability and related issues, traditional engineers concentrate on design failures (e.g., why a bridge collapsed). For financial engineers, the deep study of failures is just beginning.

Regulations have an enormous impact on both domains. With the 1936 Flood Control Act, the government created regulations that required government projects to meet minimum economic standards. Those regulations led to methods enabling the government, and companies, to compute cost-benefit analyses of proposed projects and to engage in projects only when the overall benefits outweighed the overall costs. Similarly, the 1974 ERISA Act helped U.S. pension plans analyze their assets and liabilities and compute annual pension plan surpluses. When there are deficits, contribution rules are based on these calculations. In addition, the "prudent-man rule" (required by ERISA) has had a substantial impact on how decisions are made.

Despite these significant regulations, severe difficulties can arise. In the past three years, many large U.S. companies have seen ample surpluses turn to large losses as the equity markets have plunged and interest rates have declined. The 1974 regulations should be revised to prevent this type of difficulty from recurring. Financial engineering can play an important role in developing more efficient regulations for the pension industry.

IMPROVING EFFICIENCY IN THE INSURANCE INDUSTRY

The U.S. insurance industry, another highly regulated domain, is regulated mostly through the 50 state insurance commissions. In 1998, the National Association of Insurance Commissioners completed its revisions of statutory accounting standards, the code of standards that requires insurance companies operating in the United States to evaluate their assets and liabilities according to regulatory standards. Annual assessments are made so that a company's assets and liabilities can be applied to surplus calculations. There are several methods for determining an insurance company's surplus, including GAAP, statutory surplus, and economic (market value) surplus. Each of these values helps determine the health of an insurance company in terms of its ability to pay future liabilities and make a profit along the way.

An "optimal" insurance company would not only be safe in terms of protecting itself against adverse circumstances, but would also be reasonably profitable so that shareholders benefit and the cost of capital is relatively low. An optimal insurance company would satisfy all of its policy holders, provide relatively inexpensive products and services, pay shareholders a profit, and have a low chance of bankruptcy. Company employees and customers would both be pleased with this optimal environment.

Are there insurance companies that satisfy all these criteria? Most existing insurance companies, including health care insurers, fall short on several counts. Many primary insurers have low profitability, and customers may be unhappy with existing rates. Financial engineering can play an important role in improving the efficiency of insurance companies.

An example of an efficient company is the Renaissance Reinsurance Company of Bermuda, which operates primarily in the area of catastrophic risk. This reinsurance company takes in money by selling reinsurance to insurance companies that sell catastrophic insurance—mainly for earthquakes and hurricanes. Major decisions for a reinsurance (or insurance) company are: (1) how to invest assets (called asset allocation); and (2) which businesses to insure. Other decisions include who the policy holders are, how much is charged, and how diversification is done. Once assets and liabilities are decided, the question becomes how much insurance the company buys for itself—thus insuring its own risk. This leads to what is called retrocessional insurance.

For large insurance companies, the capital structure is an important factor in these decisions. Capital acts as a buffer that protects the company against loss. How large the capital should be depends on how much risk the organization is willing to accept. The amount of risk capital generally depends on the size of losses at the left tail of the profit/loss probability distribution. As we will see, diversification reduces the tail losses thereby lowering the capital charge.

GLOBAL INSURANCE COMPANIES

In many cases, multidivisional insurance companies can operate more efficiently than single product companies. For example, AXA, the global insurance company based in Paris, France, allocates capital according to a system that projects scenarios into the future and estimates profit under each scenario for each division. The company then allocates risk capital through its headquarters (see Figure 1). This approach saves total enterprise capital because benefits are diversified and profits are gained by lower capital requirements.

Would this work for an insurance company in the health-care industry? A company with a life-insurance division and

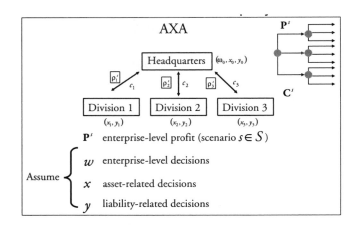

FIGURE 1 Allocation of risk for a global financial company.

a health-insurance division would have to determine how capital should be spread between the two divisions. Would it be more or less efficient to separate risks? The factors that determine risk are related to the work of both the life insurer and the health insurer. For instance, a health insurer makes less profit on elderly patients, but a life insurer makes more profit if the clients live longer. So in some sense, for an efficient operation, the enterprise risks would be lower for a merged health/life insurance company than for two separate companies. However, current regulations discourage the single organization structure and the sharing of risks between life insurance and health insurance.

PLANNING TO ACHIEVE FUTURE GOALS AND OBLIGATIONS

Financial engineering methods can be used by individuals planning their personal investment, consumption, and savings decisions. The first step is determining an individual's financial goals, for example, establishing an account for retirement purposes or saving for the purchase of a house or setting up a health care expense account.

Someone aiming for a long-term target, for example, a million dollars for retirement, could use various formulas to calculate how much to set aside each year to reach that goal. There are several ways to simplify this process, such as assigning a market value to cash flows and discounting them back to the present with a risk-adjusted rate to determine the individual's surplus value (similar to a pension plan). However, because cash flows and discount rates are generally uncertain, this approach is not usually used for future savings. Also, the decision involves long periods of time and information regarding the chances of meeting the goal at the designated time is not available.

A more comprehensive approach to help individuals make investment decisions for their future retirement would be to

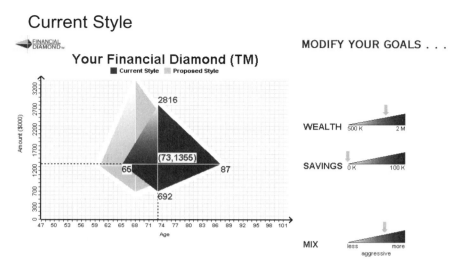

FIGURE 2 A graphical representation to help individuals make financial decisions.

project the investor's wealth for a set of plausible scenarios via a stochastic Monte Carlo simulation. In particular, we can evaluate factors, such as interest rates or inflation, and then simulate each of these factors, along with the respective performance of the assets over a planning horizon. This approach is the basis for a multiperiod asset and liability management (ALM) model for an individual. The planning model helps estimate how much capital is needed to protect against any particular set of circumstances, such as, if the equity market returns are lower than their historical 10.5 percent average annual values. As we did for the pension plan, we evaluate the assets and liabilities (and now goals) under a common framework. This analysis is similar to the analysis insurance companies use to make risk-based capital decisions—how much money the company needs to protect against adverse losses when future targets are uncertain.

LIMITATIONS OF INDIVIDUALS MAKING DECISIONS UNDER UNCERTAINTY

Financial engineering promises to help individuals make investment decisions under uncertainty. Unfortunately, individuals may not always make the most economically efficient decisions. For example, Princeton University allows employees to set aside up to $5,000 a year before taxes in a health care expense account; unspent monies are lost at the end of each year. We have observed that many Princeton faculty and staff, despite their greater than average intelligence, rarely make the best decision relative to the costs of overage and underage. In fact, most individuals do not evaluate the opportunity cost of saving from the expense account as rendering an error and, therefore, do not set aside adequate funds in the health-expense account. Even in simple cases, individuals do not address risk consistently. Nevertheless,

the U.S. government is encouraging individual responsibility for life-choice decisions.

Information to assist individuals with investment decisions can be provided based on the ALM model. One graphical approach is called the Financial Diamond™ (see Figure 2). This illustration provides an intuitive way of thinking about the risks of achieving future goals. It allows an investor planning for retirement to set a target goal and then simulate scenarios to arrive at a range of time periods to obtain the goal. A portfolio of assets, such as stocks and bonds, is simulated in conjunction with savings strategies to determine the chances of meeting the goal. The shape of the Financial Diamond™ determines the range of likely outcomes in the future, given the proposed investment and saving strategies. Thus, individuals can evaluate alternative strategies and *see the results*.

Individuals require sound, intuitive methods to understand stochastic outcomes from investment/consumption/savings strategies. Training is also important for selecting the best strategy for an individual. A barrier to improving the health-care system is getting individuals to think about health-related decisions consistently and cost efficiently. Like pension planning decisions, health-care decisions often involve long time periods and substantial uncertainties.

IMPLICATIONS FOR THE HEALTH CARE INDUSTRY

Two primary challenges relate to financial engineering and the U.S. health care system. The first involves the design of an efficient insurance industry. Deciding how risks across organizations should be diversified involves: (1) structural decisions for the enterprise; and (2) the creation of effective risk-transfer mechanisms. Because capital allocation helps determine an insurance company's future profitability, a well diversified company will not only be more profitable but will also be safer than a single-line company. Of course, the combined company must manage it risks and price its products via profitable risk-adjusted values for the enterprise. Thus, the overall structure of an insurance company should be optimized as a single enterprise.

Improving the environment for health care delivery will require determining a market mechanism, choosing a way to transfer risk across different kinds of activities, seeking stability across time, and planning under uncertainty. The insurance industry should be restructured to make greater diversification of risks possible, thus improving the profitability of companies and reducing their overall risks. Given the large losses in the past few years, insurance companies in the health care field are ripe for restructuring. Of course, a primary issue involves the rapid increase in costs for U.S. health care. Even a highly efficient insurance company cannot overcome the barriers created by rapidly rising costs. Nevertheless, well managed insurance companies can improve the environment of the health care industry.

The trend today is to give individuals greater responsibility for managing their affairs in general. The emergence of defined-contribution pension plans (Keoghs, IRAs, etc.) over defined-benefit pension plans is a significant example. A similar pattern may be emerging in health care, with proposals for increasing rollover health care expense accounts and related arrangements. Individuals will have to make significant investment decisions that may affect their future health. Unfortunately, individuals are not always equipped to make wise decisions when faced with financial choices involving uncertainty.

Financial engineers can assist by creating understandable decision-support systems. Education will also be important; for example, courses on decision making under uncertainty in health care could show how to find the best compromise between costs, efficiency, and possible states of future health. Financial engineers face similar issues on a regular basis. Many insights and methods from financial engineering can be directly applied to the health care industry.

RELATED READING

Doherty, N. 2000. Integrated Risk Management: Techniques and Strategies for Managing Corporate Risks. New York: McGraw-Hill.

Laster, D., and E. Thorlacius. 2000. Asset-liability management for insurers. Swiss Re, sigma 6: 7–11.

Mulvey, J.M., and W.T. Ziemba. 1999. Asset and Liability Management Systems for Long-term Investors: Discussion of the Issues. Pp. 3–38 in Worldwide Asset and Liability Modeling, W.T. Ziemba and J.M. Mulvey, eds. New York: Cambridge University Press.

Zaik, E., J. Walter, and G. Kelling. 1996. RAROC at Bank of America: from theory to practice. Journal of Applied Corporate Finance 9(2): 83–92.

Engineering Tools and Methods in the Delivery of Cancer Care Services

Molla S. Donaldson
National Cancer Institute

For several reasons, cancer care is an especially interesting and challenging field. First, cancer is a major cause of mortality. Second, we have a large, rapidly increasing evidence base of what works, promoted in part by strong patient advocacy groups. Third, as more patients survive for longer periods of time, cancer is changing from an acute condition to a chronic condition. Fourth, despite the existence of comprehensive cancer centers, we need new models of care delivery based on the consistent use of evidence about ways to deliver care that meet the needs and expectations of patients and their families.

This year, 1.3 million new cases of cancer will be diagnosed in the United States. Cancer is the second leading cause of death in the United States, accounting for slightly more than 23 percent of all deaths; large disparities in incidence and mortality rates have been found for different racial and ethnic groups, despite the strong evidence base that has been developed for cancer screening, diagnosis, and treatment (DHHS, 2001). Randomized controlled trials (RCTs)—cancer's working models of care—are the gold standard in cancer care. RCTs compare, for example, the best known treatments with new approaches. Based on a few simplified assumptions and a very restricted set of variables, RCTs test the efficacy of new agents or combinations of agents. Based on the results, they put forward hypotheses about how well a model will work and its effectiveness in real-world practice. Only 2.5 percent of adults with cancer are ever involved in clinical trials, and participation in trials varies by age (Sataren et al., 2002). One estimate is that more than half of children younger than 15 are in clinical trials and that findings are quickly translated into pediatric oncology practice (Bleyer et al., 1997).

The evidence base on effective cancer treatment and management has been used as the basis of guidelines that include descriptions of the strength of the evidence for treatment and supportive care for most tumor sites by stage. The guidelines developed by the National Comprehensive Cancer Network, for example, are reviewed annually by standing panels, for a large set of tumor types and are readily available to oncologists (NCCN, 2001) and patients (*www.nccn.org*). Yet, when researchers studied oncologists' compliance with these guidelines, they found a lot of room for improvement. For example, the appropriate use of guidelines depends on accurate staging, yet many patients are not accurately staged, not staged at all, or staging information is not available to treating clinicians.

The evidence base is also growing because of major advances in basic biology. The implication of the genome project is that oncologists will no longer classify cancers by tumor site (e.g., lung, prostate, pancreas, etc.) but by genetic transcription errors in the germ line (i.e., in the genetic makeup) or in somatic cells. Previously unexplainable differences in patient responses to therapy for tumors that look alike to pathologists are beginning to be understood in terms of the chemical pathways that produce various proteins. Recent advances have raised hopes that molecular profiles and individual phenotypes can be matched to the most effective therapy, something like matching antibiotics to specific bacteria, but at the molecular level.

With earlier diagnosis and more effective treatment, survival times have increased, sometimes making cancer care more like treating a chronic condition than an acute condition; thus, coordinated follow-up care and the late effects of treatment are becoming a central interest. New therapies may also require sustained treatment. Molecular therapies may mean less toxic and more targeted interventions, but they may also mean that patients will have to take pills for a very long time, perhaps even for a lifetime. Successful treatment will also mean that survivors will live much longer, which will shift the emphasis to follow-up care. Like care for other chronic diseases, long-term follow-up care is complex and requires multidisciplinary, multisetting, coordinated services. In addition, early detection may require long-term chemoprevention. Long periods of time may pass during which cells change before genetic defects become evident as tumors, and the distinction between prevention and therapy may disappear as detectable genetic errors are treated long before they are expressed as lesions.

The achievements and promise of genomics, proteomics, and molecular discoveries, however, have not been matched by advances in the organization and delivery of services. When patients are diagnosed with cancer, they often find navigating the medical care system a nightmare. A colleague I had not seen for a while said to me, "When I was diagnosed with Stage 3 melanoma, I thought everyone in the health system would swing into action and take care of me. I didn't realize until much later that no one could or would. It was up to me to make sure things happened and that my doctors knew about it." She is a patient in a world-class medical center in the Baltimore-Washington area. Despite her education, her considerable resources, her excellent insurance, and her husband who took full-time leave to help her, she was not able to make the system work.

The processes by which a patient accesses care (because of a symptom or for screening), receives a diagnosis, makes decisions, and plans for care in a hospital or outpatient facility or arranges for services from community service and support groups or home care may include initial treatment (such as surgery), follow-up treatment (such as adjuvant chemotherapy or radiation therapy), palliative care, education and information about community services, monitoring as a survivor, and treatment for recurrent disease, continuing primary care, and if needed, timely and appropriate end-of-life care in a hospital, hospice, or home. It may also involve genetic screening, rehabilitation, and support for family and others during and after serious illness. It is easy to understand why when Lee Atwater, campaign manager for Ronald Reagan, was diagnosed with a brain tumor and began treatment, he is reported to have exclaimed, "I need a campaign manager."

One hears the same complaints from the medical side of health care. *Ensuring Quality Cancer Care*, a report by the Institute of Medicine National Cancer Policy Board, states emphatically, "There is no national cancer program, care program or system of care in the United States" (IOM, 1999). A pediatric oncologist commented, "In the standard model of delivery of care to pediatric cancer patients, the onus of negotiating all aspects of treatment falls on the patient and his or her family" (Wolfe, 1993).

Figure 1 shows a very common model of health care for cancer. In this distributed model, with oncologists practicing in the community, the patient goes from one doctor and laboratory to another trying to integrate sometimes conflicting information. In addition, oncologists have difficulty obtaining information, which results in waste, duplication of effort, and delays; and the primary care physician often has little information about the patient's treatments. Care is provided in multiple settings, not only at the time of diagnosis and primary treatment, but also over time through later

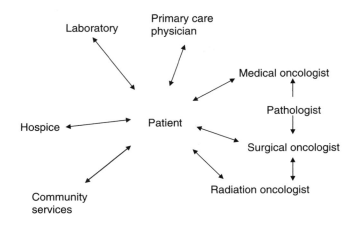

FIGURE 1 Distributed model of health care for cancer.

treatments and follow-up, as needed. Recently, interest has grown in the use of "patient navigator" programs to help patients schedule appointments and keep up with their treatment and progress, but I am not aware that such programs have been evaluated for effectiveness (American Cancer Society, 2002; Christensen and Akcasu, 1999).

Figure 2 shows a different model based on care in a comprehensive cancer center, such as M.D. Anderson, Memorial Sloan Kettering, or Dana Farber, where oncologists and other caregivers are grouped together in one facility. Even in these settings, patients may still go from one caregiver to another, and their records may be quite separate. A care coordinator, such as a nurse oncologist, might help the patient coordinate his or her care, and patients in these centers are more likely to enter clinical trials with stringent protocols and follow-up. In this model, tumor boards or multidisciplinary conferences among oncologists and pathologists develop a plan for patient care. Such conferences, which may be held

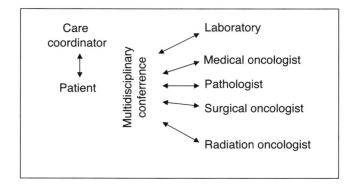

FIGURE 2 Comprehensive cancer center model.

periodically after primary treatment, may, but usually don't, include the patient and his or her family (Joishy, 2001).

Figure 3, a pediatric multisite model, was developed by Dr. L.C. Wolfe and his colleagues when he was at the New England Medical Center (Wolfe, 1993). The model attempts to remedy the boundary problems at the transitions between settings, particularly between the hospital and home, home care and some outpatient care, and outpatient care and inpatient care. When something goes wrong, people do not always know what to do or who to contact.

The model addresses these problems by having the oncologist and the nurse spend time in the hospital together with the patient and then in the outpatient setting and then, as a team, continuing to care for patients who had been in the hospital. To ease the boundary problems between hospital and home care, Wolfe devised an electronic system that enables families to transmit problems and questions to their doctors. O'Connell and colleagues (2000) have critiqued other models of care that try to integrate the hospital-community interface.

Only a few efforts to design better health care delivery systems have been reported. Last week, I attended the annual meeting of the American Society of Clinical Oncology, which drew 25,000 participants from all over the world. Of the more than 3,000 abstracts published, only two reported on programs for improving care. One was a report from France on the number of cancer patients who had attended a nutritional workshop; the other was on the costs and satisfaction of palliative care service in a hospital.

This points up a stark contrast. The knowledge base for the science of cancer care has undergone a radical transformation, but little attention has been paid to ensuring the consistent translation of this knowledge to the health care setting—not just for patients in cancer centers on protocols, but for all cancer patients all the time. Indeed, the assumption seems to be that the results of clinical trials will be translated into practice without error and without specifying how services should be organized and delivered.

The lack of well designed systems can result in the loss of benefits to patients. In many systems, failures can and do occur that could have been addressed by operational engineering. One of the most common consequences is the failure to screen patients. A research project involving health maintenance organizations found that only 50 to 83 percent of women who were expected to have mammographies in a particular year actually had them (Taplin et al., 2002). In Colorado, a risk-management study of lawsuits for failure to diagnose breast cancer found that the average length of delay from symptom to detection or detection to diagnosis was 13.4 months (Marjie G. Harbrect, M.D., personal communication, April 2001). There were many reasons for the delay, but most of them were system problems. In some cases, the primary care clinics did not have systems for tracking or follow-up. In many cases, individuals thought someone else was following up with the patient. Sometimes a lump found in an exam was not visible on a mammogram, and there was simply no follow-up. Failure to diagnose was also found in the United Kingdom, where there was on average a seven-month delay between detection and definitive diagnosis.

A study in New York hospitals on women who clearly should have had adjuvant breast therapy after treatment for early-stage breast cancer found that in hospitals that were part of the Mount Sinai system, only 18 to 33 percent of these patients, depending on the hospital, received their indicated adjuvant therapy for early-stage breast cancer (Bickell and Young, 2001; Bickell et al., 2000). This was not because of a lack of knowledge. After going through the medical records of these patients and talking to the surgeons, the study found that the surgeons simply did not know what had happened to these patients, they had simply "fallen through the cracks."

Another serious problem is failure to use the evidence base. Dr. Ezekiel Emanuel (2001) at NIH recently reported on an excessive use of chemotherapy for patients in the last months of life. He found that in the last six months, three months, and one month of life, as much chemotherapy was given for tumors that are known to be unresponsive to chemotherapy as for tumors that are responsive to chemotherapy.

Other losses of benefits include: failure to ensure that the necessary information is available at the time of decision making and at the point of care; failure to help with transitions following active treatment; failure to monitor and manage symptoms, including pain; and failure to support dying patients and their families.

A few health systems have reported their attempts to develop an integrated model of care—financially, organizationally, and in data management (Clive, 1997; Demers et al., 1998; Glass, 1998). Other reports include the development of disease-management models of inpatient and outpatient oncology care (Hennings et al., 1998; Piro and Doctor, 1998; Sagebiel, 1996; Uhlenhake, 1995), breast cancer centers (Frost et al., 1999; Kalton et al., 1997), psychosocial support services (McQuellon et al., 1996), support for

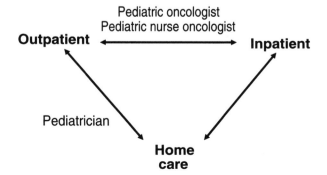

FIGURE 3 Pediatric multisite model. Source: Wolfe, 1993.

long-term cancer survivors (Hollen and Hobbie, 1995), and quality improvement teams (Frank and Cramer, 1998).

A remarkable example of what can be accomplished is the use of logistical engineering in the United Kingdom for cancer services (Kerr et al., 2002; NHS Modernisation Agency, 2001; H. Bevan, personal communication, May 2001). The story began with a major comparative study that showed that survival rates in the United Kingdom were low compared to rates in the rest of Europe and the United States. The study also found that therapy was initiated at a much more advanced stage of disease than expected, which resulted in low five-year survival rates. One reason was the seven- to eight-month delay between (1) detection and (2) diagnosis and staging. Patients were also not able to get the radiation therapy they needed, even though 20 to 50 percent of the appointment slots were not used. By the time patients were seen, the plan of care was often outdated or no longer appropriate. Although the patients' needs were predictable, they did not know what to do once they left the hospital. Further, the percentage of patients referred for abnormal exams or test results who will, in fact, have cancer can be predicted. Hence, services could be designed according to a known demand function.

Using such information, the National Health Service (NHS) made improvements in cancer care services a priority. The program began with 50 teams from nine cancer networks; the program has now been expanded to all 34 networks. The project teams tested more than 4,400 changes in the first 12 months and implemented nearly 550 of them. They instituted multidisciplinary teams that meet regularly to manage the experiences of families and caregivers. They revamped services to meet patient and family needs. For example, tests that used to require three separate hospital visits are now done in one visit.

As a result of this initiative, there was, on average, a 50-percent reduction in time to first appointment and a 60-percent reduction in radiology waiting times. The NHS believes the five-year cancer survival rate can be improved by 10 percent and is reengineering systems accordingly.

Engineering can play a major role in accelerating improvements in the quality and efficiency of cancer care. The unique skills of practicing engineers should be applied in six major arenas of cancer care:

1. Redesign care processes using engineering tools, such as the 80/20 rule, continuous flow, mass customization, production planning, and supply-chain manufacturing.
2. Use information technology to make medical information and patient-specific information available when needed. The goal is to ensure that timely, accurate information is available to clinicians and patients when they need to make decisions.
3. Redesign care to include the patient and family in decision making.
4. Encourage the continuous acquisition of knowledge and skills by all health care workers to support multidisciplinary work. The health care workforce must have the expertise to manage complex tasks, which may require changes in training, education, and protocols and rules about which tasks are permitted. Human factors analysis, which has been used in other industries for crew resource management, shift management, ensuring patient and worker safety, and ensuring high-level, reliable performance in dynamic, high-risk settings, should be applied to the health care setting.
5. Care should be coordinated across settings and over time using any engineering tools available.
6. Measurement of performance and outcomes should be used to improve care. This entails measuring the results of practice and removing the distinctions between research and clinical practice environments so that all patients and patient care can increase our knowledge.

REFERENCES

American Cancer Society. 2002. Harlem cancer screening clinic embraces the medically underserved. ACS News Today. Available online at: *http://www.cancer.org/docroot/nws/content/nws_1_1x_harlem_cancer_screening_clinic_embraces_the_medically_underserved.asp*. Accessed 9/04/03.

Bickell, N.A., and G.J. Young. 2001. Coordination of care for early-stage breast cancer patients. Journal of General Internal Medicine 16(11): 737–742.

Bickell, N.A., A.H. Aufses, Jr., and M.R. Chassin. 2000. The quality of early-stage breast cancer care. Annals of Surgery 232(2): 220–224.

Bleyer, W.A., H. Tejeda, S.B. Murphy, L.L. Robison, J.A. Ross, B.H. Pollock, R.K. Severson, O.W. Brawley, M.A. Smith, and R.S. Ungerleider. 1997. National cancer clinical trials: children have equal access; adolescents do not. Journal of Adolescent Health 21(6): 366–373.

Christensen, J., and N. Akcasu. 1999. The role of the pediatric nurse practitioner in the comprehensive management of pediatric oncology patients in the inpatient setting. Journal of Pediatric Oncology Nursing 16(2): 58–67.

Clive, R.E. 1997. Update from the Commission on Cancer. Topics in Health Information Management 17(3): 10–14.

Demers, R.Y., R.A. Chapman, M.H. Flasch, C. Martin, B.D. McCarthy, and S. Nelson. 1998. The Henry Ford Health System. Cancer 82(10 Suppl): 2043–2046.

DHHS (U.S. Department of Health and Human Services). 2001. 2001 Cancer Progress Report. NIH Publication No. 02-5045. Bethesda, Md.: National Institutes of Health. Also available online at: *http://progressreport.cancer.gov*.

Emanuel, E. 2001. Use of Chemotherapy for Advanced Disease. Presentation at the Annual Meeting of the American Society for Clinical Oncology, San Francisco, California, May 2001.

Frank, J., and M.O. Cramer. 1998. The development of an oncology services performance improvement team. Journal for Healthcare Quality 20(6): 26–32.

Frost, M.H., R.D. Arvizu, S. Jayakumar, A. Schoonover, P. Novotny, and K. Zahasky. 1999. A multidisciplinary healthcare delivery model for women with breast cancer: patient satisfaction and physical and psychosocial adjustment. Oncology Nursing Forum 26(10): 1673–1680.

Glass, A. 1998. Delivery of comprehensive cancer care at Kaiser Permanente. Cancer 82(10 Suppl): 2076–2080.

Hennings, M.N., D.S. Rosenthal, D.A. Connolly, M.N. Pollach, and M.M. Lynch. 1998. Collaborative approaches to purchasing and managing oncology services for a prepaid population. Cancer 82(10 Suppl): 2026–2034.

Hollen, P.J., and W.L. Hobbie. 1995. Establishing comprehensive specialty follow-up clinics for long-term survivors of cancer: providing systematic physiological and psychosocial support. Supportive Care in Cancer 3(1): 40–44.

IOM (Institute of Medicine). 1999. Ensuring the Quality of Cancer Care, M. Hewitt and J.V. Simone, eds. Washington, D.C.: National Academy Press.

Joishy, S.K. 2001. The relationship between surgery and medicine in palliative care. Surgical Oncology Clinics of North America 20(1): 57–70.

Kalton, A.G., M.R. Singh, D.A. August, C.M. Parin, and E.J. Othman. 1997. Using simulation to improve the operational efficiency of a multidisciplinary clinic. Journal of the Society for Health Systems 5(3): 43–62.

Kerr, D., H. Bevan, B. Gowland, J. Penny, and D. Berwick. 2002. Redesigning cancer care. British Medical Journal 324(7330): 164–166.

McQuellon, R.P., G.J. Hurt, and P. DeChatelet. 1996. Psychosocial care of the patient with cancer: a model for organizing services. Cancer Practice 4(6): 304–311.

NCCN (National Comprehensive Cancer Network). 2001. Practice Guidelines in Oncology. Available online at: *http://www.nccn.org/physician_gls/index.html.*

NHS Modernisation Agency. 2001. The Cancer Services Collaborative: Twelve Months On. Presented to the National Patients' Access Team, Leicester, England, July 18, 2001.

O'Connell, B., L. Kristjanson, and A. Orb. 2000. Models of integrated cancer care: a critique of the literature. Australian Health Review 23(1): 163–178.

Piro, L., and J. Doctor. 1998. Managed oncology care: the disease management model. Cancer 82(10 Suppl): 2068–2075.

Sagebiel, R.W. 1996. The multidisciplinary melanoma center. Surgical Clinics of North America 76(6): 1433–1439.

Sateren, W.B., E.L. Trimble, J. Abrams, O. Brawley, N. Breen, L. Ford, M. McCabe, R. Kaplan, M. Smith, R. Ungerleider, and M.C. Christian. 2002. How sociodemographics, presence of oncology specialists, and hospital cancer programs affect accrual to cancer treatment trials. Journal of Clinical Oncology 20(8): 2109–2117.

Taplin, S., M. Manos, J. Zapka, A. Geiger, M. Ulciskas-Yood, S. Weinman, S. Gilbert, and J. Mouchawar. 2000. Frequency of Potential Breakdowns in Screening Implementation among Women with Invasive Cervical and Late Stage Breast Cancer. Presented at the 8th Annual HMO Research Network Conference, Long Beach, California, April 9–10, 2002.

Uhlenhake, R. 1995. Is patient-focused outpatient cancer care on target? Journal of Ambulatory Care Management 18(4): 32–42.

Wolfe, L.C. 1993. A model system: integration of services for cancer treatment. Cancer 72(11 Suppl): 3525–3530.

Patient Trajectory Risk Management

Charles Denham
HCC Corporation and
Texas Medical Institute of Technology

This paper addresses the notion of risk trajectory of individual patients and the resultant aggregate risk trajectory of the healthcare enterprise caring for populations of patients. It also describes the use of various engineering concepts applied to medicine.

In the late 90's, working with a team from the Institute for Healthcare Improvement (IHI) and Premier Inc. a group purchasing organization of 1,800 hospitals we focused our attention on medication management. The project involved collaborators from the Cleveland Clinic, Partners System, Harvard Medical School, Mayo Health System, a number of frontline hospitals and leading experts. Our goal was to identify the idealized design for medication management to reduce adverse drug events, a major cause of preventable death and disability in U.S. hospitals. To do that, we first had to identify achievable world-class performance, then the "is state" of frontline hospital performance, and finally processes and technologies that would enable us to close the gap between the two. We were surprised by our findings and gratified by the opportunities they revealed.

Engineers are used to using process impact evaluations, risk analyses, and pattern recognition methods, however these are new to the practice of medicine at frontline institutions. Clearly, medicine has much to gain from engineering, and many benefits have yet to be realized.

The Institute of Medicine report, *Crossing the Quality Chasm* (IOM, 2001), proposes that we must redesign healthcare so that it is patient centered, evidence based, and systems focused. As such we must have a much better understanding of "integrated performance"—i.e. operational, clinical, and financial processes and outcomes—of an individual patient's care delivery through a healthcare episode. We must look at the performance/risk trajectories of common patient treatment process paths and examine the contributive impact to enterprise wide performance. Hospital administrators must step back from their traditional vertical business unit view and take into account their patient populations as they move through those vertical units so that they can recognize operational innovations that can eliminate process segment failures.

The game of golf provides a powerful metaphor. The desired outcome is to deliver the ball to the hole. For a given link one golfer may take eight strokes and another might take three. Both reach the goal if the outcome measure was just "ball in hole," however one expended more energy and time than the other. The golfer taking eight strokes has increased the risk of having mishap along the way. In a similar way, if a patient requires two or three extra days of care, the risk of having an adverse event is greatly increased due to greater exposure to the inherently dangerous hospital environment.

To come up with an ideal design for medication management, we first mapped the clinical and operational processes involved in medication use. Next, we considered the products, services, and technologies involved that enable best or better practice (technologies might include process reengineering tools, for example). Then we identified their impact on the risk of adverse events and whether they closed the gap between typical performance and best achievable performance.

Traditionally administrators and clinicians have been trained to define a medication error by violation of one or more of the "five rights"—the right patient, the right drug, the right time, the right dose, the right route. Such errors occur with virtually every patient admitted to hospital. Dr. David Classen a noted patient safety expert on our team demonstrated that the overlap between error and harm minimal using this definition of error—only a small fraction of harm is caused by error as defined by the "five rights." A great number of errors do not cause harm, and more importantly a number of adverse drug events that cause death, disability, or require treatment would not normally be counted using the classical "5 rights" framework.

During the idealized design process, we worked with a

number innovative healthcare technology suppliers; 70 to 80 percent of them were attuned to error. Few focused on harm. The deeper we explored adverse drug events it became more and more apparent that distinguishing between error and harm was critical. We focused on the most common causes of adverse drug events including transition zones between care teams and high impact intravenous infusion events. We did not ignore errors without harm, but we did not focus on them. After completing about 80 percent of a thorough, evidence-based review of integrated care and operational processes, with the guidance of a number of experts, the opportunities for mitigation started to become clear.

Subsequently IHI led a number of very successful hospital collaborative initiatives using a "trigger tool" medical record review framework that helped identify adverse drug event (ADE) risk and performance gaps.

We studied smart the Alaris smart infusion pumps that have now have the ability of capturing and even preventing the most serious IV adverse events, clearly a technology advance that will deliver dramatic speed to impact in reduction of ADEs.

To illustrate the error-harm gap and the notions of patient trajectory and hospital risk trajectory we used the example case of anticoagulation management with our teams and collaborative groups. Anticoagulant drugs are often very poorly managed by clinicians and patients resulting in severe adverse drug events. In fact this is the area of the most common drug related malpractice claims and awards.

Certain engineering concepts have great application to medicine. When engineers evaluate airplanes, they examine and discuss its performance envelope. We applied this concept to the management of anticoagulation. Warfarin is an anticoagulant drug used to manage patients. Its danger lies in the fact that the therapeutic envelope of safety relating dose to effectiveness and complications may change or shift. The patient's diet (i.e., wine or vitamin K consumption), or liver function can shift the therapeutic window. The therapeutic envelope is always changing, posing huge risk to patients for overdose or under dose leading to clotting or bleeding disorders. Currently physicians try to manage patients undergoing anticoagulation by trying to interpolate and extrapolate the relative patterns of multiple lab values and historical factors. Application of the performance envelope delivers terrific pattern recognition opportunities.

We also demonstrated the use of other aviation tools to communicate performance. For instance we created a mock up "digital dashboard," illustrating how clinicians could recognize patterns, access relevant protocols, and in the case anticoagulation decide how to manage the patient.

In collaboration with one of the nations leading anticoagulation experts we presented an example case study of a young adult admitted for treatment of a defective heart valve who experienced 11 typical and different adverse drug events, none of which was caused by a medical error (using the 5 right classification) and none of which would have

been picked up by the typical methods we use to catch medical errors. Dose adjustments unique to the patient's condition and omissions due to missed laboratory values would not typically be classified as a medication error. The patient eventually has a stroke. In this case, the potential for recognition of the risk for adverse events would have been picked up by a computerized physician order entry (CPOE), which integrates order entries with laboratory and historical information. We know from other studies that CPOE can reduce adverse events dramatically.

In the future, we will have a decision-support systems that enable clinicians who are not specialists in anticoagulation to put that part of the treatment in the hands of a pharmacy team while being able to monitor potential adverse events. That is precisely what an information integrating device that pilots use called a flight director does. Flight information is provided as an input, the crew makes sure all the instrumentation is synchronized and the director follows the plan. If the workload becomes too heavy, the autopilot can be turned on.

Today, 16 different types of specialists prescribe anticoagulants; none are specialists in anticoagulation. Orthopedists, internists, and cardiologists are all administering the drug and are responsible. The risk trajectories such patients are not being managed well and adverse events such as preventable strokes and bleeding related complications are occurring in epidemic proportions.

We used a mockup of the digital dashboard to study the young adult described earlier. His medical history and his recent history revealed a number of health problems that predisposed him to a bleeding and clotting disorder that made anticoagulation drugs extremely dangerous for him. When we asked what might have been done differently, we found that when the care data is reconstituted in a graphic it would allow us to recognize a pattern. Had the data presentation been like that presented in aircraft instrumentation we would have seen the window of safety narrowing and prevented catastrophe. Instead, we are caught by surprise driving from a view through the rear view mirror.

Clinicians could be assisted by innovations that make patterns simpler to recognize. The average doctor in an intensive care unit can interpolate three or four trends. A patient on a respirator who is very ill might have could have 60 pertinent trends. Our slowest cognitive capability is in processing data, which is exactly what computers do well.

Before retiring to focus full time on emerging technologies, I was a radiation oncologist with a very large practice, and I managed all of my patients all the way through therapy. I had a high volume of patients with common diseases, including colon, breast, lung, and prostate cancer. I had to navigate between the response of the tumor to radiation therapy and the response of normal tissue. I had to manage that patient through a safety window that would become narrower and narrower as we proceeded through care. As the dose was increased, the risk for a host of complications would increase and continue intensify through out treatment. We knew that every treatment decision had a risk-benefit balance to it. Every patient had a unique trajectory based on historical data and how certain factors had impact as therapy progressed. These patients were managed based on tacit knowledge— we could tell when a patient was headed for trouble, we could link this to certain parameters.

In working with healthcare technology suppliers, we have found that an evidence-based, patient centered, and systems performance targeted approach to "enabling" best or better practice allows innovations to be developed that improve clinical performance and reduce risk. In addition, they often deliver improved enterprise wide performance as a by-product of improved patient specific performance.

If we had continuity of information with pattern recognition support we could examine the risk trajectory of patients with very complex disorders and create scenarios and real time forecasts, as we do in aviation. In the future, we might ask a medical student to use a computer model to run scenarios for a specific patient. We could graphically portray patterns and risk trajectories to assist in decision making before patients get into trouble. Is the patient's cardiac function adequate? Will his kidneys clear everything? What-if scenarios can be run before events cascade.

Engineers already provide wonderful computational support and pattern recognition solutions for many industries. These technologies will offer physicians a terrific opportunity to "think through" treatment scenarios. With an appropriate decision-support system, we could apply the lessons learned in other industries, such as aviation and aerospace, to complex medical problems. The principles of data analysis from engineering could be tremendously beneficial for health care.

REFERENCE

IOM (Institute of Medicine). 2001. Crossing the Quality Chasm: A New Health System for the 21st Century. Washington, D.C.: National Academy Press.

Deploying Resources for an Idealized Office Practice: Access, Interactions, Reliability, and Vitality

Thomas W. Nolan
*Associates in Process Improvement and
Institute for Healthcare Improvement*

The goal of our initiative is to create an idealized design of clinical office practices (IDCOP) that offers the best possible solutions to the health care practice needs of our customers. When implemented, these solutions should lead a visiting patient to say, "They give me exactly the help I want (and need) exactly when I want (and need) it." To accomplish this goal, we have to improve measures associated with: clinical outcomes; patient satisfaction; finance; and staff satisfaction. To simplify and further systematize the systems that emerge from IDCOP, we have developed a framework of four "themes" to guide the redesign processes as a whole: access, interactions, reliability, and vitality.

Access. Timing is an essential component of health care. *When* things happen is almost as important as *what* happens. Of all forms of timing, patients almost certainly value most the timing of entry into the system—getting *to* care when the care is needed. *Care* in this context does not mean only encounters or visits. It means all appropriate forms of interaction, including access to information, support, dialogue, reassurance, treatment, and supplies, as well as all possible routes of delivery—not just face-to-face meetings, but also electronic, print, and other media of exchange.

Interactions. Health care is fundamentally interaction. Interaction is not the price of or vehicle for care; it *is* the care. Those who regard health care as a list of resources—people, medications, machines, technologies, and so forth—are merely listing the "inert" ingredients that become care only when they are combined in interactions between patients and the system. The quality of care is the quality of interaction among resources, not the quality of the resources per se.

Reliability. Reliability involves ensuring an exact match between knowledge and activity in the IDCOP practice. Ideally, "all and only" effective and helpful care is given. The IDCOP practice, therefore, aims *always* to give care that can

help a patient and *never* to give care that harms or cannot help a patient. Reliability is the conscious attempt to avoid the defects in health care that the Institute of Medicine Roundtable on Quality summarizes as "overuse, underuse, and misuse" of care. (The Roundtable defines misuse as errors in care and threats to patient safety.)

Vitality. IDCOP aims for a sustainable design. The new system would be financially viable and would provide a great workplace. In other words, the demanding performance standard is not realized at the expense of those who work in the practice and depend upon it for their livelihood. Vitality also implies renewal—continual innovation and improvement. The IDCOP practice is not a fixed, solved system; it is a learning organization with the capability, agility, resilience, and will to change over time as desires, environments, and knowledge change.

Each of these themes or aspects of IDCOP requires certain activities, some familiar and some new. One of the initial steps to redesigning the system as a whole is the systematic examination of the current premises and beliefs concerning the activities performed and the people who perform them. Meeting each of the goals requires some resource deployment and scheduling. To achieve excellent *access*, the demand for visits and other interactions must be estimated beforehand, and capacity, for example for appointments, must be available to meet the demand. Conceiving of care as *interactions* between the patient and the system via multiple media means that resources must be deployed to enable these interactions. *Reliability* requires an exact match between knowledge and activity in the practice, knowing the activities that will meet the needs of patients and ensuring that these activities are performed in an orderly manner and at the proper time. The activities that contribute to the *vitality* of a practice, such as training and process redesign, might easily be put off in the face of pressing daily demands, but these activities are essential. Hence, time must be scheduled for them.

Besides helping with the daily deployment of resources, the development of a master schedule for the practice will facilitate the fundamental rethinking of the design of the practice. The following three tasks serve as a guide to the deployment of resources consistent with the IDCOP themes:

1. Understand and define the *work* involved in caring for persons who depend on the practice.
2. Assemble a *team* of people and resources to match the work.
3. Develop a *repetitive master schedule* to optimize the use of resources relative to the needs of the population.

Defining the work involves describing activities in the practice and then assessing them in terms of the four themes. The activities can then be adjusted to ensure that the practice has all four characteristics and the appropriate clinician matched with the work. Once the work and appropriate team have been identified, the practice can match the work to the members of the team on specific days of the week using a repetitive master schedule.

REPETITIVE MASTER SCHEDULE

The work of a clinical practice is varied and complex—no two patients are alike, insurance companies have different requirements, and the external environment is changing rapidly. Designing an IDCOP practice is impossible unless some sense of order is established in the midst of increasing demands and varying conditions. Developing and using a repetitive master schedule is one method of establishing order.

Although the work varies, every practice has a natural rhythm—the length of time after which the work begins to repeat. Staff in a primary care practice often cite one week as the repetitive period. Up to a point, the work done in one week is similar to the work done the next week. Of course, the rhythm in a practice is also influenced by shorter periods, such as days, and longer seasonal periods that must also be taken into account.

The practice must first establish the period for which a master schedule will be designed. For purposes of discussion, let's assume the period is one week. That means that a master schedule for a "typical" week can be used with minor adjustments for any week. The definition of the repetitive period simplifies the task of deploying the resources of the practice because the schedule is built only for a short period of time.

Once the period has been chosen, a master schedule can answer the questions of what work will be done, who will do it, when they will do it, and where they will do it. An IDCOP practice calls for forms of interaction in addition to one-on-one visits with the doctor. Who will be using e-mail? Who will provide chronic disease management and review registries? When will training and staff development take place? The master schedule should provide answers to these questions.

The slogan for a master schedule with a period of one week is "do today's work today." Although there is some overlap in each day's work, Tuesday's work will not be exactly the same as Thursday's. The practice may hold a group visit on Tuesday, for example, and review the chronic disease registries on Thursday. Daily work should be completed on the day it is scheduled.

"Open access" requires that patients be scheduled within the master schedule cycle. Hence, practice-patient interactions are a very large component of the master schedule. Backlogs are defined as work that is not scheduled or completed within the master scheduling period. Consider a patient's initial appointment in a behavioral health practice. Because the initial appointment requires that multiple providers see the patient during the visit, a practice may designate one morning a week for initial appointments. The "open access" philosophy requires that new patients be seen within a week. Backlogs of two or more weeks for new patients are inconsistent with the repetitive master scheduling approach.

Open access and repetitive master scheduling are based on the general concept of "continuous flow," which requires that the amount of work be predicted and resources deployed to complete the work in a specified period of time without backlogs. Continuous flow principles apply to weekly scheduling and even daily scheduling. The physician who sees a patient and completes the chart before moving on to the next patient within the specified activity cycle time is using continuous flow.

Many practices already use some aspects of master scheduling. Practices with open access to visits and phone calls are well along in the development of a repetitive master schedule. For practices that wish to develop a master schedule the following steps should be considered:

1. Implement an open access system for visiting patients.
2. Define the care process for each of the top diagnoses to use as input to the master schedule. Include in the definition the desired time between when a patient first presents with the problem and when an effective plan of treatment is begun.
3. List the services required to accomplish the themes and the internal processes required to support these services.
4. Devise a master schedule of one to two weeks that addresses who, what, where, and when for the services and processes enumerated above.
5. Use the following metrics to assess success in executing the master schedule:
   a. the degree of completion of the schedule and the reasons for not achieving it
   b. the percentage of time physicians are doing work that only they can do or that only they are legally allowed to do
   c. the time from patient presentation to treatment for the top 10 diagnoses

Information Technology for Clinical Applications and Microsystems

Engineering and the System Environment

Paul C. Tang
Palo Alto Medical Foundation

I will address three questions: (1) how engineering can help determine characteristics of a desirable information infrastructure; (2) how engineering can help establish data standards; and (3) how engineering can help build an information infrastructure for health care.

Ethnography, the social science method of studying human cultures in the field, is a useful technique for understanding information needs in the health care environment. A derivative technique, video ethnography, includes the video recording of subjects in their natural state. With the consent of patients and physicians, we used observational ethnography and video ethnography to study the information-seeking habits of physicians.

Time and motion studies have shown that physicians spend up to 38 percent of their time foraging for data in the paper medical record and creating more data for the record (Mamlin and Baker, 1973). Formal studies of physicians' information needs showed that 81 percent of the time they were unable to find one to 20 pieces of information (four pieces on average) important to a specific patient visit at the time decisions were being made (Tang et al., 1994). Although physicians often spent additional time trying to track down the missing information, including asking patients what they might have heard, they often ended up making decisions without the information, even though they had the paper-based medical record 95 percent of the time. In summary, although clinical decision making depends on the availability of patient data, domain information, and administrative information, these data are routinely not available when physicians make patient-care decisions.

In *Crossing the Quality Chasm*, the Institute of Medicine stated that "American health care is incapable of providing the public with the quality health care it expects and deserves." Furthermore, "if we want safer, higher-quality care, we will need to have redesigned systems of care, including the use of information technology to support clinical and administrative processes" (IOM, 2001). There are many challenges to be overcome in transforming health care via information technology. Some of the environmental barriers to the adoption of information technology are: high capital acquisition costs for electronic medical records (EMR); an inadequate supply of fully functioning EMR systems; high training costs for EMR implementation; and uncertainty about who will pay and who will benefit.

Another challenge facing the health care system is the lack of an effective mechanism for knowledge diffusion. Even though medical knowledge is increasing very rapidly, the diffusion of medical knowledge into practice has been limited by the absence of decision support at the point of care. Compliance with the guidelines for influenza vaccinations is a good example. It is well known that administering the influenza vaccine to eligible adults can halve the death rate, halve the hospital admission rate, and halve the costs associated with outbreaks of influenza. Nevertheless, because of human oversight, physicians immunize only 50 to 60 percent of the eligible patients they see during flu season. Simple computer-based reminders at the time of a patient's visit have been shown to increase adherence to the simple clinical guideline by 78 percent compared to controls (Tang et al., 1999). Engineering techniques, such as EMR systems that remind physicians at the moment of opportunity, have been proven effective.

Another area of opportunity for engineering is in resolving cross-organizational issues that impede health care delivery. Health care is delivered in many settings, by multiple providers, and over a period of time. Yet, because of an absence of standards, neither the paper system nor computer-based systems allow for the seamless, reliable exchange of data across settings of care. The current health care delivery model is highly fragmented and poorly designed. Furthermore, current health care financing schemes create disincentives to the creation of any kind of *system* of care. Engineering could make a major contribution by applying systems design and analysis techniques to the health care delivery system.

Another area of opportunity is at the interface between devices and information systems. As living beings, patients constantly emit signals, but there is no instrumentation to capture and filter those signals. At best, information is gathered at random intervals determined by the vagaries of matching schedules rather than by clinical events. As the care of patients is transferred from one clinic to another or to a specialist or to a hospital, the inefficiency of these "handoffs" further impedes the delivery of coordinated care. We have also failed to provide patients with tools to help themselves. We must do a better job.

Engineering can help provide methods for the continuous gathering of data at patients' homes, the automatic filtering of data, and alerts to care providers when there are deviations from expected control points. EMRs with evidence-based decision support can improve the diffusion and implementation of best practices. Collaborative work technologies—among providers and between patients and providers—could be applied to patient care.

In short, twenty-first century clinicians have been practicing medicine with twentieth-century information tools. We need a National Health Information Infrastructure (NHII) to support the information-driven practice of contemporary medicine. This infrastructure would consist of standards for connectivity, system interoperability, data content and exchange, applications, and laws. The challenge is to design, develop, and implement these necessary systems in a resource-constrained environment. Financing NHII and reimbursing the costs of ongoing operation will be key to the widespread adoption of engineering and information technology that supports the delivery of care.

There are many engineering opportunities in building the NHII. First, we will need a technical infrastructure that includes standards to enable systems to interoperate technically and semantically. Second, the system must have an application infrastructure that supports mobile, secure, and robust functionality that can access patient information wherever it is stored. Third, there must be an interoperable method of storing structured, executable knowledge that can be used at the point of care by any qualified provider. Fourth, policies must be in place to protect sensitive, confidential patient information stored and transmitted by these systems. And finally, there must be a financing and incentive model that provides investment resources for the implementation and continuing operation of patient care systems.

Engineering opportunities abound to address the information-technology needs of health care. At the top of the list is the need for a systems perspective and repertoire of methods in the study and design of a rational health care system that serves the diverse needs of current and future patient populations. Monitoring technologies that process and interpret high-volume data and mine the important information therein would be useful. A secure, wireless infrastructure would support patient and provider mobility. Interoperability, for both computers and people, would be important for collaboration among providers and patients. Knowledge diffusion tools would be important to help physicians keep up with fast-paced advances in medical knowledge. Tools to assist with distributed authoring of key technical standards would help accelerate the development of essential technical standards. Methods of managing the constant queues in scheduling scarce medical resources would help distribute medical services to those who need them.

In summary, delivering patient-centered, evidence-based, safe care is an expectation of twenty-first century health care. To deliver on that expectation, we need sophisticated, computer-based tools, and an NHII. That is the engineering challenge—and the engineering opportunity.

REFERENCES

IOM (Institute of Medicine). 2001. Crossing the Quality Chasm: A New Health System for the 21st Century. Washington, D.C.: National Academy Press.

Mamlin, J.J., and D.H. Baker. 1973. Combined time-motion and work sampling study in a general medicine clinic. Medical Care 11(5): 449–456.

Tang, P.C., D. Fafchamps, and E.H. Shortliffe. 1994. Traditional medical records as a source of clinical data in the outpatient setting. Pp. 575–579 in Proceedings of the 18th Symposium on Computer Applications for Medical Care. Philadelphia: Hanley & Belfus Inc. Medical Publishers.

Tang, P.C., M.P. LaRosa, C. Newcomb, and S.M. Gorden. 1999. Measuring the effects of reminders for outpatient influenza immunizations at the point of clinical opportunity. Journal of the American Medical Informatics Association 6(2): 115–121.

Challenges in Informatics

William W. Stead
Vanderbilt University Medical Center

The ultimate purpose of information technology is to help everyone make better decisions, no matter what their role in the system. Biomedical informatics is the structuring of information into simple systems that clarify complex relationships, reveal relationships between similar or related information from disparate sources, and link that information into the work flow.

Implementing a solution can be difficult, however, because current tools were built largely to administrate and automate processes instead of to provide information to help us function more effectively. The value of information decays exponentially over time. Without effective information technology, information moves very slowly through administrative processes or publication channels. The object of information technology is to move information quickly so it can be assimilated into decision-making processes at the right time.

Let me give you an example from Vanderbilt. A few years ago, we noted that physicians were ordering many more tests than could be justified. They did this for one simple reason—the tests were routine. We put an intervention in place to address this problem. Physicians now have a decision-support tool that shows them patient data and local and national guidelines at the time they are making ordering decisions. When a physician tries to order basic chemistries, for example, a screen pops up showing graphically the results of previous tests for that patient and highlighting which chemistries are stable. With that information, physicians may choose to order tests just for the chemistries that are changing or the ones they think need to be done. With this change, we reduced the number of basic chemistries ordered by 60 percent.

Two trends in information technology will be particularly important for the management and provision of knowledge in health care. First, with the convergence of media, computing, and communication, all information will be available in digital form. The information will be easily accessible and available at minimum cost, which means we will be able to provide the most appropriate information organized to meet an objective. Second, the continuing movement toward smaller, cheaper, faster technology will result in better user interfaces and embedded, context-sensitive sensors that can identify the time, location, and function of a technology. This will eliminate a large number of data entry problems.

When data displays in fighter cockpits became too big, too numerous, and too fast for pilots to react, virtual reality displays were developed to create patterns they could recognize. Thus, data were turned into useful signals, and overload was eliminated. The same kind of advancements will be made in health care.

One of the trends in informatics is the development of an architecture that allows you to separate the content from the tools. Historically, information systems have held information about how we practice hostage. When we separate the content from the tools we use to automate processes, the information becomes scalable and much more useful. We will have to figure out how to protect information about patients and about how we practice. This will require a system that keeps the information separate and encapsulates it in digital rights technology, so that the patient can always pull the key. Caregivers, however, are not trained to protect privacy, so unless "We shall not violate privacy" becomes their Hippocratic oath, we will not be able to reap the benefits of new information technologies.

A second trend concerns process redesign. We are working on new approaches based on constant communication between the different parts of a distributed system process. This will lead to changes in the educational system based on a model of continuous education in which teaching is done with tools and techniques that students use as they move forward. Instead of credentials being based on completion of a curriculum, credentials would be based on competencies built up over time and on learning records and outcome records. This will lead to changes in traditional roles. The role of the physician would change from intermediary and prescriber to coach. Our current concept of patient compliance is backwards. If a physician prescribes something that doesn't fit in with a patient's life style, the patient probably won't follow it. Instead of working with the patient to develop a regime the patient is likely to follow, we label the patient noncompliant.

One of the challenges facing informatics designers is the need for standard structures for representing biomedical knowledge, data, and patient data. We will also need people who can certify that products are in compliance with various standards. We will need a payer system with incentives for installing the informatics infrastructure and for people to use it.

People will need new skills, such as data-driven practice improvement, to perform well in this new environment. Physicians at Vanderbilt were surprised when they were presented with data about how they actually practice. They suddenly realized the variability in how they practice. Another new skill will be learning at "teachable moments" instead of trying to learn "just in case." If a physician reads two articles every night, he will be 800 years behind at the end of the first year. Physicians will have to learn new ways to learn. Physicians and other care providers will also, of course, continue to provide traditional care and comfort.

SUMMARY

Some of the challenges facing the developers of informatics for health care delivery are listed below:

- standard structures for representing biomedical knowledge, protocols, and patient data
- techniques for modeling diversity
- digital certification and rights technology
- decision-support tools that reduce the caregiver's workload
- certification of products for compliance with standards
- incentives

Some of the new skills caregivers will require are listed below:

- data-driven practice improvement
- privacy, confidentiality, security
- learning at teachable moments
- distributed clinical trials
- licensing of intellectual property

Traditional skills that all caregivers will need are listed below:

- comforting patients
- observing patients
- reflecting patients' values
- knowing what one needs to know
- recognizing patterns

A National Standard for Medication Use

David Classen
First Consulting Group

The unsafe use of medication is not the only safety problem in the health care system, but it is certainly one of the most significant. Most published studies about patient safety relate to the use of medication, and a lot of attention has been focused on improving the safety of medication use (Classen, 1998, 2000, 2003; Classen and Metzger, 2003; Classen et al., 1991, 1992a,b; Evans et al., 1994). Ensuring a safer medication system at an organizational level, as well as at the national level, is a major challenge that involves engineering, information technology, and the overall health care system. The creation of a national standard is very much a work in progress.

Engineers tend to think in terms of process, and this is also one way to approach the issue of medication management. From a process perspective, medication management is multidisciplinary and highly complex. Interestingly enough, in most organizations it is also a largely manual process. Even if the process of providing medications goes well, the system must be monitored prospectively to detect when things begin to go wrong. Surveillance will be one component of an improved system.

Most studies have shown that the use of medications is very risky for patients. We must incorporate what we know from the literature about risks—especially two kinds of risk. One is medication errors—errors that occur in the medication process but usually do not lead to harm to the patient. For instance, one common medication error is giving medication a few minutes late, which rarely causes harm to the patient. Another kind of risk is adverse drug events—events that actually do cause harm to patients. These two kinds of risk overlap but are not concurrent (Classen et al., 1997).

A process model showing where and how errors occur reveals that at least a quarter of the events that harm patients occur during the administration phase of the process. Many of these errors involve IV fluids rather than pills. Interventions to improve the safety of the medication process should initially be focused on the events that harm patients, rather than on the more numerous events that do not. The process model also shows that interventions in the prescribing and transcribing phases of the process could affect almost 60 percent of events that adversely impact patients (Classen et al., 1997).

One change that could affect a substantial percentage of events that harm patients is computerized physician order entry (CPOE), which is being adopted all across the country. My company, First Consulting Group, is working on a national safety standard for CPOE (Kilbridge et al., 2001; Metzger and Turisco, 2001). Another group, the Leapfrog Group, a large employer group dedicated to improving health care, is aggressively pushing for the implementation of standards (Leapfrog Group, 2003). So far, Leapfrog has focused on three proven safety practices it believes could markedly improve the safety of health care (Classen, 2003). A fourth standard, which will touch on CPOE and will be the first ambulatory standard, is about to be issued. The new standard will relate to the electronic retrieval of laboratory results and the electronic prescribing of medications for outpatients. Leapfrog intends to introduce standards in certain regions of the country and engage business leaders to pressure health care organizations to adopt the standards. But these standards have also stimulated interest in a national standard for CPOE (Classen, 2003).

The Leapfrog CPOE standard has several components. First, it will require physicians to enter medication orders for inpatients via a computer system linked to error-prevention software. Second, it will require documented acknowledgement by the prescribing physician of any interception (warning or alert) prior to an override. Third, the hospital or health care organization will be required to demonstrate that the CPOE system picks up at least half of the most common serious errors. There has been a great deal of debate about the third component (Kilbridge et al., 2001).

An organization cannot simply put in a CPOE system and say it meets the standards, because the literature shows that there is a great deal of variability in the safety impact of CPOE systems (Bates et al., 1995; Classen et al., 1997; Evans et al., 1998; Kilbridge et al., 2001; Leape et al., 1995). The debate has centered on whether a national standard should require that CPOE systems be tested for safety using simulations. The literature shows that CPOE systems can have a wide range of effects on safety. One study of a CPOE system at Brigham and Women's Hospital in Boston showed there was a significant decrease in medication errors, but a much smaller decrease in actual harm to patients (Bates et al., 1998). A study at another hospital showed there was a much larger decrease in adverse drug events with CPOE (Evans et al., 1998). The differences between these two studies have raised a number of questions (Classen, 2003).

The Institute of Safe Medicare Practices conducted another study of a CPOE system testing electronically ordered medications at the pharmacy level, the level at which most medications are ordered (ISMP, 1999). For the test, 10 unsafe orders were created posing 10 different problems. For instance, a drug toxic to the kidney was ordered for a patient with markedly elevated kidney function. The 10 unsafe orders were sent to 304 pharmacies around the country. Some of them caught a few of the errors, but only four of the 304 picked up all 10. And remember, these sites had systems designed to pick up errors.

A second study focused on the drug Cisapride, which was withdrawn from the market after six or seven years because it was found to interact adversely with a number of commonly used drugs (Jones et al., 2001). The FDA issued three very strong warnings that prescribing Cisapride with contraindicated drugs could be fatal. This study of how Cisapride was being prescribed in a managed care system showed that the drug was often prescribed for patients taking contraindicated drugs. Half of the time, the contraindicated drugs were ordered by the same physician; 90 percent of the time, the prescriptions were filled by the same pharmacy. When the pharmacies were investigated, it was discovered that pharmacists had turned off aspects of the safety systems in the interest of saving time.

As these studies show, having a system in place does not equal safe operation. Both studies created a lot of angst about the value of a national standard in this area. Another test, a simulation of installed CPOE systems that evaluated if they met safety standards, has led to some changes (Kilbridge et al., 2001). A variety of categories were developed, based on the points at which very common errors occurred (e.g., therapeutic duplication, ordering too high a dose, and ordering a drug to which the patient is allergic). Other areas that were tested included corollary orders (Overhage et al., 1997). For instance, if a patient is admitted with a seizure disorder, a physician may put the patient on a seizure drug but not specify the dosage. Cost was also tested. For instance, sometimes within an hour or two the same test was ordered twice. Another area tested was nuisance alerts (Kilbridge et al., 2001). If safety systems have too many warnings, physicians

tend either to ignore all of them or refuse to use the system. Deception analysis was also tested (i.e., orders intended to test safety) (Kilbridge et al., 2001).

The 12 organizations tested in the first round showed a very high degree of variability in impact on medication safety. This is still a work in progress, however. The test I just described was designed for inpatients; a test for outpatients is being designed (Classen, 2003).

So far, we have learned three major lessons from testing this national safety standard. First, the impact on safety depends on how a system is installed and used rather than on which system is used. Second, CPOE had the greatest impact on safety in organizations with the most clinical decision support. Third, organizations with highly disparate systems (clinical applications from several different vendors) did not score well.

REFERENCES

Bates, D.W., D.J. Cullen, N. Laird, L.A. Petersen, S.D. Small, D. Servi, G. Laffel, B.J. Sweitzer, B.F. Shea, R. Hallisey, et al. 1995. Incidence of adverse drug events and potential adverse drug events: implications for prevention: ADE prevention study group. Journal of the American Medical Association 274(1): 29–34.

Bates, D.W., L.L. Leape, D.J. Cullen, N. Laird, L.A. Petersen, J.M. Teich, E. Burdick, M. Hickey, S. Kleefield, B. Shea, M. Vander Vliet, and D.L. Seger. 1998. Effect of computerized physician order entry and a team intervention on prevention of serious medication errors. Journal of the American Medical Association 280(15): 1311–1316.

Classen, D.C. 1998. Clinical decision support systems to improve clinical practice and quality of care. Journal of the American Medical Association 280(15): 1360–1361.

Classen, D.C. 2000. Patient safety, thy name is quality. Trustee 53(9): 12–15.

Classen, D.C. 2003. Medication safety: moving from illusion to reality. Journal of the American Medical Association 289(9): 1154–1156.

Classen, D.C., and J. Metzger. 2003. Improving medication safety: the measurement conundrum and where to start. International Journal for Quality in Health Care. Accepted for publication, Fall 2003.

Classen, D.C., J.P. Burke, S.L. Pestotnik, R.S. Evans, and L.E. Stevens. 1991. Surveillance for quality assessment IV: surveillance using a hospital information system. Infection Control and Hospital Epidemiology 12(4): 239–244.

Classen, D.C., R.S. Evans, S.L. Pestotnik, S.D. Horn, R.L. Menlove, and J.P. Burke. 1992a. The timing of prophylactic administration of antibiotics and the risk of surgical-wound infection. New England Journal of Medicine 326(5): 281–286.

Classen, D.C., S.L. Pestotnik, R.S. Evans, and J.P. Burke. 1992b. Description of a computerized adverse drug event monitor using a hospital information system. Hospital Pharmacy 27(9): 774, 776–779, 783.

Classen, D.C., S.L. Pestotnik, R.S. Evans, J.F. Lloyd, and J.P. Burke. 1997. Adverse drug events in hospitalized patients: excess length of stay, extra costs, and attributable mortality. Journal of the American Medical Association 277(4): 301–306.

Evans, R.S., S.L. Pestotnik, D.C. Classen, S.D. Horn, S.B. Bass, and J.P. Burke. 1994. Preventing adverse drug events in hospitalized patients. Annals of Pharmacotherapy 28(4): 523–527.

Evans, R.S., S.L. Pestotnik, D.C. Classen, T.P. Clemmer, L.K. Weaver, J. Orme Jr., J.F. Lloyd, and J.P. Burke. 1998. A computer-assisted management program for antibiotics and other anti-infective agents. New England Journal of Medicine 338(4): 232–238.

ISMP (Institute for Safe Medication Practices). 1999. Over-reliance on pharmacy computer systems may place patients at great risk. ISMP Medication Safety Alert 4(3). Available online at: *http://www.ismp.org/MSAarticles/Computer.html*.

Jones, J.K., D. Fife, S. Curkendall, E. Goehring Jr., J.J. Guo, and M. Shannon. 2001. Coprescribing and codispensing of Cisapride and contraindicated drugs. Journal of the American Medical Association 286(13): 1607–1609.

Kilbridge, P., D.C. Classen, and E. Welebob. 2001. Overview of The Leapfrog Group test standard for computerized physician order entry. Report by First Consulting Group to The Leapfrog Group, November 2001. Available online at: *http://www.fcg.com/research/serve-research.asp?rid=40*.

Leapfrog Group. 2003. Factsheet: Computer Physician Order Entry. Available online at: *http://www.leapfroggroup.org/FactSheets/CPOE_FactSheet.pdf*.

Leape, L.L., D.W. Bates, D.J. Cullen, J. Cooper, H.J. Demonaco, T. Gallivan, R. Hallisey, J, Ives, N. Laird, G. Laffel, et al. 1995. Systems analysis of adverse drug events: ADE prevention study group. Journal of the American Medical Association 274(1): 35–43.

Metzger, J., and F. Turisco. 2001. Computerized physician order entry: a look at the vendor marketplace and getting started. Report by First Consulting Group to The Leapfrog Group, December 2001. Available online at: *http://www.informatics-review.com/thoughts/cpoe-leap.html*.

Overhage, J.M., W.M. Tierney, X.H. Zhou, and C.J. McDonald. 1997. A randomized trial of "corollary orders" to prevent errors of omission. Journal of the American Medical Informatics Association 4(5): 364–375.

Obstacles to the Implementation and Acceptance of Electronic Medical Record Systems

Paul D. Clayton
Intermountain Health Care and
University of Utah

If an investigator could come up with a big yellow pill that would reduce the length of hospital stays by 10 percent for all patients across the board, then that investigator would be a serious candidate for the Nobel prize. The issue in this paper is whether "information intervention" can accomplish the same goal as a big yellow pill.

The benefits of electronic medical records systems have been highlighted in several reports released by the Institute of Medicine (IOM, 1991, 1997, 2001):

- convenient, rapid access (by legitimate stakeholders) to organized, legible patient data
- links from displayed information to pertinent literature
- automated generation of alerts, reminders, and suggestions when standards of care are not being met
- analysis of population databases for clinical research, epidemiological assessments, quality measures, and outcomes
- lower costs
- better service to providers and patients

Although good examples of electronic medical records exist, the industry in general has not yet implemented systems that can routinely provide all of the desired functionality. In this paper, I describe the obstacles keeping us from enjoying the potential benefits of these systems. There are high-level obstacles, such as the absence of institutional commitment and the lack of capital, and low-level obstacles that have more to do with engineering, functionality, and technical issues.

The biggest obstacle is the lack of institutional commitment. Many hospitals in the United States are losing money and cannot afford all of the technologies and services they would like. Because it takes at least a decade to select and implement a comprehensive clinical information system, beleaguered executives are often reluctant to initiate a long-range strategic project that they might not be able to see through to fruition. Lack of commitment may also be attributable to concerns about demonstrable returns on investment in information technology, and there are some examples of wasteful failures (Littlejohns et al., 2003). However, the number of well documented examples of financial savings and improved quality is increasing (Pestotnik et al., 1996; Wang et al., 2003). Even if the cost and quality benefits of clinical information systems are appreciated and the institutional leadership is committed to the idea, the lack of capital remains an issue both for hospitals that are losing money and for private practices.

In fact, the benefits of investments in information systems often accrue to the payer rather than to the care provider. For example, if the blood glucose levels of a patient with diabetes can be monitored remotely, the patient may require fewer office or hospital visits to treat complications of the disease. Some payers now offer a premium for care provided with the assistance of competent information systems. The Leapfrog Group, for example, pays extra to hospitals that have computerized physician order entry. The problem is that there are many payers, and all of them want to lower costs for the patients they insure by having providers use information systems that support standards of care. If United Health Care promotes one standard for people with diabetes and Intermountain Health Care (IHC) supports a slightly different standard that requires additional data, how does a physician know which standard or information system to use? Another challenge is keeping standards of care up to date on a national basis (Shekelle et al., 2001).

A nontechnical obstacle is the lack of people who understand clinical practice, project management, and software technology and who have practical strategic vision, wisdom, and experience. We need people with both education in medical informatics and a sense of economic considerations. We currently have openings for such people that we cannot fill.

A partly technical, but mostly sociological, obstacle is maintaining a longitudinal medical record for patients being cared for by multiple parties. If the care is episodic, the benefits of an electronic medical record may not accrue. One provider may enter allergies and prescriptions into a system, but when the patient visits a second provider, that information may not be available. Patients often switch insurers (on average, once every four years); they may see a primary care physician, multiple specialists, and be treated at different hospitals, nursing homes, and emergency rooms. In the 1980s and 1990s, the Hartford Foundation attempted to build community health information networks, but as of 1995, with one or two exceptions, when the grant support diminished, these models disintegrated because of complex legal, organizational, funding, and control issues (Duncan, 1995). The problem was not only the reluctance of competitors to facilitate easy switching of providers by patients, but also the question of how to identify individual patients. Even in communities that have networks (e.g., state childhood vaccination registries), when a patient goes from provider to provider, it is difficult to consolidate information because duplicate versions of the same patient contain fragments of the record; often merged information from more than one patient creates an inaccurate composite. Some have suggested that we use a national patient identifier akin to a Social Security number. But cost and privacy implications have impeded progress in that direction, even though such an identifier was mandated in the original Health Insurance Portability and Accountability Act of 1996 (P.L. 104-191). Standards for providers and payers have been established, but individual patient identifiers have not. Then, in 1998, Congress rescinded the original requirement and forbade the U.S. Department of Health and Human Services from issuing ID numbers. Several approaches to this problem have been identified (Appavu, 1997). For obvious reasons, countries in which government is the single payer for health care have been more successful in addressing the problems of unique identifiers.

The problems discussed to this point have been addressed by IHC in Salt Lake City. However, few organizations in the country can emulate them. IHC is an integrated health delivery network with 21 hospitals, 400 physicians who practice in 90 ambulatory clinics, and a health insurance plan that has affiliations with another 2,500 physicians. IHC provides health insurance for a half-million people and brokers insurance for another half-million; we provide care for more than 50 percent of the population of the intermountain region. The IHC patient population and facilities are distributed over a 400 mile geographic area connected by high-speed networks. But even in this organization, in which investment in information systems (3.9 percent of gross revenues) is considered a key to the delivery of high-quality, cost-effective care, we still have problems. In the remainder of this paper, I will discuss the technical problems facing IHC.

In the 1960s, work began on an electronic medical record system for hospitals. This system, known as HELP, generates automatic alerts, reminders, and suggestions based on logical criteria used to evaluate coded data recorded in the patient database. The suggestions have been well received by clinicians and have been shown to improve care (Pryor et al., 1983). In 1992, IHC realized the need for a longitudinal medical record that could provide for continuity of care, regardless of where the patient was located (e.g., hospital, clinic, or home).

Figure 1 shows the basic architecture of our current approach. The system is based on: (1) a master patient index, in which local medical record numbers/identifiers for each person are mapped to a unique, persistent identifier; and (2) a longitudinal patient database (clinical data repository) that includes as much health-related information as we are able to capture for each of 1.45 million patients. This clinical repository is designed for optimum retrieval of data for a single patient.

A separate enterprise data warehouse (that includes cost information as well as clinical data) is used for population research, quality improvement, and cost analysis. About a dozen people are devoted full time to analyzing the data in this population-oriented warehouse.

Data are entered using a variety of applications and are transmitted to the clinical data repository. Necessary data captured in one application are shared via interfaces with other applications that may need particular data items. For example, when a patient encounter is created in one of our registration systems, the information is fed to the billing system, the laboratory system, the operating room scheduling system, and other relevant systems. The interfaces are complicated, because even simple things like the concept of gender are not standardized (radiology uses M and F, pharmacy uses one and zero, and laboratory uses zero and one). A dictionary contains coded identifiers for medical concepts and mappings from the canonical description of that concept to the analogous vocabulary used by other systems that have been developed by vendors independently of our nomenclature. This mapping allows us to build interfaces that communicate with independent systems using their native languages and still maintain a canonical representation of information for generating alerts and reports, regardless of the origin of the data. Eight people are devoted full time to management of the dictionary content and data models.

Implementing each interface costs us as much as $50,000 because there are no universally accepted vocabularies or data models in the health care industry. We currently employ 22 people to implement and maintain our 60 or so interfaces. Under current conditions, the interfaces are just as expensive for smaller organizations, which do not have our level of resources. In 1997, the interface issue was identified as a major obstacle by Clem McDonald (1997), one of the leaders trying to develop standards for vocabulary and messaging formats. A group known as Health Level 7 (HL7) is trying to promote standards, but vendors are resistant because of their investment in existing product platforms and because they do not want to make it easy for purchasers to

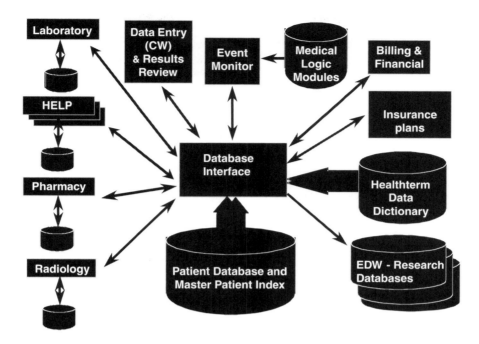

FIGURE 1 An overview of the IHC information architecture. This architecture reflects the philosophy that data should be entered only once regardless of the source and that multiple independent components can be integrated. The entry of data or the passage of time evokes the event monitor, which evaluates medical logic to produce, when warranted, alerts, reminders, and suggestions. Source: Clayton et al., 2003.

switch vendors or to buy components from multiple vendors. Few institutions have the resources to drive market demand for interoperability (HL7, 2003).

The IHC system also has a rules engine triggered by the arrival of new data or the passage of time. Logical criteria are used to evaluate patient data to generate patient-specific alerts, reminders, and suggestions, when appropriate. Because these alerts must be generated in real time, the design of the data dictionary and the clinical data repository has extremely challenging requirements (Bakken et al., 2000; Huff et al., 1998; Johnson 1996). New data items must be stored without adding new tables. Response time for queries generated by users and the rules engine must be minimal (up to 500 queries per second). The database should not be taken down for maintenance, but because the system is very complex, we have trouble keeping it up 24 hours a day, seven days a week. Therefore, we have redundant hardware. Despite our best quality-assurance efforts, however, we still have problems, especially when we make software changes. We need better tools for managing complex systems.

All of our coded medications, problems, and laboratory values, can be linked via an "info button" to five or six standard questions about a particular patient diagnosis/problem, medication, or laboratory test result (Cimino, 1996; Reichert et al., 2002). With three clicks of a button, one can be reading a paragraph that provides a concise answer to the question at hand. The problem is that publishers publish books,

not paragraphs. We need reference literature that is marked up and searchable quickly.

The most vexing unsolved problem involves data capture. When we link instruments, such as infusion pumps, respirators, spirometers, labor and delivery monitors, or ICU monitors to our system, the devices need to "know" the identity of the subject and must transmit data in a way that can be easily accommodated. As more and more monitoring takes place in the home, these challenges will become more difficult. We have documented that monitoring (blood glucose, blood pressure, weight in heart failure patients, etc.) patients at home is cost effective, especially for patients with certain chronic diseases. The effectiveness of therapy would be greatly improved if we had unobtrusive ways to ascertain whether people were routinely taking their medications.

Studies have shown that nurses spend one-third of their time at work dealing with documentation. For every hour of direct patient care, they spend up to an hour documenting that care (PricewaterhouseCooper, 2001). Estimates for physicians are not as high, but the time required is still significant. Individuals can enter data by typing text, dictating and having someone else transcribe the dictation, using bar codes or other scanning devices, filling in forms by clicking with a mouse, or letting the computer understand the spoken commands and narrative dictation. We have 20 to 30 physicians who use voice recognition, but many users (about 225 of our 400 employed physicians) prefer to use "hot text" (macros created for certain types of patients and certain types of visits that enable clinicians to change only the items that are exceptional/remarkable). We have found that this approach is much faster than dictation or clicking and that physicians in the ambulatory setting change only 3 percent of the standard text. Overall, we need to reduce the amount of required documentation, reduce the amount of duplication in documentation, and derive billing information from data collected at the point of care (rather than asking people to fill out separate billing-oriented forms).

Natural language processing is emerging as a valuable means of extracting coded, machine-processable data from narrative text (Hripcsak et al., 2002). Much of the documentation burden stems from regulatory requirements to ensure that we have provided the care for which we generate bills. In essence, regulators have added a 25-percent overhead to catch the 1 or 2 percent of crooks who abuse the system. If we could use sampling techniques instead, the 99 percent would not be punished.

Wireless mobile devices would be very convenient, but many problems would have to be overcome: battery life, screen size, the need for individualized devices (e.g., individual profiles for voice recognition), and the propensity to lose information.

Authentication is another challenge. Proximity cards, biometric markers, and other tokens present logistical challenges for rotating medical students, residents, interns, and per diem nurses. Once we have accurately identified the user, we believe that the confidentiality of patient information can be preserved, but no system, paper or electronic, is absolutely secure in the face of a truly determined investigator. At IHC, we have five criteria for allowing someone to see patient information: (1) an established *patient/provider relationship* (these relationships can often be established automatically via scheduling or registration systems); (2) other people with a *relationship to the provider* (e.g., covering partners, nurses who work with physicians, etc.) who assist in the care of that provider's patients; (3) *patient location* (if the patient is in one of our facilities); (4) *user location* (clinicians in the same facility); and (5) *user's role* (revealed information may be limited in scope). These criteria narrow the number of patients whose information can be seen by a particular user from more than a million to a few thousand. We also keep audit trails of who has looked at what data and terminate individuals who violate their agreement by looking at data when there is no legitimate need.

In the emerging Web-based, desktop paradigm, one should ideally be able to switch seamlessly from application to application (e.g., literature server, image browser, registration process), even if the applications have been developed by different vendors and run on different servers. The goal is to preserve user authentication and privileges and patient context without requiring the user to re-authenticate or reselect the patient. The approach in medicine has been to establish a standard (CCOW) (HL7, 2003). The World Wide Web consortium is addressing these same issues, and it would be nice to end up with a universal standard.

The final obstacle is facilitating best practices based on evidence, rather than on recent experience or premonition. Our approach at IHC is to create a knowledge base of problem-specific standards of care and measurable expected outcomes. After a clinician enters a problem, we generate a patient-specific work list and suggested order sets for the patient. We find that it is easier for physicians to use these order sets (modified, if appropriate) than to write their own list of 15 or so items, which may not be complete or justified. We recognize that managing this knowledge base for every individual institution will be very expensive.

I hope this brief summary of the challenges we face will stimulate those of you with applicable expertise and accomplishments in the engineering domain to help us find solutions. In the end, we hope to provide better, more cost-effective care.

REFERENCES

Appavu, S.I. 1997. Analysis of unique patient identifier options: final report. Available online at: *http://ncvhs.hhs.gov/app0.htm*.

Bakken, S., K.E. Campbell, J.J. Cimino, S.M. Huff, and W.E. Hammond. 2000. Toward vocabulary domain specifications for Health Level 7-coded data elements. Journal of the American Medical Informatics Association 7(4): 333–342.

Clayton, P.D., S.P. Narus, S.M. Huff, T.A. Pryor, P.J. Haug, T. Larkin, S. Matney, R.S. Evans, B.H. Rocha, W.A. Bowes, F.T. Holston, and M.L. Gundersen. 2003. Building a comprehensive clinical information system from components: the approach at Intermountain Health Care. Methods of Information in Medicine 42(1): 1–7.

Cimino, J.J. 1996. Linking patient information systems to bibliographic resources. Methods of Information in Medicine 35(2): 122–126.

Duncan, K.A. 1995. Evolving community health information networks. Frontiers of Health Service Management 12(1): 5–41.

HL7 (Health Level Seven, Inc). CCOW. Available online at: *http://www.hl7.org/special/Committees/ccow_sigvi.htm*.

HL7. 2003. HL7 Standards. Available online at: *http://www.hl7.org/*.

Hripcsak, G., J.H. Austin, P.O. Alderson, and C. Friedman. 2002. Use of natural language processing to translate clinical information from a database of 889,921 chest radiographic reports. Radiology 224(1): 157–163.

Huff, S.M., R.A. Rocha, H.R. Solbrig, M.W. Barnes, S.P. Schrank, and M. Smith. 1998. Linking a medical vocabulary to a clinical data model using Abstract Syntax Notation 1. Methods of Information in Medicine 37(4-5): 440–452.

IOM (Institute of Medicine). 1991. The Computer-Based Patient Record: An Essential Technology for Health Care, R.S. Dick and E.B. Steen, eds. Washington, D.C.: National Academy Press.

IOM. 1997. The Computer-Based Patient Record: An Essential Technology for Health Care (Revised Edition), R.S. Dick, E.B. Steen, and D.E. Detmer, eds. Washington, D.C.: National Academy Press.

IOM. 2001. Crossing the Quality Chasm: A New Health System for the 21st Century. Washington, D.C.: National Academy Press.

Johnson, S.B. 1996. Generic data modeling for clinical repositories. Journal of the American Medical Informatics Association 3(5): 328–339.

Littlejohns, P., J.C. Wyatt, and L. Garvican. 2003. Evaluating computerized health information systems: hard lessons still to be learnt. British Medical Journal 326: 860–863.

McDonald, C.J. 1997. Barriers to electronic medical record systems and how to overcome them. Journal of the American Medical Informatics Association 4(3): 213–221.

Pestotnik, S.L., D.C. Classen, R.S. Evans, and J.P. Burke. 1996. Implementing antibiotic practice guidelines through computer-assisted decision support: clinical and financial outcomes. Annals of Internal Medicine 124(10): 884–890.

PricewaterhouseCoopers. 2001. Patients or Paperwork?: The Regulatory Burden Facing America's Hospitals. Paper prepared for the American Hospital Association (AHA). Chicago, Illinois: AHA.

Pryor, T.A., R.M. Gardner, P.D. Clayton, and H.R. Warner. 1983. The HELP system. Journal of Medical Systems 7(2): 87–102.

Reichert, J.C., M. Glasgow, S.P. Narus, and P.D. Clayton. 2002. Using LOINC to link an EMR to the pertinent paragraph in a structured reference knowledge base. Pp. 652–656 in Proceedings of the American Medical Informatics Association Symposium 2002. Bethesda, Md.: American Medical Informatics Association.

Shekelle, P.G., E. Ortiz, S. Rhodes, S.C. Morton, M.P. Eccles, J.M. Grimshaw, and S.H. Woolf. 2001. Validity of the Agency for Healthcare Research and Quality clinical practice guidelines: how quickly do guidelines become outdated? Journal of the American Medical Association 286(12): 1461–1467.

Wang, S.J., B. Middleton, L.A. Prosser, C.G. Bardon, C.D. Spurr, P.J. Carchidi, A.F. Kittler, R.C. Goldszer, D.G. Fairchild, A.J. Sussman, G.J. Kuperman, and D.W. Bates. 2003. A cost-benefit analysis of electronic medical records in primary care. American Journal of Medicine 114(5): 397–403.

Automation of the Clinical Practice: Cost-Effective and Efficient Health Care

Prince K. Zachariah
Mayo Clinic Scottsdale

According to the American Society of Testing Material, the purpose of the health record is to present a unified, coordinated, and complete repository of genetic, environmental, and clinical health care data (ASTM, 1991). It has been estimated, however, that as much as 30 percent of the information an internist needs is not accessible during a patient's visit because of missing clinical information and missing laboratory reports (Covell et al., 1985). At the very least, this lack of information can be considered inconvenient; at worst, it may have a negative impact on patient care.

The health care record becomes highly fragmented over the life of an individual patient as care is sought from multiple practitioners with various subspecialties practicing at numerous health care institutions. For each practitioner to have a complete record, there must be frequent duplication, reiterations by multiple practitioners with potential recording or transcription errors, which, over time, affects the reliability of the information. These inherent weaknesses in the system hinder the tracking of clinical problems and often result in duplicate testing, which makes it difficult to evaluate outcomes and reduce the cost of health care.

Although the complexity of health care has increased exponentially, the patient medical record has remained essentially the same. The paper record, historically consisting of pages of handwritten notes, is archived and stored in medical records departments or warehouses managed by each health care organization that provides care. Although this antiquated method has obvious limitations, health care professionals have been reluctant to change. Now, however, pressures to change are increasing from external and internal sources because of concerns about the quality of the record, its inaccessibility to patients and health care providers, declining reimbursements, increasing medicolegal and regulatory agency reporting requirements, and many others.

At the Mayo Clinic, patient records have a long history of being well organized, thorough repositories of information. Originally designed in Rochester, Minnesota, around 1907 by Henry Plummer, M.D., the Mayo Clinic record was planned to be a comprehensive compendium of patient medical information that spans the life of the patient. Upon arrival at the clinic, each patient is registered and assigned a unique serial number. Dr. Plummer developed a central file consisting of an envelope (called a "dossier") bearing that identification number in which all of the patient's records are placed for the first and subsequent visits. Upon completion of a visit, the record is cross-indexed according to disease, surgical technique, surgical result, and pathologic findings to make record archiving and data gathering at a later date simpler. Patient number one was registered on July 19, 1907 (Clapesattle, 1954). With 88 years of experience and more than 4.5 million patient records, this invaluable database daily complements our practice. The record is designed to include a variety of forms filed in a certain order that can be easily identified by color. Today, the Mayo Clinic uses more than 350 different color or coded forms that span both outpatient and inpatient care (*Mayo Magazine*, 1989).

Historically, an elaborate manual system has been used to maintain this record. Large numbers of people are required to sort, organize, and transcribe data, as well as to file and retrieve records. Beyond organizing charts, clinic personnel manually transcribe all laboratory and x-ray results. "Green sheets" provide in one location in the record a summary of all laboratory and radiological test results arranged in chronological order. This design has allowed for a consolidation of results into a concise summary format, which reduces the bulk of the record and makes it easier to use. Patient care is both more efficient and, at the same time, simpler because of this summarization. Another benefit is that the Mayo Clinic record easily complements research activities by allowing quick access to needed information.

Over time, patient demands, as well as our own administrative and clinical work flow, have required us to increase our level of service in the midst of a changing health care system that has experienced significant reductions in reimbursements. In response to these influences, Mayo Clinic has an opportunity to improve the quality of the patient record through automation, at the same time increasing the efficiency of the physician's use of time, decreasing the patient's waiting time, and reducing expenses. We believe that the implementation of a clinical information system can improve not only the patient chart, but also our integrated practice by automating the processes of ordering, billing, scheduling, and result inquiry.

Historically, because of the limitations of computer-based patient records (CPRs), physicians have resisted using them. Concerns have included the organization of data, security, and most important, how data are entered and retrieved (Barnett, 1984). A CPR should provide patient information in a clear, intuitive format concurrently from any terminal. It should automate charge capture and improve the use of institutional resources. Finally, the process of entering data should require no more time than the manual method. In fact, it should require less time because data entered in a single, online location are automatically available in a variety of electronic formats.

According to C.J. McDonald, M.D., physicians want automated clinical records that provide access to appropriately organized patient information when they want it, in a format tailored to their needs. They also want pertinent data trends and patterns displayed, the ability to organize subsets of information, flexible reporting requirements, and order entry capability (IOM, 1991).

For Mayo Clinic to continue to provide high-quality health care with a high degree of patient satisfaction based on an integrated practice model, the shift to a CPR (the electronic medical record [EMR]) is not an option; it is a mandatory change dictated by declining revenues at a time of increased demand. A true CPR provides the automated management of a comprehensive, longitudinal health record (IOM, 1991). EMR is designed to meet this definition. Using a common format via a central system, EMR incorporates all of the elements necessary for a lifetime of care for each patient. These elements are: the medical record, laboratory reports, surgery and pathology reports, dictation and transcriptions, consultations, hospital records, radiology reports, and radiology images.

Not only are these basic components represented in an intuitive, easy-to-use graphical interface, they are accompanied by the tools necessary to customize the display to suit each user's practice style and personal preferences. The user interface integrates automated support services for ordering, scheduling, and coordinating the activities of a business office. These features are incorporated into a system that can be expanded and adapted to accommodate varied specialty care needs.

With the EMR, most of the limitations of our practice have been streamlined or eliminated. A physician's ordering and scheduling requests are automatically and immediately processed by the computer alone. The patient's schedule can be printed out almost instantly on the floor, and the patient promptly sent on his or her way. The billing information is also immediately processed and, in an electronic billing arrangement, is ready to be sent to the payer. Mayo Clinic's management will have the ability to access current clinical and financial data instantly as a basis for making practice decisions. And the record, the fixture that started this all, is legible, accessible, and reliable—in fact more accurate. In addition, there is less room for error because the radiology and laboratory reporting systems have direct data links to the EMR. The record is also more organized through the use of standardized dictation templates, whose contents vary according to the level of service, which makes billing and the justification for billing straightforward and simple.

We believe with EMR we will achieve our goal of increasing efficiency and reducing cost. The Mayo Clinic sites (Jacksonville, Rochester, and Scottsdale) are at different stages of EMR implementation because of differences in the size and complexity of the organizations. Through further automation, Mayo will meet its commitments to patients and enhance its academic mission.

The system security arrangement makes it possible to assign different levels of access to individuals, based on the information required by each care provider. System managers are granted the highest level of security access, followed by physicians, and so on, down the security ladder. Each security level restricts user access to specified documents, thereby allowing graduated access to the record but not necessarily to privileged clinical information. This approach to system security has alleviated physicians' concerns about maintaining the confidentiality of patient information.

Even though there is a strong desire to share EMR data with patients, differences in medical institutions and clinical practices and the lack of standardized data elements, common clinical vocabularies, and formatting have hampered the portability of EMR and the acquisition of data for research. However, attempts are being made to achieve commonly accepted recommendations of diagnoses and open-standard clinical vocabularies, such as SNOMED and formats like XML. To meet the challenges facing the health care system, significant automation of operational processes has become imperative, and we are attempting to meet these challenges without compromising the quality and efficiency of care.

In this discussion, I have outlined the history of the Mayo Clinic patient medical record, as well as the motivation for change at Mayo Clinic. We acknowledge that our past policies and procedures have been labor intensive, but a review of medical records practices at most other medical facilities will show that they too have tremendous operating costs for moving and managing patient medical records. From the outset, our goal has been to maintain, if not improve, patient satisfaction and the efficiency of patient care delivery. We believe that if we can achieve this goal, physician satisfaction will also be enhanced. Where EMR is available, almost instantaneous access to patient records, laboratory results, ordering, and billing services has become a practice asset to which physicians have eagerly responded.

Nevertheless, although physician acceptance has been high, there is a price. Using the EMR requires significant physician procedural rewiring. It requires significant, sometimes painful, changes in the methods and habits physicians have developed over years of clinical training and practice. Physicians have become comfortable and dependent upon the paper record, and adapting to its absence requires time and patience. In our experience, after four to eight weeks of training, physician workloads are reduced and practice volumes return to their normal levels.

The Institute of Medicine concluded that CPR should be the heart of the health care information system (IOM, 1991). It should form an individual's longitudinal health record and provide a terminal-based system that supports text and graphics, requires minimal training time, and includes a private and secure form of data entry that takes no longer to create than the paper record. The Mayo Clinic EMR meets these goals and builds upon the history of the CPR by establishing an expandable, open architecture as a foundation for future progress.

REFERENCES

ASTM (American Society for Testing and Materials). 1991. Standard Guide for Description for Content and Structure of an Automated Primary Record of Care. Standard E1384-91. West Conshohocken, Pa.: ASTM.

Barnett, G.O. 1984. The application of computer-based medical-record systems in ambulatory practice. New England Journal of Medicine 310(25): 1643–1650.

Clapesattle, H.B. 1954. The Doctors Mayo. Minneapolis, Minn.: University of Minnesota Press.

Covell, D.G., G.C. Uman, and P.R. Manning. 1985. Information needs in office practice: are they being met? Annals of Internal Medicine 103(4): 596–599.

IOM (Institute of Medicine). 1991. The Computer-Based Patient Record. Washington, D.C.: National Academy Press.

Mayo Magazine. 1989. Old records never die: medical records at the Mayo Clinic. Mayo Magazine 4(1): 2.

The eICU® Solution:
A Technology-Enabled Care Paradigm for ICU Performance

Michael J. Breslow
VISICU, Inc.

This presentation describes a broad-based effort to redesign a complex clinical environment, the intensive care unit (ICU). ICUs account for about 10 percent of inpatient beds nationwide, although in tertiary-care centers the percentage is higher. ICU patients have the highest acuity of all patients in the hospital; their mortality rate exceeds 10 percent, and their daily costs are four times higher than those of other inpatients. As a result, the ICU represents an ideal target for quality initiatives. ICU patients experience a high incidence of medical errors (1.7 per patient per day in one study), and because of their inherent instability, they are particularly vulnerable to harm from suboptimal care (Donchin et al., 1995). Improvements in care delivery can lead to substantial improvements in outcomes, both clinical and financial.

ICUs also provide major support for other areas of the hospital. Many key functional areas (e.g., emergency department, operating room) send patients to the ICU. If ICU patients are not well enough to leave the ICU, the unit becomes a bottleneck—a common problem in many urban centers—and the operation of other service areas is adversely affected. Thus, improving clinical outcomes in the ICU can improve the overall efficiency of the hospital.

Several trends in ICU care suggest a need for new systems. First, the number and acuity of ICU patients is increasing rapidly, driven primarily by the aging of the population. It is estimated that the number of patients requiring ICU care will double in the next 10 to 15 years. These changes in ICU volumes and the severity of problems are increasing demands on care providers and adversely affecting the operating effectiveness of ICUs and the throughput of patients. At the same time, there are major problems with the clinical workforce. The number of nurses choosing to work in ICUs is decreasing, and the average level of experience of the nursing force is lower than in years past.

In addition, physician coverage is inadequate to meet patient needs. ICUs with intensivists in constant attendance have been shown to have clinical outcomes superior to those of ICUs with other staffing models. The value of these specialists derives both from their expertise and from their constant monitoring and altering of care plans in response to changes in patients' clinical status. Intensivists also serve as the leaders of care teams, coordinating the activities of the many different physicians and ancillary staff who contribute to the care of ICU patients with complex conditions. Despite the clear advantages of this staffing model, less than 15 percent of U.S. hospitals have dedicated physicians in the ICU. There are many reasons hospitals do not have dedicated intensivist staffs, but the biggest problem is a severe shortage of these specialists. Fewer than 6,000 intensivists are currently in active practice. Staffing ICUs nationwide, 24 hours a day, seven days a week, would require 30,000 intensivists. Therefore, most ICUs depend on nurses to detect new problems, assess their severity, identify the appropriate physician, track him or her down, and communicate the nature of the problem—just to get a treatment order.

Despite the shortage of intensivists, the Leapfrog Group, a health care purchasing organization created by Fortune 500 companies to improve the quality of health care, has called for dedicated intensivist staffing for all nonrural U.S. hospitals within the next two years. Leapfrog estimates that broad implementation of this staffing pattern would save 50,000 to 150,000 lives annually. Although the call for intensivist staffing is controversial—after all, how can hospitals meet this performance standard if the resources aren't there—the corporate leaders of the Leapfrog Group want to change behaviors and expectations by sending a strong message that businesses do not trust the health care system to maintain the health of their workers and control the costs. Don Berwick, of the Institute for Healthcare Improvement and a longtime proponent of fundamental changes in health care, put it this way, "Every system is perfectly designed to get the results it achieves."

There are many points of failure in our current system. The Institute of Medicine (IOM) created quite a stir with the publication in 2000 of *To Err Is Human*, a report that estimated there were as many as 100,000 deaths each year in American hospitals from medical errors. IOM focused almost exclusively on errors of comission. In ICUs, errors of omission outnumber errors of comission by a large margin. When these errors are included, the number of unnecessary deaths is even higher. *Crossing the Quality Chasm*, the follow-up report by IOM in 2001, outlined the need for fundamental changes in the way health care is delivered. The basic message was that outcomes will improve only when new systems of care are introduced.

In the remainder of this presentation, the eICU solution, a systematic reorganization of ICU care focused on improving patient safety and operating efficiency, is described. The reengineering of ICU care was initiated by two intensivists (the author and Brian Rosenfeld, the other founder of VISICU, Inc.) who ran a large tertiary-care center ICU for almost 20 years. The eICU solution has two main components. First, technology is used to leverage the expertise of intensivists. A telemedicine-type application bridges the manpower gap by creating networks of ICUs and linking them to centralized command centers (eICU facilities) that are continuously staffed by intensivists and support personnel. eICU care teams, led by intensivists, provide continuous monitoring and timely interventions when intensivists cannot be available on site. The second feature of the eICU solution is the use of technology tools to help both on-site and remote intensivists do their jobs better, more safely, and faster. Specifically, information technology systems are used to identify problems, guide decision making, and improve operating efficiency.

Figure 1 is a schematic drawing of an eICU network, which usually links multiple hospitals within an integrated delivery system (or any geographically proximate aggregation of hospitals) to an eICU facility. The participating hospitals generally care for different types of patients, and the availability and sophistication of on-site physicians and the organization of their ICUs vary. Tertiary-care centers usually have multiple ICUs with very high acuity patients and some dedicated intensivist presence during daytime hours. They frequently have step-down units with unstable patients but minimal physician presence. They also often care for similar patients in the emergency department, at least until they can be transferred to the ICU. Community and rural hospitals generally have fewer ICU beds, less acutely ill patients, and fewer intensivists. Rural hospitals, which often do not have sophisticated ICU resources, attempt to stabilize sick patients and transfer them to larger hospitals. All of these sites may be included in an eICU network, but their needs are different, and the role of the off-site team varies accordingly.

The physical network connecting an eICU to participating hospitals and ICUs must be secure and robust and must have adequate bandwidth to support real-time video. Some hospitals already have such networks, but most do not. In the

absence of an existing network, dedicated T-1 lines can be used. Each patient room has a high-resolution camera and a two-way audio system so the eICU care team can see the patient and communicate directly with on-site personnel. In addition, "hot" phones provide ICU staff with immediate access to the intensivist-led staff in the eICU. Other equipment in the eICU includes real-time bedside monitor viewers, an electronic data system, note-writing and order-entry applications, an alerting system, and a computerized decision-support tool. High-resolution scanners are used for x-rays and other images, unless a digital x-ray system is already in place.

Some have suggested that it would be helpful to provide remote patient access to physicians in their offices or at home. We see many advantages to a dedicated staffing center instead. When I (as a physician) am at home, in my office, or on the golf course, I am doing something else, and the staff person in the ICU (usually a nurse) has to detect a problem and decide whether or not to contact me. I then have to stop what I am doing to address that problem. Once the problem has been dealt with, I probably will return to my preferred activity, without providing follow-up. Acutely ill patients need continuous monitoring by people who have the expertise and the authority to initiate therapies and who have nothing to do but oversee the care of patients in the network.

Experience suggests that eICU personnel often detect patient problems before the on-site nurses. We have noticed that nurses in traditional ICUs often are reluctant to ask for help—usually because they don't want to "bother" the physicians (a reaction that may be conditioned by prior inappropriate physician responses to such calls). In addition, ICU nurses today are less experienced than they were in the past, and they may not recognize problems early. Prompt detection is very important because appropriate interventions at an early stage often can restore stability and prevent complications.

The eICU program uses a suite of information technology tools to support the remote team and the on-site team. The core information system collects data from a variety of sources and reconfigures it to optimize data presentation and facilitate physician work flow. The goal is to organize data in a format that makes the information easily accessible so clinicians can see temporal and other associative relationships. As part of this application, we provide note-writing and order-writing applications that allow physicians to initiate therapies and document their actions. We also provide real-time decision support designed for succinct data presentation and real-time use in guiding patient care decisions. Computer-based algorithms provide patient-specific assistance. These decision trees solicit key clinical information and, based on the data entered, provide clinicians with concrete recommendations suited to the situation. Another major focus has been on the creation of an early warning system that provides timely alerts designed to ensure that appropriate actions are initiated as soon as problems begin to develop.

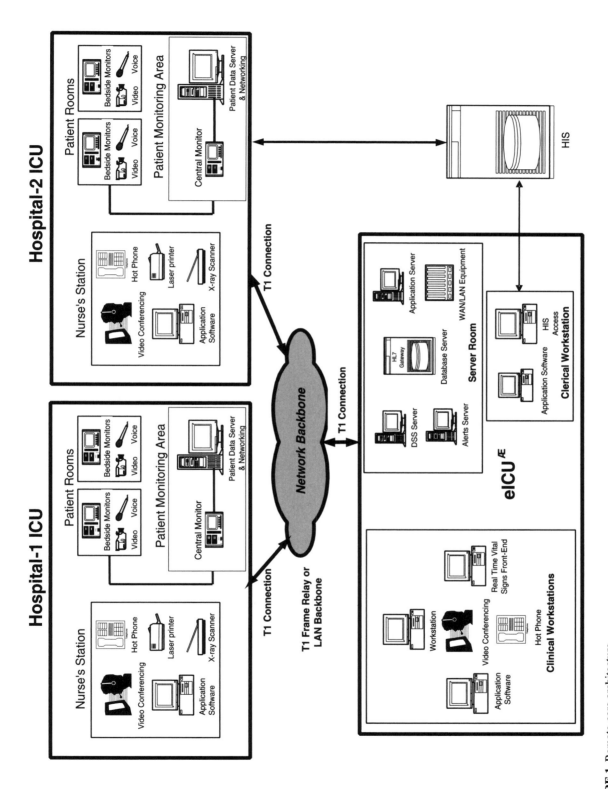

FIGURE 1 Remote-care architecture.

The goal is to move away from a system in which correct decisions depend solely on flawless behavior of busy clinicians.

Four key applications have been developed to achieve these goals. The first, called eCareManager, is a physician-focused ICU electronic medical record and tool set for executing routine tasks (e.g., monitoring, note and order writing, care planning, communication, etc.). eCareManager was designed to support the key functions of an intensivist, on site or off site. Data display screens are organized by organ system to provide context, and data are formatted to show changes in key parameters over time. The data density is high to highlight important relationships. Other screens show more detailed information (e.g., laboratory results, medications, etc.) with icons that announce the presence of new information. The overall acuity of the patient is prominently displayed, and this is tied to specific care processes. For example, the most acutely ill patients are reviewed comprehensively at least once every hour by the eICU team. Another screen contains all details of the care plan. ICUs have many different caregivers (e.g., intensivists, consultants, nurses, nutritionists, respiratory therapists, pharmacists, etc.) all providing care to the same patients. Often each member of the care team carefully documents his or her activities, but other members of the team do not take the time to process the information. As a result, communication and coordination are less than optimal. For better integration, we created a single site to document the inputs of team members. The goal is to facilitate information transfer. Our decision support tool, called The Source, was created with the assistance of more than 50 physicians around the country. The Source, which includes approximately 160 acute medical problems, provides succinct summaries of the literature, with an emphasis on diagnosis and therapy. Links to source material are provided for additional detail, but the primary goal is to provide real-time assistance with decision making.

A second important feature is the presence of clinical algorithms that help physicians deal with a specific patient. These algorithms are generally based on published best practices or, if evidence is not definitive, major consensus reports, such as recent publications by the American Thoracic Society and the American Society of Infectious Diseases on the empirical treatment of hospital-acquired pneumonia. These comprehensive review articles have been deconstructed and a series of decision trees created. Based on physician-provided, patient-specific answers to key questions, the user is directed to appropriate recommendations for prescribing antibiotics.

The third major application, Smart Alerts, functions as an early warning system. Remember that all relevant clinical data (e.g., vital signs, laboratory results, medications, etc.) are being stored in a relational database. Whenever new data are entered, they are run against a complex set of rules to determine whether the ICU team (on-site or remote) should be notified of an impending problem. These rules can identify values that are out of range or parameters that have changed by a predetermined amount over a fixed period of time. One example flags patients on heparin if their platelet count drops. The rationale is to alert clinicians to the possibility of an infrequent (but life-threatening) complication.

The fourth application, Smart Reports, also capitalizes on the robust information stored in the database. Smart Reports provides detailed information about outcomes, practice patterns, resource utilization, and clinical operations. For example, a report on the use of deep-venous thrombosis prophylactic therapies identifies the population at risk, shows when preventative treatments were begun during the ICU stay (if at all), and shows which agents were used. These reports, which can detail individual physician practice patterns, become an effective tool for managing change.

The eICU solution is currently being used in five health care systems. The impact on outcomes has been studied formally at Sentara Healthcare, a six-hospital system in Virginia, where the program has been up and running for two years. This detailed study showed a 25 percent reduction in hospital mortality, a 17 percent reduction in ICU length of stay (LOS), and a 13 percent reduction in hospital LOS. The decrease in ICU LOS is attributable entirely to a reduction in the number and LOS of the outliers, which strongly suggests that early, appropriate interventions can prevent complications that prolong ICU stay and lead to outliers.

Cap Gemini Ernst & Young, which performed a detailed analysis of the financial impact of the program, found that hospital revenue went up because of the reduction in ICU LOS, which made room for 20 percent more patients to be admitted to the ICU. Costs of care also fell, through a combination of decreased LOS and improved use of resources. Practice standardization and a reduced illness burden, as a result of fewer complications, are thought to have contributed to the latter benefit. A number of ancillary benefits were also noted: nursing turnover was lower; intensivist lifestyle improved; and the hospital was able to market an innovative patient-safety initiative.

In conclusion, ICUs represent an ideal target for quality improvement efforts because of the high acuity of ICU patients and the high cost of caring for them. Substantial improvements in outcomes are possible, but they require a comprehensive reorganization of existing systems of care. Technology solutions can provide meaningful increases in operating efficiency and quality if they can be integrated effectively into physician work flow. The eICU Solution represents a new paradigm for ICU care that treats the management of acutely ill patients as an enterprise-wide priority and uses a suite of technology applications to reduce errors, standardize practice patterns, and improve operating efficiency. Early results suggest promising changes in clinical and economic performance.

REFERENCES

Donchin, Y., D. Gopher, M. Olin, Y. Badihi, M. Biesky, C.L. Sprung, R. Pizov, and S. Cotev. 1995. A look into the nature and causes of human errors in the intensive care unit. Critical Care Medicine 23(2): 294–300.

IOM (Institute of Medicine). 2000. To Err Is Human: Building a Safer Health System, L.T. Kohn, J.M. Corrigan, and M.S. Donaldson, eds. Washington, D.C.: National Academy Press.

IOM. 2001. Crossing the Quality Chasm: A New Health System for the 21st Century. Washington, D.C.: National Academy Press.

Wireless Biomonitoring for Health Care

Thomas F. Budinger
Lawrence Berkeley National Laboratory and
University of California, Berkeley

Biomonitoring methods have developed substantially since 1965, and wireless technologies of the last few years promise major advances in efficiency by simplifying hospital and home health care. Improved technology has led to better sensors for monitoring pulse, heartbeat (ECG), blood pressure, blood oxygenation, physical activity, falls, vascular compliance, and even endoscopy. But what about communication between the patient and caregiver and between the patient and the environment (e.g., brain-computer interfaces)? If we could do anything we wanted with wireless technology for health care, what would we choose? This analysis argues for inexpensive engineering technologies that improve health care and substantially improve the quality of life for patients who are severely disabled from spinal cord injury or aging processes.

TRACKING FALLS

A few commercial medical-alert networks provide communication between the subject and a remote communication center, similar to contemporary fire and burglar alarm systems. These systems are designed to be used by a conscious subject to alert loved ones or caregivers in case of a fall, trauma, or cardiac arrest. Of some 300,000 falls a year in the United States, 10 percent happen to people at home alone who are not discovered for more than an hour after the fall. One-third of people over 65 who fall and are not found for more than an hour are seriously disabled or die (Gurley et al., 1996). This is a very serious problem.

Current devices for monitoring falls have some serious flaws, and innovations are urgently needed. Commercial devices are costly, bulky, and not scalable to contemporary communications. They rely on a type of fire-alarm system that is commercially operated at a monthly cost of $20 and depends on an answering operator putting the subject in contact with the appropriate response team or person. Indeed, a variety of monitors currently on the market have limited range and a layered communication system that is not flexible enough to meet the needs of patients and loved ones at home alone. We need wearable systems that can communicate through a local low-power communications system to a module that then connects to the Internet, land lines, or specified cell phone numbers.

There are more than 400,000 cases of sudden cardiac death (SCD) each year. The key element in resuscitation is the time interval between the cardiac event and the administration of professional aid. We need a reliable communication interface to a patient-friendly device that can detect falls or irregular heart action (e.g., a wrist-worn device that monitors pulse or a chest-strap device that monitors electrical events) to ensure against SCD, particularly when the patient is sleeping.

Commercial tracking devices also need improvement. Commercial systems advertised for tracking elderly patients with Alzheimer's disease are available, but they are expensive and not scalable at low cost to a wide variety of situations. It is possible, using GPS with a combination of modern communication networks (e.g., 802.11, ultra-wideband) to create a wireless system that monitors not only location but also the health status of individuals, just as we monitor the location and status of automobiles. In fact, there is no barrier to engineering customized tracking systems that can locate a wandering family member or a lost pet and, in addition, provide information on some physical signs, such as activity, pulse, temperature, and so on.

TRACKING THE AGED, CHILDREN, AND PETS

A commercial system that can track people or pets over a distance of 1.5 miles from a base station has been developed by Wheels of Zeus Inc. (WoZ). The system operates at about 900 Mhz and uses small poker-chip-like tags attached to the subject. Each tag has a GPS and local wireless device and an option for storing data related to the subject. The system

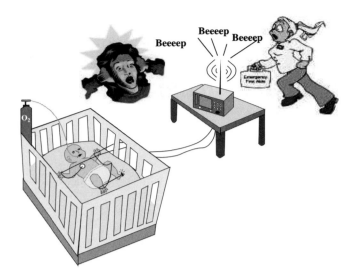

FIGURE 1 A wired system to monitor oxygenation by pulse oximetry.

requires a base station (a few base stations could serve an entire town). In field trials in February 2005 (evaluated by me), the system proved to be highly reliable in most terrains. A commercial version should be available in late 2005 (WoZ, 2005).

HOME CARE

Patient-centered home telecare and health systems have shown great promise, but little modern engineering is being used to develop them. Wellness promotion now focuses on bringing patients home and caring for them at home, a very practical idea. Improved monitoring systems could greatly facilitate the objective of caring for patients at home.

A study has been going on in Australia for the last few years to monitor the physiological condition of patients at home (Wilson et al., 2000). This study is of great interest to the National Cancer Institute, which is looking for a way to monitor the drug therapy of cancer patients in a home setting. Participants in the study wear a radio connected to a number of sensors, including a blood-pressure monitor. The information is sent through a modem to a central location. The results of this and other studies on child monitoring (Neuman et al., 2001) have shown that remote sensing is reliable and can replace home visits. However, wireless communication methods are still not standardized.

Wireless technology that can transmit images of patients, as well as monitor vital signs, via radio or TV frequencies has existed since 1965. Years ago when home monitoring was first considered, the available technologies were encumbered by FCC regulations. In 2005, however, wireless technologies can reach almost anywhere on the planet via the Internet, cell phones, or other hand-held devices, and

WEBCAM technology can visualize patients and health care monitors or situations. Many physicians would agree that the number-one priority for patient in-home care is ready access to a video of the patient or the patient's bedside monitor. At this point, however, although the technology exists (e.g., WEBCAM), it is not adaptable to a scalable system. Improving video monitoring of home-care patients will require the participation of engineers, physicians, and nursing support institutions.

RESPIRATORY MONITORING

A recent example illustrates the need for wireless monitoring in a hospital. In February 2003, 60 percent of the patients admitted to Children's Hospital in Oakland, California, a major hospital in the Bay Area, were admitted for infections with respiratory syncytial virus. Treatment for this condition is mainly by oxygen delivery, and oxygenation is monitored by pulse oximetry. Patients being monitored must wear a wire connected to a bedside unit from a toe or finger. Figure 1 shows the chaotic scene on the wards using this wired system.

With a wireless system, false alarms due to motions of wires and disconnects would be eliminated (Figure 2). In addition, hospital stays could be shortened from four days to one and one-half days with reliable respiratory monitors and pulse oximeters with oxygen controls appropriate for home care. The engineering agenda for creating the monitoring device is a lightweight, reliable power supply for the pulse oximeter and wireless transmitter.

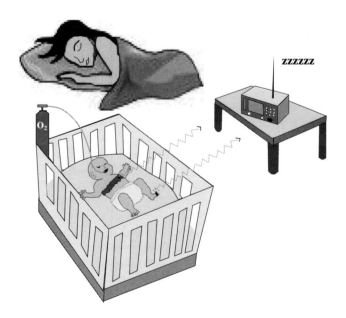

FIGURE 2 A wireless system for monitoring oxygenation by pulse oximetry.

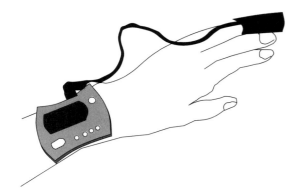

FIGURE 3 A Minolta Pulsox™ system.

My group has built a small pulse oximeter that can be worn on the forehead and that uses the Bluetooth or another system (802.11, 802.15 "mote") for local wireless transmission. Pulse oximeters already on the market could be used if they were adapted for wireless transmission (e.g., the Minolta Pulsox™ system that can be worn on the hand and costs about $240) (Figure 3). The device would communicate with a modem or router situated within 10 meters of the subject through which the data would be uploaded to the Internet where it would be available to caregivers.

Sleep apnea is a serious health problem related to cardiovascular disease. Yet, for many people with sleep apnea, the only monitor is a sleeping partner. The gadgets now sold to monitor episodes of sleep apnea are bulky, expensive, and complicated. If they were re-engineered to be wireless, they would be much simpler and smaller (Figure 4).

Another wireless device is a breathing sensor incorporated into a strap around the chest similar to the device used to monitor pulse in athletes. Wireless transmission to a local receiver can facilitate recording, alarms, and further transmission to data archives.

One of the newest ideas for wireless monitoring is to use ultra-wideband frequency technology. For example, one could use a crib-installed radar device to monitor a baby's breathing. An electronic signal-processing system would set off an alarm if lung motion were abnormal or absent (Budinger, 2003).

MONITORING ACTIVITY

Accelerometers used to evaluate how much activity an individual expends during a day could be used to monitor the activity of patients at home. Current accelerometers (produced by four different companies) are all one dimensional. A three-dimensional accelerometer could potentially pick up both the activities and pulse rate of a patient who has fallen or who is lying down. The same system could also detect a fall reliably with a low rate of false alarms. A reset button could be pushed in case the fall alarm was triggered accidentally. In addition, 3-D accelerometers the size of a nickel could improve GPS tracking systems.

BLOOD PRESSURE AND VASCULAR COMPLIANCE

High blood pressure is one of the major risk factors for heart attacks and heart failure. But of the 50 million people in North America with high blood pressure, 30 percent do not know that their pressure is abnormally high and that they would benefit from medical treatment (Mensah, 2002). A single blood pressure measurement during a visit to a doctor's office or clinic is extremely unreliable. A simple, inexpensive ($75) blood pressure monitor that can be worn on the wrist was manufactured in 2003 by Omron, and based on tests by the author, the device is reliable. Other devices available in 2005 are 60 percent less expensive, but their reliability has not been verified.

However, a wireless device must await the establishment of a practical communication network for convenient transmission to caregivers. Such a system could be combined with the WoZ network, or a router could send transmissions from the blood pressure or other monitoring device to the Internet.

Another monitor for measuring compliance of the vascular system could possibly be developed within five years.

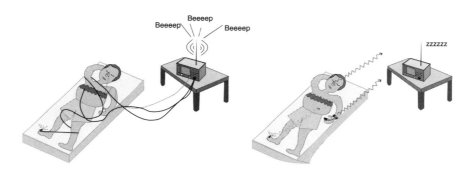

FIGURE 4 Wired (left) and wireless (right) systems for monitoring sleep apnea.

Ideally, this would be a simple wrist-worn device that transmits the arrival of a pulse and a chest strap that transmits the time of the R wave (Figure 5). The time difference between these measurements is proportional to the compliance of the vascular system and reflects endothelial function. This device would require a wireless timing signal between the heart electrical event and the pulse arrival at the wrist. The system could take repeated measurements to demonstrate vascular response to psychological stress and changes associated with drugs and foodstuffs. This wireless unit could also transmit information to a permanent record or to a caregiver (Budinger, 2003).

Another device now under investigation is a wireless colonoscopy that can monitor for signs of colon cancer. The subject swallows a little disposable transmitter that takes pictures as it travels through the colon and transmits them to a recorder worn on a belt (Appleyard et al., 2001). A problem with this device is that a clinician has to look through all of the pictures.

WIRELESS TECHNOLOGIES FOR PARALYZED PATIENTS

The incidence of spinal cord injuries in the United States is 11,000 cases per year, and there are currently about 250,000 patients. The annual medical cost of caring for these patients is $9.3 billion (NSCISC, 2004). The cost could be substantially reduced and the quality of life for these patients improved by new techniques of wireless communication. Electronic equipment and wireless communications can make it easier for quadriplegic patients to control powered wheelchairs, light switches, heating devices, televisions,

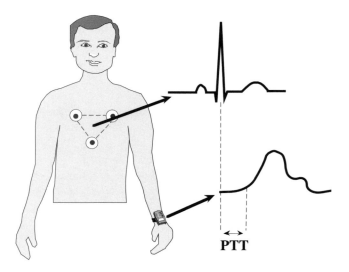

FIGURE 5 Wireless system for measuring vascular system compliance.

radios, telephones, and computer systems for learning, entertainment, and communications (Friehs et al., 2004; Keirn and Aunon, 1990).

An array of small electrodes implanted into the brain of a 25-year-old quadriplegic man was programmed through wired connection signals to control a computer cursor (Figure 6A). After a short learning period, the patient was able to check his e-mail and control aspects of his environment by moving a cursor on a computer screen with his thoughts alone. The system, called BrainGate™, is an investigational device being tested clinically by Cyberkinetics Inc. (2005). At this point, Brain Gate is not an approved device and is available only through a clinical study. The innovations are the implanted electrode system and the module that interprets brain signals and translates them into control of devices. The system could potentially be used to help people with disabilities become more independent by allowing them to control various devices with their thoughts.

Monkeys with similarly implanted electrodes have shown that brain signals can move robotic arms in two dimensions (Taylor et al., 2002). More recently, an array of external electrodes have been used as a brain-computer interface that can translate externally detected brain signals (Figure 6B) into both horizontal and vertical movements of a computer cursor (Wolpaw and McFarland, 2004).

Another approach that does not require invasive electrode implantation or an array of electrodes on the surface of the scalp is to use the tongue to control a cursor, just as one would use a touch pad or a mouse. The idea of using an intra-oral device with tongue switching dates back to 1990 (Parker and White, 1990), but a fully wireless implementation has not yet been developed.

Nevertheless, this idea has many practical advantages over other systems that have been proposed for quadriplegic patients (Figure 6C). The tongue-operated intra-oral remote controller consists of an acrylic plate fitted to the roof of the mouth. A capacitor-based platform on the plate is similar to the touch pad of a laptop. The electronics of the pad are in resonance with a loop antenna around the head or neck that senses the tongue activations by a power drop. This information can then be sent wirelessly to a computer or other pickup device to control light switches, a television, and even movement of a wheel chair.

The device could also be used to send messages by tongue taps for transmitting Morse code (Yang et al., 2003). Alternatively, the intra-oral wireless signaling device could be used in conjunction with a head-mounted pointing system that employs a laser or infrared beam (Chen et al., 1999).

Another method is to use an infrared-controlled human-computer interface with a laser pointer and infrared-transmitting diode mounted on the patient's eyeglasses. Using the laser, the patient could point to a computer cursor control panel and keyboard equipped with an infrared receiver. With his or her tongue, the patient would key a switch on the side of the cheek suspended from an arm also mounted

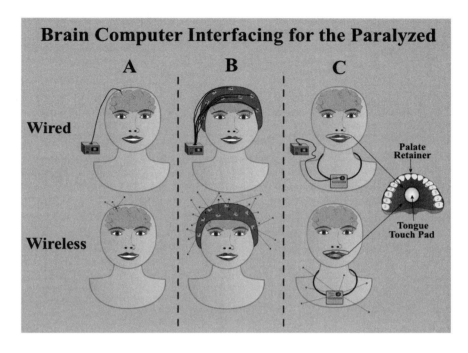

FIGURE 6 Brain-computer interfacing. A. Implanted electrodes. B. External electrodes. C. Tongue-operated intra-oral remote controller.

on the eyeglasses. When the laser points to the desired target on the computer control board, the patient would key a switch "to send" the infrared signal (Chen et al., 1999).

WIRELESS SYSTEMS FOR HEALTH CARE

Many wireless systems operate with low power at 2.45 gigahertz; thus, they have very short range (e.g., 10 meters or less). Even though these systems are not regulated by the FCC, their use in hospitals has been limited. The purpose of the prohibition against using cell phones in hospital environments is not only to prevent voice interference out of respect for patients, but also, in some cases, to prevent interference by high-power wireless transmissions with devices used in acute care, such as monitors and infusion systems. This problem now seems to be coming under control, and wireless systems are being widely used in hospitals across the country.

In February 2003, the FCC finally endorsed a new ruling loosening restrictions on unlicensed ultra-wideband radio transmissions. In principle, this technology enables one to see through walls, monitor patients, and implement communications in radiofrequency-busy environments without interference, thus opening enormous possibilities for wireless transmissions in hospitals and in homes with devices that do not interfere with each other. Thus, the limitations of wireless communications for medical sensor devices have disappeared, and opportunities for improving health care abound.

ACKNOWLEDGMENTS

This paper was prepared with the assistance of Kathleen Brennan, Jonathan Maltz, Thomas Ng, and Dustin Li. The work was supported by the U.S. Department of Energy Office of Biology and Engineering Research.

REFERENCES

Appleyard, M., A. Glukhovsky, and P. Swain. 2001. Wireless-capsule diagnostic endoscopy for recurrent small-bowel bleeding. New England Journal of Medicine 344(3): 232–233.

Budinger, T.F. 2003. Biomonitoring with wireless communications. Annual Review of Biomedical Engineering 5: 383–412.

Budinger, T.F. 2005. Wireless Biomonitoring for Health Care. Report No. 57043. Berkeley, Calif.: Lawrence Berkeley National Laboratory.

Chen, Y.L., F.T. Tang, W.H. Chang, M.K. Wong, Y.Y. Shih, and T.S. Kuo. 1999. The new design of an infrared-controlled human-computer interface for the disabled. IEEE Transactions on Neural Systems and Rehabilitation Engineering 7(4): 474–481.

Cyberkinetics Inc. 2005. Brain Gate. Available online at: *http://www.cyberkineticsinc.com/braingate.htm*.

Friehs, G.M., V.A. Zerris, C.L. Ojakangas, M.R. Fellows, and J.P. Donoghue. 2004. Brain-machine and brain-computer interfaces. Stroke 35(11 Suppl 1): 2702–2705.

Gurley, R.J., N. Lum, M. Sande, B. Lo, and M.H. Katz. 1996. Persons found in their homes helpless or dead. New England Journal of Medicine 334(26): 1710–1716.

Keirn, Z.A., and J.I. Aunon. 1990. A new mode of communication between man and his surroundings. IEEE Transactions on Bio-medical Engineering 37(12): 1209–1214.

Mensah, G.A. 2002. The global burden of hypertension: good news and bad news. Cardiology Clinics 20(2): 181–185.

Neuman, M.R., H. Watson, R.S. Mendenhall, J.T. Zoldak, J.M. Di Fiore, M. Peucker, T.M. Baird, D.H. Crowell, T.T. Hoppenbrouwers, D. Hufford, C.E. Hunt, M.J. Corwin, L.R. Tinsley, D.E. Weese-Mayer, and M.A. Sackner. 2001. Cardiopulmonary monitoring at home: the CHIME monitor. Physiological Measurement 22(2): 267–286.

NSCISC (National Spinal Cord Injury Statistical Center). 2004. Facts and Figures at a Glance, August 2004. Available online at: *http://www.spinalcord.uab.edu/show.asp?durki=21446* (accessed 11/11/04).

Parker, C.B., and S.P. White. 1990. Intra-oral remote control: an access device for the severely disabled. British Dental Journal 169(9): 302–303.

Taylor, D.M., S.I. Tillery, and A.B. Schwartz. 2002. Direct cortical control of 3D neuroprosthetic devices. Science 296(5574): 1829–1832.

WoZ (Wheels of Zeus). 2005. Introducing: low-cost, reliable GPS. Available online at: *www.woz.com*.

Wilson, L.S., R.W. Gill, I.F. Sharp, J. Joseph, S.A. Heitmann, C.F. Chen, M.J. Dadd, A. Kajan, A.F. Collings, and M. Gunaratnam. 2000. Building the Hospital without Walls—a CSIRO home telecare initiative. Telemedicine Journal 6(2): 275–281.

Wolpaw, J.R., and D.J. McFarland. 2004. Control of a two-dimensional movement signal by a noninvasive brain-computer interface in humans. Proceedings of the National Academy of Sciences 101(51): 17849–17854.

Yang, C.H., L.Y. Chuang, and C.H. Luo. 2003. Morse code application for wireless environmental control systems for severely disabled individuals. IEEE Transactions on Neural Systems and Rehabilitation Engineering 11(4): 463–469.

Rehabilitation Redefined

Mindy L. Aisen
Department of Veterans Affairs

The Department of Veterans Affairs (VA) has redefined rehabilitation as everything done to address chronic impairment, and, therefore, disability, including hearing loss, vision loss, problems with ambulation, and sensory impairment. The VA's needs encompass a great many engineering areas, and the VA is looking to engineers to provide better wheelchairs made of lighter weight materials, better implant technologies, and so forth.

The VA is the third largest agency in the federal government; only the U.S. Department of Defense and the Department of Homeland Security are bigger in terms of human capital. The Veterans Health Administration (VHA) is the largest academic health care system in the world. Every state in the union has at least one VA hospital, and many have more than one. The VHA also has clinics, nursing homes, and a research program. It provides medical care to about four million of the ten million veterans living in the United States. The agency also has a statutory obligation to affiliate with academia, and almost every VA hospital is affiliated with a medical school, a university, or both. The VA also provides professional training and has numerous programs that dovetail with educational programs at the Ph.D. level; VA hospitals provide training for medical students, interns, and residents.

VA engineering research is focused on the development of cutting-edge rehabilitation technology and the translation of that technology from the workbench to patient use. The VA takes an active role in the development of patented technology. Rehabilitation engineers create environmental control units and replace and/or restore lost function through functional electrical stimulation that helps people make the most of the abilities they still have.

The VA is very supportive of engineering research, especially on neuroprostheses—devices that are activated by outputs of the brain. Work at other institutions has shown that picking up motor directions from the brain does not require a massive number of electrodes; studies on nonhuman primates have shown that very small patches of electrodes can pick up signals for volitional movement. The results of these experiments have clear implications for the development of peripheral stimulators. The VA also vigorously supports work on retinal prostheses.

The VA already keeps entirely paperless electronic records; telemedicine and, more broadly, e-health programs are critical to the VA. We hope to provide better care—including better visualization, more electronic connectivity, and electronic records—to rural veterans via telemedicine. One of the persistent problems in treating veterans who live in remote areas is determining when a clinician is needed. e-Health has been very successful in a few areas, such as psychiatry, but it could be useful in dozens of other areas, including post-stroke follow-up. We need technology that can perceive the severity of a patient's problems when a clinician cannot be there in person. So far, no technology or combination of technologies can provide even a prototype test of such a system. One can imagine remote sensors that can monitor many parameters, such as strength and range of motion.

The VA is eager to explore uses for the global positioning system, activity monitors, and temperature sensors for vulnerable patients with psychiatric problems and major disabilities. Some patients, particularly quadriplegics, have trouble regulating their body temperature on hot days, and even some very young patients have died of hyperthermia. Technology could help these patients stay healthy and lead more independent lives.

Rehabilitation following stroke has undergone a revolution in our lifetime. Formerly, when a patient lost control of a body part, that part would be immobilized during rehabilitation, and the patient would be taught to compensate with the other side of the body. Now we understand that the body has a great capacity for plasticity, and rehabilitation now focuses on constrained, induced therapy—in other words, patients are taught to move the weakened limb. There are many possibilities for assistive devices, including imaging, to quantify sensory, motor, and cognitive recovery.

Outcomes research is critical. After engineers create a design, it must be tested clinically. Unfortunately for the engineer, this entails a lot of drudgery, from compiling data through determining whether an outcome is reproducible in clinical trials. Outcomes research requires a blending of cultures and seamless interaction between the engineers who create the design and clinicians who treat the patients. Because clinicians and engineers may have very different expectations about what a device should do, the engineer must observe the clinician and the patient to determine their needs. It is essential that we know what patients and doctors want before we invest in development. A product created without input from the clinical world may do little to improve a patient's quality of life.

The VA in Pittsburgh, working with the University of Pittsburgh and Carnegie Mellon University, is funding work to improve wheelchair design and technology. Dr. Rory Cooper, who is a veteran and a paraplegic, is leading the research. One chair under investigation uses built-in gyroscopes to climb stairs and can climb in and out of a van. The chair is collapsible and can be folded into a backpack. But it does have drawbacks. It is very heavy, is not entirely stable, and is extremely conspicuous.

The VA has also funded a virtual reality program to train people who are newly confined to a wheelchair to handle rapid turns and curves—a virtual driving experience. The program has also been modified for other purposes—for instance, to help people in a chair who have problems with visual perception. This work could also potentially help patients with brain disease overcome perceptual problems.

Another area of interest is in body-weight-supported treadmill training, which began with work by Reggie Edgerton at UCLA; it was initially used for patients with spinal-cord injuries. The idea is to place people who cannot support their own weight over a treadmill with their feet in contact with the treadmill and to move them through the ambulation sequence. Many patients develop appropriate sequential firing of electromyogram signals, or messages between nerves and muscles. The meaning of the findings remains cloudy, however, and more studies are necessary before we will know if adding this activity to conventional rehabilitation will be helpful. One persistent finding so far is that stroke victims who are put in this device regularly learn to walk sooner and better. The current technology is very labor intensive and uncomfortable, involving at least three therapists. But one new system that is commercially available now, a robotic system from Switzerland, requires only one therapist and has a number of safety features. The VA plans to purchase some of these apparatuses.

The VA in Palo Alto is working on a device based on the idea of aggressive stimulation of a limb. The device enables a good arm to direct a weak arm—a mirror image experience.

Prosthetics is a wide-open field. Our main concerns are limb preservation and best-function preservation after loss of a limb. Research is desperately needed in this area, as well as on the manufacture of prostheses. Prosthetic devices are currently made largely by hand and are, therefore, labor intensive; they are only as good as the prosthetist who makes them. We believe the process could be automated, and the VA has tried to promote the idea of computer-aided design. Electronic or e-health could also come into play. Take, for example, two VA patients who use prosthetics who live in rural Nevada and Colorado. Right now, doctors must fly out to see them to get their measurements. With e-health, we could provide their measurements to a centralized manufacturer.

Current prosthetics could be greatly improved. People with upper limb loss suffer greatly because they have to wear big harnesses that are creaky, itchy, and uncomfortable. Lower-extremity prosthetics, particularly above the knee, are also less than optimal. At the moment, engineers are not working on these problems, even though the VA has money to support this kind of research.

Another area for research is osseointegration to eliminate the need for heavy harnesses. Osseointegration is the direct attachment of inert metal to bone, giving the prosthetic limb an anchor or clip. Because limbs are not built to accept metal implants, infections are common, and impedance matching can be difficult, more research is needed before osseointegration will become commonplace. There is a great need for engineers to determine how to provide comfortable, durable prostheses that do not cause infection. In implants that have been successful, patients report better perception and no skin irritation or swelling at the end of the day. Work in this area with accident victims in Scandinavia has been successful. The VA believes we need more fundamental research in this area and is eager to invest in it.

One of the programs the VA is funding now is on a device called BION™, a tiny, implantable, neural and muscular stimulation device being developed by the Alfred Mann Foundation. BIONs are battery-powered, radio-controlled devices that are implanted subcutaneously alongside a nerve to facilitate coordinated functional stimulation. In a Cooperative Research and Development Agreement with the Mann Foundation, the VA provides subjects for study, scientists, and work space; the Mann Foundation provides technological and engineering support. We are in the midst of the first Request for Abstracts (RFA)—requests for research plans using BION. RFAs that are deemed scientifically meritorious and applicable to rehabilitation issues facing veterans are awarded grant support.

The VA is eager to work in partnership with industry on similar studies. Our goal is to enrich the intellectual environment of VA hospitals and make them vibrant, academic institutions.

Evaluating the Potential of New Technologies

Carolyn M. Clancy
Agency for Healthcare Research and Quality

On a recent tour of the Baltimore VA Hospital with Tommy Thompson, the secretary of Health and Human Services, Anthony G. Principi, secretary of Veterans Affairs, and Senator Barbara Mikulski, I was struck by how much information technology (IT) has improved the health care process. And it occurred to me that such improvements are figured out only after investments in IT have been made, rather than up front.

Some of this is inevitable, of course, and after-the-fact improvements *are* beneficial. Nevertheless, one can imagine a process in which technology-induced changes in care delivery are anticipated prior to and throughout the implementation of interventions. In addition to targeting problems at the point of care, it could also be useful to anticipate the effects of new technologies on the larger health care system. For instance, as a result of some changes now being put in place at many hospitals, the future system may require fewer cardiologists, and cardiologists may also face very different challenges. These changes could influence medical education and increase the return on investment for innovations in care.

The mission of the Agency for Healthcare Research and Quality (AHRQ) is to support and conduct research to improve the safety and quality of health care. In short, we produce evidence-based information and ensure its effective use. A very high priority of the agency is patient safety. In 2001, Congress appropriated $50 million for AHRQ to work on this issue, and the agency's safety portfolio is very diverse, including many investments related to human factors, IT, and human psychology. This work is incredibly exciting and, in some ways, is a striking departure from traditional research paradigms. Applying human factors research to improving patient safety, for example, is based on a research model that looks more like continuous quality improvement (i.e., iterative testing of interventions) than classical hypothesis testing.

As a steward of public resources, the agency must be careful that breakthrough findings from research investments in patient safety and quality can be put to wider use. An investigator who develops and evaluates a brilliant idea but fails to consider how it will be used in current settings is not an unmitigated success. This happened with the shared-decision-making software programs that emerged from the agency's outcomes research. These are fabulous programs, but if the software were given to many hospitals today, it would not be helpful. First of all, patients and residents would have no idea how to use it. Second, there is no place to store the paperwork. And, third, no one knows when to use the software in the flow of practice. Should a patient use it before or after a primary care encounter? Before or after seeing a specialist? Is a coach necessary? Will some patients hesitate to use it at all? The program is terrific, but no one appears to have thought through how it might interfere with the psychology of interactions between clinicians and patients or where it fits in conceptually.

Although we are proud of our track record in producing evidence-based information, we now recognize that an essential and underdeveloped part of our mission is to identify strategies for making that information useful at the point of care. Making this transition will require insights from a broad array of disciplines, including engineering. But what other changes can be anticipated in this regard as more systems take up IT? Why have hospitals like Cedars-Sinai, which have made huge investments in IT, encountered enormous problems when it was implemented?

The answer, in part, is that no one thought about how the new system would change the work process. Doctors were being asked to use a brand new information system that added hours to their workday. So the dislike of new systems may be only partly because people resist change. It may also be because they know from experience that new systems do not always improve the work process. And, in fact, many of these systems, often designed with little or no input from clinicians, do not make things better.

In terms of using technologies to make human error less likely, health care is way behind most other industries. Starbucks has more built-in checks for errors in making a cup of coffee than the health care system does for treating a patient. It is hard to grasp that health care is based mostly on intuition and a common knowledge base rather than on a built-in system.

Having said this, it is important to say also that there are many, many opportunities to bring disciplines together and improve the situation. Improvements in care delivery through the wise application of innovations are within our reach—if we bring in the right disciplines and support the right research. Statisticians and others who are poised to make real breakthroughs in terms of improving health care delivery should be working alongside health care researchers.

This will require that specific changes be put in place. How can these people be brought together? How should current training programs be changed? What about career paths? Are we willing to provide academic rewards (in addition to peer-reviewed publications) to people whose contributions make "smart" applications of knowledge and technologies to improve care? A senior researcher recently challenged us with the following questions, "Would you advise a young person to get into the improvement arena? Is it a viable career path?" As the National Institutes of Health turn attention to reengineering clinical research, they will also confront the issues of academic incentives.

Another major challenge facing us is how to accelerate knowledge transfer. In the old model, a researcher conceives a study, carries out the study, and publishes the results. Then the results trickle down, and people eventually change their practices. The old model works much too slowly.

There are many opportunities for improving the safety and quality of health care. We must rigorously evaluate the potential of new technologies so that the improvements that are possible are realized and so that we avoid costly investments in applications that yield little gain, and may actually impede progress.

Barriers and Incentives to Change

Political Barriers to Change

Nancy-Ann DeParle
JP Morgan Partners, LLC and
The Wharton School

The United States spends more than $200 billion a year to provide guaranteed health care to some 39 million Medicare beneficiaries. The federal government, through Medicare, supplies one-third to one-half the revenues of every hospital in the country and a substantial proportion of the revenues of each and every physician, nursing home, and other health care provider and vendor of every stripe. Medicare is one of—if not the—most popular government programs ever invented, at least among its beneficiaries, if not among hospitals and physicians. So it might be reasonable to think that if the federal government can run such an effective, popular program, it could also lead the charge to reengineer health care delivery systems to promote better quality of care. Reasonable, but naive. I hate to be the skunk at today's party, and no one wants to improve health care quality more than I do. But I guess I am here to provide the realpolitik. Based on my experience as a health-policy official in the federal government, I believe that not only do we have a very long way to go to achieve acceptable levels of clinical quality (as others today have persuasively argued), but also that it will not be easy for the federal government to be involved appropriately in moving the system in the right direction.

We are gathered here under the auspices of the National Academy of Engineering, and I imagine there are some rocket scientists in this room, so I hesitate to say this. But I think it is important to understand that changing health care is not rocket science. It is harder. This morning I will talk about my experiences as a health-policy official in the Clinton administration that have led me, regrettably, to a fairly pessimistic assessment of what we can reasonably expect the government to do in reengineering health care delivery systems to improve the quality of care.

Last October, the Health Care Financing Administration (HCFA) (now the Centers for Medicare and Medicaid Services, or CMS), the agency that administers Medicare, finally published the first state-by-state assessment of the quality of care Medicare provides to beneficiaries (Jencks et al., 2000). I say finally both because it took us a long time to get the sign-offs from the U.S. Department of Health and Human Services and from "down the street" (the way we referred to the White House and the Office of Management and Budget) to release the study and because it had taken Medicare more than 35 years to get around to making this assessment.

To do this first-ever qualitative assessment, we began by assembling a group of experts to decide which areas should be included. The group decided to focus on process measures rather than outcomes, which would be more controversial. According to the clinicians who worked on the study, the measures were very basic; one told me they were practically at the level of washing one's hands before surgery. In other words, all of the measures were supported by clinical consensus, and, in an ideal world, they should all have been at or near 100 percent. The beauty of the study is that it clearly indicates where we are and what needs to be done.

We chose to assess processes in the six most significant areas for Medicare beneficiaries: acute myocardial infarction, heart failure, stroke, pneumonia, breast cancer, and diabetes. For some measures, we did a systematic, random sample of up to 750 patient records in each state; for others we looked at all Medicare claims.

For pneumonia, for example, the study showed that the 39 million Medicare beneficiaries are not getting some of the basic things they need to treat them when they are sick or to prevent them from getting sick. The study focused on errors of omission rather than errors of commission (in this sense, it was slightly different than the focus of *To Err Is Human* [IOM, 2000], the ground-breaking study documenting 50,000 to 100,000 death annually from preventable medical errors). Overall, it wasn't a very pretty picture. The individual indicators ranged from a low of 11 percent to a high of around 95 percent. Some of the data suggest major problems in medical education and care processes. Practice patterns showed physicians were not providing some very basic treatments in roughly 50 percent of the cases.

The report was published the week I left HCFA, and this timing was not accidental. It required a great deal of effort to get it published, and in fact, I think some of the career clinicians and policy analysts who worked on the assessment and the article we published began to doubt whether it would ever see the light of day. The agency did not publicize it widely, in part because of a concern that the information might make Medicare, or some physicians or hospitals, look bad, and in part because it might be embarrassing to some states. We did not have a political agenda when we undertook the study. We wanted to know where we stood and how effective Medicare was in translating insurance coverage into high quality care so we could assess how well we were doing in purchasing good care on behalf of Medicare beneficiaries and taxpayers.

The silence that greeted our efforts was deafening. I remember that New Jersey ranked near the bottom of the 50 states on an aggregate basis. The day after the data were released, the New Jersey Medical Society held a press conference. Surprisingly, the physicians at the press conference did not question the data or criticize HCFA (a popular pastime). Instead, they said they were concerned and would work to improve the quality of care provided to Medicare beneficiaries in New Jersey, which seems like an entirely proper and laudable reaction. But except for that press conference, I heard nothing about the report. I have since quizzed clinicians in other states—and found, totally unscientifically but, I fear, very reliably, that almost no one had heard of it. In fact, let me see a show of hands in this room of those who have heard about this report. So that is the bad news.

The good news is that just because no one has heard of the report doesn't mean that it won't have an impact. HCFA's plan is for the peer review organizations that conduct quality improvement projects (called "QIOs" or Quality Improvement Organizations) to work with the providers in each state to develop a plan to improve their scores on each of the quality-of-care indicators. Over time, the plan for New Jersey might raise some indicators by 10 or 20 percent, which would make a real difference in the lives of Medicare beneficiaries. That, I think, is the best we can hope for.

Don't get me wrong. I think that result would be terrific. But I think this example illustrates why changing health care is so hard—it is personal, and it challenges people's assumptions, and it forces them to think about things they would prefer not to think about, like what happens when loved ones get sick. It is really difficult to get a consensus about what constitutes quality health care. And I guarantee you, most clinicians believe they are providing high quality care.

Consider an anecdote that illustrates why changing health care is so hard. In the late 1980s and early 1990s, Medicare tried a demonstration program in which we designated "centers of excellence," which were hospitals that had demonstrated consistently high quality care and good outcomes for

certain procedures and were willing to accept a capitated payment and meet other standards. Beneficiaries could still go wherever they wanted to have their cataracts removed or to undergo coronary artery bypass grafting surgery, but they were offered lower copayments if they chose a center of excellence. We wanted to see if giving beneficiaries incentives to choose hospitals that had demonstrated a better quality of care would improve outcomes and save beneficiaries (and Medicare) money.

The results were even better than we expected. The outcomes for patients improved, and Medicare and the beneficiaries saved money. Therefore, we proposed extending the centers of excellence program to include other procedures and make it a permanent feature of Medicare. Great idea, right? Not so fast.

Our proposal was included in several versions of the Balanced Budget Act but was rejected by congressional conferees in the end because of heavy lobbying against it. You might assume, as I did, that the lobbying was on behalf of a group of mediocre hospitals that were threatened by the notion of providing information about outcomes and quality and offering beneficiaries incentives to choose higher quality care. You would be wrong, however. The intense opposition came from one of the premier academic health centers in this country. As it was explained to me, this facility felt it was already considered a center of excellence and did not want Medicare to put its "Good Housekeeping Seal of Approval" on other facilities. Amazing, but not that unusual! It seems that everyone wants a market-based health care system where competition is allowed to drive prices down and quality up—unless it affects them. When there's this much money involved, and when providers view it as a zero-sum game—"if hospital X gets the patients and the money, hospital Y loses"—markets do not (or are not allowed to) function as they are intended to function.

Another reason changing health care is harder than rocket science is that there is no real consensus about its goals or the laws that govern it. When you're faced with a vexing scientific or technical problem, you can go back to first principles, theorems, settled laws, and formulas. There is nothing like that in health care. Other than the vague principle that promoting the public health is a good thing and laws that say certain Americans are entitled to Medicare and Medicaid coverage, there are no rules and no entity with the authority to enforce them.

This may strike you as a strange insight coming from the person who used to run Medicare, the 900-lb. gorilla. And yes, it is true that the government, because Medicare controls about one-third of health care spending, can have a great deal of influence over what happens in health care. But in Medicare's nearly 40-year history, I think our record of using Medicare and its huge dollar impact to affect the quality of the health care delivery system is mixed at best. Medicare has shown that it can set prices. Medicare has shown that it can set minimal conditions of participation (which in some cases are proxies for quality, or at least, in the aggregate, a basis for concern if they are not met). And in recent years, the federal government has shown that it can control waste, fraud, and abuse in Medicare by aggressively (some would say too aggressively) prosecuting and punishing wrongdoers.

What is less clear is whether Congress or the public would tolerate Medicare using its market leverage and its authority to purchase health care for 40 million elderly and disabled people to affect broad changes in the delivery system. I am skeptical that this would be allowed—or for that matter, seriously attempted by any administration. The Clinton administration did make some efforts in this direction, but it was never anything we went to the mat for. When all is said and done, I am not convinced the country is ready to invest in the kind of assessments and distinctions based on quality that would force us to implement the changes we need. Certainly, Congress is not ready to support it. The government is a powerful purchaser and could be a powerful force for change. However, after eight years, I have learned that there is a good deal of opposition in Congress to giving HCFA, or any agency, the kind of authority it needs to make meaningful changes in the way health care is delivered in this country.

There are too many entrenched interests, and there is too much money at stake.

Even though this conference is asking the right questions and represents a step in the right direction, except for the adoption of some basic technologies that, despite their widespread adoption in other industries, are not yet widely used in this country, there is no consensus about what the government, or anyone else, should do to improve the quality of health care. For these reasons, I think we need to be realistic about how difficult reengineering health care delivery systems will be and how difficult it will be for the government to play a leadership role.

REFERENCES

IOM (Institute of Medicine). 2000. To Err Is Human: Building a Safer Health System, edited by L.T. Kohn, J.M. Corrigan, and M.S. Donaldson. Washington, D.C.: National Academy Press.

Jencks, S.F., T, Cuerdon, D.R. Burwen, B. Fleming, P.M. Houck, A.E. Kussmaul, D.S. Nilasena, D.L. Ordin, and D.R. Arday. 2000. Quality of medical care delivered to Medicare beneficiaries: a profile at state and national levels. Journal of the American Medical Association 284(13): 1670–1676.

Lessons from Financial Services

Ralph Kimball
Babson College

Financial services and medical services have many similarities. They are both data intensive. They are both service industries with high-stakes costs. Both have a mix of large and small providers. And both are opaque, meaning that consumers generally have a limited understanding of how they work. For both, as procedures and processes become more complex, the number and extent of system vulnerabilities increases. In other words, the more complex a system is, the more likely it is that something will go wrong. Innovations are simultaneously a source of risk and a means of avoiding risk. A new test, for example, may help identify a condition and treat it, but the test itself may involve risks.

Financial services and medical services also have many dissimilarities. Risks in financial services tend to be symmetrical; they have an up side and a down side. Many medical risks, however, have only a down side.

How much can be learned from financial services depends on how much you can learn from failure. In the last five years, there have been multi-billion-dollar failures among very sophisticated organizations; losses have been on the order of $2 billion to $3 billion, which can wipe out a major institution overnight.

The causes of those dramatic failures fall into two major categories. The first is errors in risk mitigation; a risk was identified but the attempt to reduce or manage the risk failed. Errors in risk mitigation come from three areas: agency risk, risk migration, and risk degradation. The second cause of failure is errors in risk measurement. One of the most common errors is the assumption that all risks are normally distributed. We tend to know a lot about the middle of a bell-shaped curve, but we have a very poor idea, based on historical data, of what is in the tails.

In financial services, returns are the outcome, and returns are not normally distributed. There are fewer outcomes in the middle of the curve and more at the extremes. In risk management, that means that the 100-year storm is going to occur every 50 years. The analogy in medical services is that your mitigation efforts will depend on how frequently you believe extreme adverse circumstances in the tails will occur. If you base your strategy on normal distributions, you will underinvest in risk management.

Another error in risk measurement is a failure to take covariances into account. We have found that risk is driven much more by covariances than by standard deviations. The poster child for this error is Long-Term Capital Management. Despite sophisticated models, Nobel laureates on the board, and bright employees, the company concluded that many adverse circumstances would not happen at once, that diversification would provide protection. It did not. In financial services, in periods of real stress or meltdown, the correlations tend to change. If you don't include covariances in the model, you will have a very difficult time modeling the risk. You cannot use normal periods as a basis for modeling crises; in addition, covariances and correlations may not be stable.

Another cause for error is risk ignorance, failure to recognize that a risk exists. Risk ignorance tends to be associated with innovations, a lack of familiarity with the characteristics of new products, new drugs, new surgical processes. If you are unfamiliar with what is likely to happen, it is very difficult to know how to mitigate the risk.

A risk mitigation plan itself can have risks because it provides a sense that risk has been addressed. If you haven't addressed the risk correctly, the risk can be higher than if you had no mitigation strategy. Perhaps the most common form of risk is what we in financial services call agency risk. In aviation, it is called pilot error. In medical terms, it is called medical malpractice. The employee or the staff member fails to follow established procedures.

Risk migration is another problem. Most risk mitigation efforts do not eliminate risk; they simply transform it into another form of risk or transfer it to another area. A new medication, for example, may reduce risk, but may raise the risk of administering an incorrect dosage. An example in financial services was during the meltdown in 1998, when many U.S. banks did foreign exchange swaps with Russian banks to protect themselves against the decline in the Russian ruble. That worked fine until the Russian banks failed.

That is a very clear example of risk migration. If you fail to recognize risk migration, you end up with risk ignorance. You assume you have protected yourself against a risk, when all you have done is transfer it to another site. You can't simply take the first step. You have to take the second step and know what to do if the backup system fails. What happens if this happens? What happens if that happens?

Now consider risk degradation. Case studies of major industrial disasters and major financial disasters have shown that over time there is a gradual degradation of the risk management process because systems are not maintained and audits are not done. These systems fail incrementally, and for a while as they fail, nothing seems to change. When the first light bulb goes out in your house, you may not change it because other lights are still on.

When one system fails and there are no obvious adverse circumstances, people may conclude that redundant systems are not necessary. The organization becomes desensitized to risk so that, over time, the probability that the degradation in the risk system will be addressed actually declines. Finally, a minor incident creates an interaction among these various failing systems that results in a major disaster, such as the disaster in Bhopal, which could have been prevented if the risk management systems had been maintained.

Risk management is an ongoing process that must be cared for and tended to as you go forward. Most financial services now are very humble about their ability to measure risk. We know that it is "fat-tailed," but we haven't come up with distributions that reflect how it actually behaves. Instead, we try to allow for very large margins of error. We do a lot of stress testing; we run the worst possible conditions through the model and see if anybody is left standing at the fault line. For example, a large life insurance company can stress its portfolio by assuming simultaneous 8.5 earthquakes in Los Angeles and Tokyo. Risk migration and risk ignorance can be addressed through risk mapping, a reengineering process that asks what could possibly go wrong at every point in the process.

The best way to manage risk is through real-time audits. That is the only way you can control agency risk. Real-time audits often reveal degradation in the risk management processes. Auditors have never been liked because they seem to be second guessing or interfering with procedures. However, financial services organizations with an "audit culture" are among the best trading houses on Wall Street. Some star traders have very aggressive auditors who walk the floors and call traders off the floor at any time to question their actions. Traders who make millions of dollars a year for their organizations and for themselves are not afraid to be second-guessed.

Another approach is what the aviation industry calls a "cockpit culture," in which there are frequent communications and discussions in the cockpit. Cockpit cultures are based on the idea that any member of the team can challenge what is going on at any time. I think that type of team culture can be substituted for an audit, basically relying on internal challenges rather than external challenges.

Can Purchasers Leverage Engineering Principles to Improve Health Care?

Arnold Milstein
Pacific Business Group on Health and
The Leapfrog Group

Most purchasers wish we didn't have to think about the question in the title of my presentation. Most purchasers would like the health care industry to adopt quality engineering methods as a natural expression of professional responsibility; and we would like our health insurance beneficiaries to select only quality-engineered providers as an expression of informed consumerism. However, the three Institute of Medicine (IOM) reports on quality and rapidly increasing health care costs have persuaded large purchasers to consider how they might use their unique role to accelerate American providers' journey to engineered care delivery.

Waiting for other stakeholders to solve the problem is not a promising option. When I ask consumers, like my mother, why she isn't a prudent buyer, she replies, "When I am well, I don't want to think about health care. When I am sick, I want to be able to trust that my treatment will be error-free. When I go to doctors' offices and hospitals, big white certifications with gold seals are hanging on the wall. I'd prefer to rely on them rather than be skeptical."

When I remind regulators that "Our moms are relying on you," they reply, "It's the tax cuts. We don't have the budget to ensure quality, so we rely on accreditors."

When I ask accreditors about the IOM reports and the hospitals they certify, they reply, "You force us to rely on providers to pay us for our accreditation activities. If we become too demanding, they will find a more tolerant accreditor."

When I ask hospitals and doctors about high average national rates of quality failure and the IOM reports, they reply, "We don't believe that our personal error rates are as bad as the national average. To achieve perfect care, we'd probably have to hire quality engineers and buy complex clinical information systems. Where is the money for that? Insurers don't pay us any more for these things."

When we then turn to each other in the purchaser community, we agree that we have to do something about this. But many of us are understandably cautious, reasoning, "If we begin to get aggressive and limit our insurance plan networks to providers that are engineering high quality into their care, we will surely receive many complaints from our insurance beneficiaries that we are restricting their access to the doctors and hospitals they know and love. Then our careers will be at risk. We can only go as far as our beneficiaries/consumers will let us go."

So we are back to our starting point in the "circle of nonaccountability" with consumers. Apparently, everyone is responsible for improving quality via better engineered care delivery methods, but no one feels accountable for its occurrence. Until every stakeholder has more responsibility for solutions, we aren't likely to make much progress. How can purchasers leverage engineering principles to advance the interests of all stakeholders?

Several options are available. First, purchasers can use various purchaser-mediated rewards to encourage health plans and providers to adopt engineering methods. Differential rewards could be offered to plans and providers who widely apply general engineering methods, such as the 80/20 principle, design for safety, mass customization, continuous flow production, and other methods that have worked well in other complex, high-risk industries. The most practical method of implementation may be to develop a meaningful ISO-type certification in health care and to make comprehensive, publicly released performance measurements available. We are very far from having anything like that today, at least not at a level that inspires confidence.

Another approach would be to use systems analysis to identify narrow, high-yield single "ingredients" (e.g., uptake of electronic clinical information systems or implementation of robust disease registries to provide continuous, stratified population risk scores). We could select a menu of tangible, multifaceted "best-operating practices," based on nationally distinguished care redesign efforts, such as the idealized design of clinical office practice or RWJ's Pursuing Perfection winners, and reward other providers that adopt them or health plans that encourage their adoption. The Leapfrog Group implemented a variant of the "single ingredient" approach by initially adopting three tangible operating practices, including computer physician order entry (CPOE), which improvement experts predicted would lead to big leaps in the safety of American hospital care.

However, rewarding single or multiple structural ingredients carries the risk of not fitting all providers equally well, and they are subject to implementation flaws. Accordingly, they may not lead to better performance. We may best use them as a stopgap until robust provider performance measurements are routinely available, if our prioritization of the structural ingredients that we encourage is evidence-based and strategic. One of the attractive features of tangible improvements like CPOE is that a purchaser or insurer can easily determine if a provider has implemented it. It is much harder to assess implementation of broad engineering principles, such as continuous flow production. For this reason, purchasers understandably favor narrow, less flexible, tangible engineering advances over the implementation of broad engineering principles.

Besides purchaser-mediated rewards, purchasers can apply engineering principles to their own purchasing processes. In the world of health care purchasing, there is no clear consensus on intermediate outcomes or the best way to pursue them. We operate in what systems engineers call a "zone of complexity," so we must focus on simple rules, good-enough vision, and room for innovation. The Leapfrog Group's approach of focusing on tangible operating practices aligns well with this heuristic from complex, adaptive systems thinking. The Leapfrog Group advocates a few simple, good-enough purchasing rules:

1. Hold purchasers responsible for rating their highest volume providers directly or via their plans.
2. Offer purchasers multiple methods for rewarding higher provider performance and creating a "business case" for quality and quality improvement.

3. Test each purchaser member's aggregate improvement incentives by applying Leapfrog's criterion that every year the percentage of the patient population receiving care from a provider that adopts the three Leapfrog safe practices must increase at a statistically significant rate. If not, the Leapfrog purchaser must notch up its provider rewards until this rule is met or drop out of the group.
4. Encourage consumers to take an interest in differences in quality of care ratings for providers.
5. Make the "back bencher purchasers" visible. We want Leapfrog purchasers to be clearly distinguished from other purchasers. It has been easy for purchasers to talk about quality, but to do very little about it.

Obviously, the application of complex, adaptive systems thinking to the purchase of health care is still in an embryonic stage. Leapfrog purchasing principles illustrate an intuitive, initial application. The concept of engineered purchasing warrants further development.

Let me close by briefly addressing a pivotal engineering challenge for all institutional stakeholders—the need for consumers and physicians to recognize the magnitude of current quality failure in health care in their own work. Research in social science by Kahneman, Tversky, and others is available on which to base new approaches, but applications have been few. As long as we continue to permit poor quality to remain invisible, purchasers and consumers will have trouble becoming robust advocates for quality care, and providers will only slowly incorporate engineering knowledge into their work. Today, quality defects are largely invisible to most stakeholders. Until we find a better way of addressing the invisibility problem, it is going to be hard to motivate any of the key stakeholders to apply the rich resources of engineering knowledge to improving health care.

Shibboleths in Modeling Public Policy[1]

Richard P. O'Neill
Federal Energy Regulatory Commission

Over the last 25 years, the principal direction of the government's modeling of public policy in the energy area has been to analyze the effects of more market-driven and incentive-driven outcomes. Similar efforts have been made in health care. Many of the regulations hastily put in place in the 1970s after the oil embargoes and price run-ups are still being unraveled today. As a result, paradigms that have been accepted for more than a century are changing.

People consume some services and commodities without knowing the price, then pay the bill without fully understanding how the price was determined. One of those commodities has been electricity. Attempts to create market forces in this area have been made since the 1970s, when legislation was passed to begin to open up natural gas and electricity markets. But paradigms shifts are not easy.

One of the most interesting paradigm shifts in history took place during the tenure of Pope Urban VIII. In 1530, Copernicus published a book stating that the earth revolved around the sun. At the time, Church theology held that the earth was the fixed, immovable center of the universe. But Galileo read Copernicus, looked at the skies through his newly invented telescope, and agreed with him. Soon after, Galileo published the *Dialogue*, his most controversial work, which presented the arguments for and against heliocentrism. The Inquisition banned the book, and Galileo was found guilty of heresy and condemned to spend the rest of his life under house arrest (in a palace). Writings by Copernicus and Galileo were placed on the Church's index of forbidden works, where they remained for more than 200 years. All of this happened despite the fact that the Church had been debating the truth of Copernican discoveries for decades and despite Pope Urban VIII's admiration for Galileo.

Western science doesn't always get things right the first time. Priestley, who is usually credited with discovering oxygen, went to his grave believing in the phlogiston theory of combustion. History shows that paradigm shifts are difficult.

In our day, the move from a centralized, regulated system of energy to a more decentralized system based on competitive incentives has been very difficult. In some ways, the electricity system is like a hospital, a centrally run institution with many agents (e.g., doctors, nurses, and administrators) operating with different incentives—some of them at odds with the overall mission of the organization. In the energy system, a key goal has been getting the incentives right. Very quickly, one realizes that entrenched cultural beliefs present major barriers to change. Some social scientists believe that cultural paradigm shifts can take several generations.

Modelers are often compared to carpenters with hammers looking for nails; if they find a screw instead of a nail, they pound it anyway. Many in the energy field assume that the market was in a Nash equilibrium (i.e., entities may not collude explicitly, but they do collude implicitly) in part because of a popular book, successful movie and Nobel prize on Nash's life and work. Much modeling was done based on Nash's theory, but it turned out that there was explicit collusion in Western markets.

Different jargons and market dialects often present barriers to paradigm shifts. Enormous efforts have been made to introduce competition and competitive market paradigms over the last quarter century, but many people in the field have been trained to think and speak in cost-of-service or cost-base dialect. In fact, a huge segment of the industry still talks and thinks in this dialect. Like Eskimos who have many words for snow but few words for heat stroke, market participants trying to talk about auctions and market processes do not have the appropriate grammar or vocabulary to discuss the topic.

Small, unwritten rules matter. In New Zealand, unwritten rules for government-owned electricity corporations were an

---

[1]This report does not necessarily reflect the view of the Federal Energy Regulatory Commission.

important factor in market outcomes. In other countries, when government-owned electric assets were sold to private interests, often one of the first things the CEOs did was increase their own salaries and buy private jets—hardly a confidence builder for competition.

Some popular analogies in policy discussions about electricity market reforms are to the natural gas market and the air traffic control system. Natural gas is a poor analogy for the electricity market, because natural gas can be economically stored. There is no simple equivalent of a valve in the electricity system. Some have argued that the electricity system controller should be like an air traffic controller, meaning there should be no central market-control process. These same people seem to want rules that direct behavior with no regard for cost. Most of these analogies are misleading because, even though they argue for market forces, they also lead either to greater socialization or easier manipulation of the market.

The California electricity market is an interesting case study. In the early 1990s, there was a great deal of discussion about liberalizing the California market. Technical people spent two years designing the new market, but when politicians got involved, they threw out all of the market designs and cut a deal that emerged as legislation (AB1890), which was passed unanimously. Environmentalists agreed to support the plan if they could be given money for their programs. Marketers pushed for a bad market design to ensure more profits for themselves later.

Employees of utilities who had been involved in the discussions before the compromise were told not to discuss the previously proposed market designs. A number of staff at the Federal Energy Regulatory Commission noted that the model did not provide good incentives and that the process could get out of control. For two years, the legislatively mandated market design underwent constant changes. Confusion and gaming masked what was to happen—no new generators, demand growth, and a drought. In the end, the state risked everything on a model designed by a legislative committee.

Prices in the wholesale electricity market are typically in the range of $30 to $50 per megawatt-hour. In California and most of the west, spot prices remained more than $100 per megawatt-hour for months. Then, suddenly, prices dropped, for a number of reasons: the utilities lost their credit ratings; the governor bought power under high-priced, long-term contracts; new generators came on line; and the weather changed.

Since then, hundreds of thousands of dollars have been spent on litigation to determine what went wrong and who should be punished. Interestingly, the smartest people turned out to be the consumer representatives who had been skeptical about the program and had called for a retail rate freeze and guaranteed rate reductions. Initially, they came out looking good, but in the end, the rate freeze contributed to the market disequilibrium. Consumers will be paying for these mistakes for years to come.

In retrospect, it can be seen that another player in this market caused a lot of the mischief. That player constantly proposed and funded campaigns for market designs that would not work, but that it could take advantage of. That player supported an array of approaches that all eventually failed. That player was Enron, the darling of Wall Street at the time. After Enron went bankrupt, it released a memo outlining the strategies it had used to manipulate the market in California. Wall Street lost its exuberance and abandoned its desire for Enron clones.

Some interesting questions have been asked about the California experience. For instance, was this a six-sigma event (i.e., was the outcome a low-probability event)? Or was this a one-sigma or two-sigma event (i.e., the wrong paradigm)? If we look at the debacle as an enormous experiment, some good may come of it. Theory can predict performance, and theory predicted that the market design in California would fail under stress. The California experiment cost billions of dollars, but it did prove the strength of the theory.

Another lesson we learned from California is that incentives matter. Financial incentives are very important, in energy markets and in the health care market. Fee-for-service versus salary systems can change the incentives significantly. You always have to ask what incentive a doctor or dentist has to cure a problem; non-monetary incentives are far more important in health care than in the energy industry. Dedication is a very important factor in health care and hard to model. Another issue is the principal agent problem—who acts on the patient's behalf? Programming this behavior into a model is difficult.

Bad incentives yield bad practice. Enron is a case in point in the energy market. Good accounting theory is mark-to-market accounting. In theory, mark-to-market accounting is theoretically correct, but in practice, in thin markets the market price is prone to manipulation. In fact, it can often simply be made up. Enron took advantage of this gap and produced a grossly distorted set of accounts.

In energy and health care markets, good market designs can yield benefits. Here are some don'ts in market design: don't oversimplify; don't create gaming opportunities; don't favor large players; don't use market jargon or model jargon to explain things; don't ignore the extreme model outcomes, because outliers often provide interesting information and stories. The modeler should be immersed in the problem. Outsiders may be brought in to help, but somebody must intimately understand the model, as well as the process being modeled.

Clients should understand that models provide insights. Forecast are often wrong, but everyone must forecast. Forecasting often involves insight into possible outcomes, rather than numbers. The model must be tuned based on experience. A model should not be a black box. It should be available to people; it should be testable; and it should be auditable.

A lesson for health care modeling is that modeling can be a useful tool, but a healthy skepticism is necessary for success.

Matching and Allocation in Medicine and Health Care

Alvin E. Roth
Harvard University

Many of the previous speakers have considered hospitals analogous to factories. But, unlike factories, hospitals are highly decentralized, and many of the important decision makers, including doctors (not to mention patients), aren't employees of the hospital; they come to the hospital on their own patient-care missions, and they have their own objectives.

To efficiently allocate resources to serve these different objectives, it becomes necessary to elicit information from the people who have it. But eliciting information isn't always simple, because the information we can elicit depends in part on what we plan to do with it. When you ask me about something I know, I want to ask you why you are asking. What you intend to do with my answers will influence the way I answer you.

That is, what information we can reliably obtain depends in part on how we use it and what incentives this gives the people from whom we must get the information. My own most relevant experience of these issues in a medical context comes from redesigning the resident match, so I'll start my discussion there. Then I'll suggest how similar "strategic" issues might arise in organ transplantation, scheduling operating rooms, etc.

Hospitals only began offering internships about a hundred years ago. Typically, a student graduated from medical school, then looked for a job at a hospital. By the 1920s, interns had become a significant part of the labor force in hospitals; and internships had become an important part of the career path of doctors. Hospitals began to try to get good interns by hiring them a little bit earlier than their competitors. Gradually, hiring began earlier and earlier, and by 1945, hospitals were hiring medical students as early as the end of their sophomore year of medical school for internships that would begin only after graduation. As a result, residents were being hired so early in their education that it was very hard for residency programs to distinguish the best candidates, or even for candidates to be sure what kind of residency program they would be interested in. In 1945, medical schools intervened by refusing to release any student information before a certain date—no transcripts, no letters of recommendation, no confirmation that a student was in good standing in medical school. It may have been risky to hire someone just on the basis of sophomore-year grades, but it was even riskier to hire someone just because he said he was a medical student. So, this intervention was successful at controlling the dates of appointment, and as this became apparent, the date of appointment was successfully moved later, into the senior year of medical school, when more information about students' abilities and preferences was available for finding appropriate matches of students and hospitals.

But, between 1945 and 1950, a new problem appeared. In 1945, hospitals were all supposed to wait until a given day to make offers and give students 10 days to accept or reject those offers. What happened? Consider a student who got an offer from his third-choice hospital and had 10 days to decide. Suppose that student also heard from his first- or second-choice hospital, saying they liked the student but were not making an offer yet; the student had been placed on a waiting list in case some of the offers they had made were rejected. So, the student waited, which was easy to do because he had 10 days to decide about the offer from his third-choice hospital. If all students waited those 10 days, the waiting lists didn't move, and on the tenth day bad things happened. The student might have accepted his third-choice offer and then, later in the day, received a more preferred offer. The student might have accepted that too. If, after even only a modest delay to gather his courage, he informed his third-choice hospital of his change of heart, students whom that hospital would have liked to hire may have already committed to other hospitals. (Obviously the hospital's problem could be even worse if a long time passed before they realized they had an unfilled position.) On the other hand, even if the student felt honor bound to decline a late, more preferred offer, he might have spent the next year very unhappily at his third-choice hospital, explaining to all his colleagues why a talented doc like him shouldn't have been working in a place like this. Either way, there was a lot of unhappiness.

Given that all these troubles had occurred on the tenth day, in 1946 hospitals agreed to allow only *eight* days for offers to remain open. As you might imagine, this didn't solve the problem. By 1949, residency programs were giving exploding offers—students had to accept or reject immediately, without knowing what other offers might be forthcoming. So, once again, decisions were being made without all the information that might be available.

In the early 1950s, a radical innovation was tried—a centralized clearinghouse. Graduating medical students submitted to the clearinghouse a list, in order of preference, of the residency programs at which they had interviewed. Residency programs similarly ranked students they had interviewed. These rank order lists—that is, the information elicited from the participants in the market for residents—were then used to match students to residency programs. And although this system has evolved over the years to take account of changes in the medical marketplace, it has survived to the present day in something close to its original form, as the National Resident Matching Program. (I had the privilege of directing the most recent redesign of the matching algorithm.)

The surprising thing that was observed in the 1950s is that most positions were filled as matched: that is, students and residency programs submitted their rank order lists and then went on to sign the employment contracts suggested by the match. We now understand that this wasn't inevitable, but it came about because the match algorithm that was chosen in the 1950s produced matches that were *stable*, in the sense that there were never "blocking pairs" consisting of a student and a residency program that were not matched to one another but that would both have preferred to be matched to one another rather than matched to their actual partners.

It is easy to see in principle why a clearinghouse that produces *un*stable matches might not succeed. A student who receives a match with her third-choice hospital, for example, only has to make two phone calls to find out if she is part of a blocking pair. She calls her first- and second- choice hospitals and says, "before I accept my match outcome, I just wanted to check if you might have a position for me." If she is part of a blocking pair, then one of the hospitals will see that they prefer her to someone with whom they are supposed to match. They might say something like, "by chance we have an extra position . . ." and then call up the candidate they liked less and say they've had a budget shortfall and are one position short. But if the match is stable, when the hospital looks at the list of people with whom it is supposed to match, it sees that it would prefer to go ahead with the match. To put it another way, if the match is stable, no candidate can find a hospital that she would prefer to go to that is willing to take her.

One way the importance of stability became evident had to do with the growing number of couples graduating from American medical schools who wanted to find two residency positions in the same city. The number of couples increased in the 1970s, as medical schools stopped being overwhelmingly male. An attempt was made to accommodate couples by allowing them (after being certified by their deans as a "genuine" couple) to indicate that they wished to be matched to residencies in the same city. Then each individual submitted a rank order list, as if they were single, except that they were asked to specify one member of the couple as the "leading" member. The leading member went through the match as if single, and the rank order list of the other member was then edited to remove options that were not in the same city as the residency to which the leading member had matched.

Although this procedure did give couples two jobs in the same city, many couples started to find their residencies outside of the match, and it is easy to see why. Suppose that my wife and I have as our first choice two particular, good positions in Boston. Our second choice would be to get two particular positions in New York. If instead we get one good job in Boston and one bad one, we're not going to be very happy (because of the Iron Law of Marriage, which says you can't be happier than your spouse). So an instability may exist: when we call the two residency programs in New York, they may be happy to take us, which now leaves the Boston jobs unfilled and some people who were matched to the New York jobs scrambling to find new ones.

So, a failure to elicit the right kind of information (the preferences of couples) contributed to a decline in the effectiveness of the match by giving couples incentives to circumvent the clearinghouse. The present match deals with that by allowing couples to submit rank order lists of *pairs* of positions. Last year about 550 couples (1,100 people) participated in the match as couples.

Another way the importance of stability became clear was through the experience of British doctors. In the 1960s, the British began to experience the same kind of troubles the American medical market had experienced before 1945. But in Britain, different regions of the National Health Service adopted different kinds of centralized clearinghouses. Some produced stable matches, and some did not. The stable systems are still working; but most of the unstable ones failed, sometimes quite dramatically, even though the National Health Service can mandate that jobs be filled through the centralized clearinghouse.

But participants learned to circumvent unstable clearinghouses. In the Birmingham area, for example, after a few years, the majority of the rank order lists submitted by students contained only a single position, and hospital programs in turn listed only the students who listed them in this way. In other words, by the time the lists were submitted, the matching of students to positions had already been determined privately, in advance, by the parties, and they wrote each other's names down and that was that. That is, people can often find ways to circumvent even compulsory systems, if they have incentives to do so. In contrast, stable mechanisms that do not give people incentives to get around them can function efficiently for years.

Before I move on to topics more directly related to patient care, let me just mention that no design of an allocation or matching system can be successful unless it is first adopted for use. So part of the design process is the adoption process. The question of how radical changes are adopted is ultimately political. Those who want to see their work implemented need to understand the objections to it, the fears it may arouse, and what constituencies are concerned. Because complex systems in which information is decentralized are subject to being gamed and circumvented, these "political" concerns need to be addressed carefully.

What are the lessons of these kinds of matching processes for allocation issues more directly concerned with patient care? People don't get sick because of incentives, so you might think that incentives, which are such a big deal in labor markets, won't play a big role in allocation decisions directly concerned with health care.

But consider organ transplants. There are about 80,000 candidates on various waiting lists for organs. Last year, about 22,000 organs were harvested from 11,000 donors. There is scarcity here and real questions about allocation. Over time, the United Network for Organ Sharing has made many modifications in the system allocating these scarce organs. There are waiting lists, with priorities based on criteria such as time on the list and current health.

While the details of the allocation rule will certainly affect who gets which organ (or who gets an organ and who does not), it might not be clear how the incentives created by different allocation rules can affect the overall efficiency of allocation. To get an idea of this, consider the case of pediatric heart transplants.

Congenital heart defects can now be discovered *in utero*. When priority started to be given to patients with greater time on the waiting list, pediatric cardiologists began to put their patients on the waiting list while they were still in the womb. If a heart became available before the pregnancy was full term, it was often nevertheless in the patient's interest to perform a C-section, so that the baby would get the heart. That meant that donor hearts started going into babies who were not full term and were lower birth weight, which isn't good for the overall survival rate. Now the system has been modified so that fetuses can be on a waiting list, but in a

different category than already born pediatric patients. But giving more priority to time on the waiting list changed the incentives of pediatric cardiologists and changed the flow of hearts into babies in an unanticipated and not necessarily positive way.

This brings me back to the game theory observation with which I began—when agents have different objectives (e.g., when each doctor is concerned with managing his own patients), how information is used to make allocations affects the incentives of those who have the information in ways that can alter the allocations in unintended ways. Many aspects of the allocation process for organs involves these issues, from the debate over regional versus national waiting lists to the priorities that should be given to different kinds of candidates (e.g., chronic versus acute illness). And patients, as well as doctors, can act strategically based on their incentives, as when a given patient may be able to place himself on multiple regional lists, for example.

Similarly, other medical allocation issues involve information that must be elicited from interested participants. For instance, one of the big issues in scheduling an operating room that is used by many surgeons is how long a given operation will take. How an operation is described can influence its estimated duration, which in turn influences what resources it is allocated. To make appropriate allocation and scheduling decisions, it is first necessary to elicit information, and what information is delivered depends on how that information will be used.

This is of course a common issue in markets. And because doctors often run their own businesses, the business of the hospital interacts with the business of the market. So we need to remain aware that anything done inside a hospital interacts with all of the other things that go on in the medical marketplace outside of the hospital.

In summary, to do allocation well, information is needed. When information is decentralized, it still must be found. One of the things that makes systems in which information is decentralized different from those in which it is centralized is the importance of incentives and the constraints that incentives put on what can be done. In the medical market for residents, there is a lot of evidence to support the contention that the stability constraint is binding. As we start to think about how to elicit information to make allocation decisions in other systems, we will have to pay attention to the incentive constraints.

Appendixes

Appendix A

Agenda for First Workshop

WORKSHOP ON ENGINEERING AND HEALTH CARE DELIVERY SYSTEMS

May 21–22, 2001
Cecil and Ida Green Building
2001 Wisconsin Avenue, N.W.
Washington, D.C.

May 21

9:15 a.m.	Welcome and Opening Remarks *Kenneth I. Shine, M.D., President, Institute of Medicine*
9:25 a.m.	Session I: Transforming Health Care Delivery Systems: Realizing the Potential of Radical Advances in Engineering, Science, and Technology Moderator: *W. Dale Compton, Lillian M. Gilbreth Distinguished Professor of Industrial Engineering, Purdue University*
9:30 a.m.	Opening Keynote Address *Jeff Goldsmith, President, Health Futures Inc.*
10:15 a.m.	Panel Presentations and Discussion "Crossing the Quality Chasm: A New Health System for the 21st Century": Key Findings of the Quality of Health Care in America Committee *Janet Corrigan, Director, Quality of Health Care in America Project and Division of Health Care Services, Institute of Medicine* Evidence-Based Medicine/Outcomes Assessment: Invitation to Engineering Process Redesign *Brian Haynes, M.D., Professor and Chair, Clinical Epidemiology and Biostatistics and Medicine, McMaster University*
Break	
	Systems Engineering: The Logistics Revolution and Opportunities for Health Care Delivery *Jennifer K. Ryan, Assistant Professor of Industrial Engineering, Purdue University* Informatics and Information Technology: Foundations for Decision Support and Process Improvement *William W. Stead, M.D., Professor of Medicine and Biomedical Informatics, Director of the Informatics Center, Associate Vice Chancellor for Health Affairs, Vanderbilt University*
1:00 p.m.	Lunch
2:00 p.m.	Session II: Transforming Health Care Delivery Systems: Exploring Potentially High-Yield Areas for Engineering/Medicine Collaboration and Innovation Moderator: *Jerome H. Grossman, M.D., Senior Fellow, Center for Business and Government, John F. Kennedy School of Government, Harvard University* Modeling the Total Delivery System: Simulation Modeling Applied to Population Health Management and Distributed Health Care Delivery Systems *John K. Taylor, M.D., Medical Director, and Seth Bonder, Chairman and CEO, Vector Research, Inc.* Modeling Disease: Cancer Services in Transformation *Molla S. Donaldson, Health Policy Analyst, National Cancer Institute, and Codirector, IOM Quality of Health Care in America Project*

Modeling the Hospital
  Robert S. Dittus, M.D., M.P.H., Director of General Internal Medicine and of the Geriatric Research, Education and Clinical Center, Vanderbilt University
Modeling the Clinic: Toward the Idealized Practice
  Thomas W. Nolan, Chief Executive Officer, Associates in Process Improvement, and Faculty Member, Institute for Healthcare Improvement

5:30 p.m.   Adjourn
5:45 p.m.   Reception and Dinner
                 Keynote Speaker: *David M. Lawrence, M.D., Chairman and CEO, Kaiser Foundation Health Plan Inc.*

May 22

8:00 a.m.   Session III: Transforming Health Care Delivery Systems: Human Factors and Risk Management in Distributed Delivery Systems
                 Moderator: *Marshall L. Fisher, Heyman Professor of Operations Management, University of Pennsylvania*
                 Disruptive Innovation in Healthcare: Implications for Patient and Provider Roles and Responsibilities
                   Richard Bohmer, M.D., M.P.H., James M. Collins Fund Senior Lecturer in Business Administration, Harvard Business School
                 Patient Risk Management Systems
                   Charles R. Denham, M.D., Cofounder, Premier Innovation Institute
                 Enhancing Delivery System Accountability and Performance: Insights from Social and Behavioral Sciences
                   Dana Gelb Safran, Director, The Health Institute, New England Medical Center
                 Failures in Risk Management: Lessons from Financial Services
                   Ralph C. Kimball, Associate Professor, School of Management, Babson College
10:30 a.m.   Session IV: Identifying Priority Areas for Health Care Delivery System Research and Innovation
                 Moderator: *Paul F. Griner, M.D., Professor Emeritus, University of Rochester School of Medicine and Dentistry*
                 Identifying Priority Areas: A Payer Perspective
                   Christopher Stanley, M.D., Medical Director, UnitedHealthcare of North Carolina
                 Improving Health and Health Care: Priority Areas for Research and Innovation
                   Lewis G. Sandy, M.D., Executive Vice President, Robert Wood Johnson Foundation
                 Can Purchasers Leverage Engineering Principles to Improve Health Care?
                   Arnold Milstein, M.D., M.P.H, Managing Director, William M. Mercer Inc., and Medical Director, Pacific Business Group on Health
                 Commentary
                   Nancy-Ann DeParle, Former Administrator, Health Care Financing Administration, U.S. Department of Health and Human Services
12:15 p.m.   Closing Remarks
                   Jerome Grossman, M.D., Senior Fellow, Center for Business and Government, John F. Kennedy School of Government, Harvard University
12:45 p.m.   Adjourn

Appendix B

Participants in First Workshop

Workshop on Engineering and Health Care Delivery Systems
May 21–22, 2001

John A. Alic, Ph.D.
Consultant
Washington, DC 20024

Neeraj Arora, Ph.D.
Outcomes Research Branch, ARP, DCCPS
National Cancer Institute

Philip Aspden, Ph.D.
Senior Program Officer
Board on Science, Technology, and Economic Policy
Policy and Global Affairs Division
The National Academies

James P. Bagian, M.D., P.E.
Director, National Center for Patient Safety
Department of Veterans Affairs
Veterans Health Administration

John E. Billi, M.D.
Associate Dean for Clinical Affairs
Associate Vice President for Medical Affairs
University of Michigan

Richard Bohmer, M.D., M.P.H.
Senior Lecturer
Harvard Business School

Seth Bonder, Ph.D.
Chairman and CEO
Vector Research Inc.

David A. Burnett, M.D., M.B.A.
Vice President
University HealthSystem Consortium

Kathryn Ciffolillo, M.A.
Writer
North Easton, MA 02356

W. Dale Compton, Ph.D.
Lillian M. Gilbreth Distinguished Professor of Industrial
    Engineering
School of Industrial Engineering
Purdue University

Janet Corrigan, Ph.D.
Director, Quality of Health Care in America Project
    and Board on Health Care Services
Institute of Medicine
The National Academies

Lance A. Davis, Ph.D.
Executive Officer
National Academy of Engineering
The National Academies

Donna J. Dean, Ph.D.
Acting Interim Director
National Institute of Biomedical Imaging and
    Bioengineering
National Institutes of Health

Charles R. Denham, M.D.
Co-founder
Premier Innovation Institute

Nancy-Ann DeParle, J.D.
Former Administrator
Health Care Financing Administration
U.S. Department of Health and Human Services

245

Robert S. Dittus, M.D., M.P.H.
Joe and Morris Werthan Professor of Investigative
    Medicine
Director, Center for Health Services Research
Vanderbilt University Medical Center

Molla S. Donaldson, M.S.
Health Policy Analyst
Outcomes Research Branch, ARP, DCCPS
National Cancer Institute

Thomas L. Garthwaite, M.D.
Under Secretary for Health
Department of Veterans Affairs
Veterans Health Administration

Jeff Goldsmith, Ph.D.
President
Health Futures Inc.

Paul F. Griner, M.D.
Professor Emeritus
University of Rochester School of Medicine and Dentistry

Jerome H. Grossman, M.D.
Senior Fellow
Center for Business and Government
John F. Kennedy School of Government
Harvard University

Diwakar Gupta, Ph.D.
Associate Professor
Department of Mechanical Engineering
University of Minnesota

Craig M. Harvey, Ph.D., P.E.
Assistant Professor of Industrial and Human Factors
    Engineering
Wright State University

Brian Haynes, M.D., Ph.D.
Professor and Chair
Clinical Epidemiology and Biostatistics and Medicine
McMaster University

Ralph C. Kimball, Ph.D.
Associate Professor
School of Management
Babson College

David M. Lawrence, M.D.
Chairman and CEO
Kaiser Foundation Health Plan Inc.

Thomas C. Mahoney, M.A.
Director, WV-MEP
University of West Virginia

Donald J. Marsh, M.D.
Dean of Medicine and Biological Sciences
Brown University

Stephen A. Merrill, Ph.D.
Executive Director
Board on Science, Technology, and Economic Policy
Policy and Global Affairs Division
The National Academies

Howard Messing
Executive Vice President
Medical Information Technology

Arnold Milstein, M.D., M.P.H.
Managing Director
William M. Mercer Inc. and
Medical Director
Pacific Business Group on Health

Thomas W. Nolan, Ph.D.
Chief Executive Officer
Associates in Process Improvement

John A. Parrish, M.D.
Director, Center for Integration of Medicine
    and Innovation Technologies
Harvard Medical School
Massachusetts General Hospital

James Phimister, Ph.D.
Postdoctoral Fellow
Risk Management and Decision Processes Center
The Wharton School
University of Pennsylvania

Ronald L. Rardin, Ph.D.
Program Director for Operations Research and Production
    Systems
National Science Foundation

Proctor P. Reid, Ph.D.
Associate Director
Program Office
National Academy of Engineering
The National Academies

Brian Rosenfeld, M.D., FCCM
Chief Medical Officer and Cofounder
VISICU

Jennifer K. Ryan, Ph.D.
Assistant Professor
School of Industrial Engineering
Purdue University

Dana Gelb Safran, Sc.D.
Director
The Health Institute
New England Medical Center

Lewis G. Sandy, M.D., M.B.A.
Executive Vice President
Robert Wood Johnson Foundation

Adam L. Scheffler, M.A., LSW
Policy Researcher/Consultant
Chicago, Illinois

Alan Scheller-Wolf, Ph.D.
Associate Professor of Manufacturing and Operations
    Management
Graduate School of Industrial Administration
Carnegie Mellon University

James C. Sherlock, B.A.
Program Manager
Science Applications International Corporation

Kenneth I. Shine, M.D.
President
Institute of Medicine
The National Academies

Warner V. Slack, M.D.
Professor of Medicine and Psychiatry
Center for Clinical Computing
Harvard Medical School

Harry J. Smolen, M.S.
President
Medical Decision Modeling Inc.

Christopher Stanley, M.D.
Medical Director
UnitedHealthcare of North Carolina

William W. Stead, M.D.
Professor of Medicine and Biomedical Informatics and
    Director, Informatics Center
Associate Vice Chancellor for Health Affairs
Vanderbilt University

John K. Taylor, M.D.
Medical Director
Vector Research Inc.

Eoin W. Trevelyan, D.B.A.
Lecturer in Management
Department of Health Policy and Management
Harvard School of Public Health

Lawrence M. Wein, Ph.D.
DEC Leaders for Manufacturing Professor of Management
    Science
Sloan School of Management
Massachusetts Institute of Technology

Mark J. Young, M.D.
Chair, Department of Health Evaluation Sciences
Penn State College of Medicine and
Chairman, Department of Community Health and Health
    Studies
Lehigh Valley Hospital

Appendix C

Agenda for Second Workshop

WORKSHOP ON ENGINEERING AND HEALTH CARE DELIVERY SYSTEMS

February 6–7, 2003
Arnold and Mabel Beckman Center
National Academies of Sciences and Engineering
100 Academy Drive
Irvine, California

February 6

7:30 a.m.	Breakfast	
8:15 a.m.	Welcome and Review of Agenda	
	Co-chairs Dale Compton and Jerome Grossman	
8:30 a.m.	Round-the-Room Introductions	
9:00 a.m.	Session I:	Engineering and the Health Care System
	9:00–9:20	*Brent James, Executive Director, Institute for Health Care Delivery Research*
	9:20–9:40	*Richard Coffey, Director, Health System Planning, University of Michigan Health System*
	9:40–10:15	Q&A
10:15 a.m.	Break	
10:30 a.m.	Session II:	Engineering and the Patient-Care Team
	10:30–11:45	Panel Presentations
		Dave Gustafson, Professor of Industrial Engineering, University of Wisconsin, Madison
		Bryan Sexton, Postdoctoral Fellow through the University of Texas Center of Excellence for Patient Safety Research and Practice
		Ann Hendrich, President, Ann Hendrich and Associates
	11:45–12:00	Q&A
12:15 p.m.	Lunch	
1:00 p.m.	Engineering and the Patient-Care Team Breakout Session	
1:45 p.m.	Plenary: Group Presentations and Discussion	
2:45 p.m.	Break	
3:00 p.m.	Session III:	Engineering and the Organization
	3:00–4:15	Panel Presentations
		Paul Clayton, Chief Medical Informatics Officer, Intermountain Health Care
		Prince Zachariah, Professor of Medicine, Mayo Clinic Scottsdale
		Vinod Sahney, Senior Vice President, Planning and Strategic Development, Henry Ford Health System
	4:15–4:30	Q&A
4:30 p.m.	Engineering and the Organization Breakout Session	
5:15 p.m.	Plenary Session: Group Presentations and Discussion	
6:15 p.m.	Reception	
6:45 p.m.	Dinner	
7:45 p.m.	Keynote Speaker: *Denis Cortese, President and CEO, Mayo Clinic*	
8:45 p.m.	Adjourn	

February 7

8:00 a.m.	Breakfast	
8:30 a.m.	Welcome and Overview of the Day	
	Co-chairs Dale Compton and Jerome Grossman	
8:45 a.m.	Session IV:	Engineering and the System Environment
	8:45–10:00	Panel Presentations
		Paul Tang, Chief Medical Information Officer, Palo Alto Medical Foundation
		Seth Bonder, Founder, Vector Research Inc.
		David Classen, Vice President, First Consulting Group
	10:00–10:15	Q&A
10:15 a.m.	Break	
10:30 a.m.	Engineering and the System Environment Breakout Session	
11:15 a.m.	Plenary Session: Group Presentations and Discussion	
12:15 p.m.	Closing Remarks by Co-chairs	
12:30 p.m.	Adjournment and Lunch	

Appendix D

Participants in Second Workshop

Workshop on Engineering and the Health Care System
Irvine, California
February 6–7, 2003

Rebecca M. Bergman
Vice President, Science and Technology
Medtronic Inc.

John R. Birge (*by phone*)
Dean, McCormick School of Engineering and Applied
    Science
Northwestern University

Seth Bonder
Retired Chairman and CEO
Vector Research Inc.

J. Mark Campbell
Director, Western Region
PROMODEL Corporation

David C. Classen
Vice President
First Consulting Group

Paul D. Clayton
Chief Medical Informatics Officer
Intermountain Health Care

Richard J. Coffey
Director, Health System Planning
University of Michigan Health System

W. Dale Compton
Lillian M. Gilbreth Distinguished Professor of Industrial
    Engineering
School of Industrial Engineering
Purdue University

Janet Corrigan
Director, Board on Health Care Services
Institute of Medicine
The National Academies

Denis Cortese
President and CEO
Mayo Clinic

Matthew Cottle
Director, Major Gifts
Office of Development
The National Academies

Robert S. Dittus
Director, Center for Health Services Research
Vanderbilt University Medical Center

Gary Fanjiang
Fellow, National Academy of Engineering Program Office
The National Academies

G. Scott Gazelle
MGH Institute for Technology Assessment

Jerome H. Grossman
Senior Fellow
Center for Business and Government
John F. Kennedy School of Government
Harvard University

David H. Gustafson
Professor of Industrial Engineering
University of Wisconsin-Madison

Randolph Hall
Professor, Chairman, and Associate Dean for Research,
    Industrial and Systems Engineering
University of Southern California

Carol Haraden
Vice President
Institute for Healthcare Improvement

Ann Hendrich
Robert Wood Johnson Fellow and President
Ann Hendrich and Associates

Brent C. James
Executive Director
Institute for Health Care Delivery Research
Intermountain Health Care Inc.

Ernest G. Ludy
EGL Investments LLC

Richard J. Migliori
Chief Executive Officer
United Resource Networks

Woodrow Myers
Executive Vice President and Chief Medical Officer
WellPoint Health Networks

Robert M. Nerem
Parker H. Petit Professor and Director
Institute for Bioengineering and Bioscience
Georgia Institute of Technology

James Phimister
J. Herbert Hollomon Fellow
National Academy of Engineering Program Office
The National Academies

William P. Pierskalla
John E. Anderson Professor of Management and Former
    Dean
The Anderson School at UCLA
University of California, Los Angeles

Ronald L. Rardin
Program Director for Operations Research and Service
    Enterprise Engineering
National Science Foundation

Proctor P. Reid
Associate Director
National Academy of Engineering Program Office
The National Academies

Frances Richmond
Director, Regulatory and Clinical Science
Alfred E. Mann Institute of Biomedical Engineering
University of Southern California

Denise Runde
Vice President
Foundation for Accountability (FACCT)

Vinod K. Sahney
Senior Vice President
Planning and Strategic Development
Henry Ford Health System

Laurence C. Seifert
Retired Executive Vice President
AT&T Wireless Group
AT&T Corporation

J. Bryan Sexton
Postdoctoral Fellow through the University of Texas Center
    of Excellence for Patient Safety Research and Practice

Andrei M. Shkel
Assistant Professor
Biomedical Engineering
University of California-Irvine

Stephen M. Shortell (*by phone*)
Blue Cross of California Distinguished Professor of Health
    Policy and Management
School of Public Health
University of California-Berkeley

Paul Tang
Chief Medical Information Officer
Palo Alto Medical Foundation

Kensall D. Wise (*by phone*)
J. Reid and Polly Anderson Professor of Manufacturing
    Technology
University of Michigan

David D. Woods
Professor in Industrial and Systems Engineering
Institute for Ergonomics
Ohio State University

Jonathan Young
Program Manager, Safety and Risk Assessment
Environmental Technology Division
Pacific Northwest National Laboratory

Prince K. Zachariah
Professor of Medicine
Mayo Clinic Scottsdale

Appendix E

Agenda for Third Workshop

WORKSHOP ON ENGINEERING AND THE HEALTH CARE SYSTEM

March 10–11, 2003
National Academies Room 201
500 Fifth Street, N.W., Washington, D.C.

March 10

8:30 a.m.	Continental Breakfast
9:15 a.m.	Welcome and Review of Agenda
	Dale Compton, Lillian M. Gilbreth Distinguished Professor of Industrial Engineering, Purdue University
9:30 a.m.	Round-the-Room Introductions
9:45 a.m.	Designing Health Care Systems That Are Caregiver and Patient Centered
	Kent Bowen, Professor of Technology and Operations Management, Harvard Business School
10:15 a.m.	Session I: Engineering as Part of the Patient Care Team
	Moderator: *Rebecca Bergman, Vice President of Science and Technology, Medtronic Inc.*
	10:15–11:30 Panel Presentations
	The Human Factor in Health Care Systems Design
	Kim Vicente, Professor, University of Toronto
	Practical Biomonitoring Using Wireless Technology
	Thomas Budinger, Head, Center for Functional Imaging, Lawrence Berkeley National Laboratory
	The eICU® Solution—A Technology-Enabled Care Paradigm for Improved ICU Performance
	Michael Breslow, Executive Vice President of Research and Development, VISICU
	11:30–11:45 Q&A
11:45 a.m.	Lunch
12:30 p.m.	Lunch Presentation
	Carolyn Clancy, Director, Agency for Healthcare Research and Quality
1:15 p.m.	Breakout Session
2:15 p.m.	Presenter Preparation Time and Break
2:30 p.m.	Plenary Session: Group Presentations and Discussion
3:15 p.m.	Session II: Engineering, Modeling, and the Health Care System
	Moderator: *John Birge, Dean, Robert R. McCormick School of Engineering and Applied Science, Northwestern University*
	3:15–4:30 Panel Presentations
	Shibboleths in Public Policy Modeling
	Richard O'Neill, Chief Economic Advisor, Federal Energy Regulatory Commission
	Matching and Allocation in Medicine and Health Care
	Alvin Roth, George Gund Professor of Economics and Business Administration, Harvard University
	Supply Chain Management: Pursuing a System-Level Understanding
	Reha Uzsoy, Professor of Industrial Engineering, Purdue University
	4:30–4:45 Q&A

5:00 p.m.	Shuttle to NAS Building
5:30 p.m.	Reception
6:00 p.m.	Dinner
7:00 p.m.	Keynote Speaker

Engineering in the Service of Health Care: An Example
David Eddy, Senior Advisor for Health Policy and Management, Kaiser Permanente

March 11

7:30 a.m.	Breakfast	
8:00 a.m.	Opening Presentation	

Mindy Aisen, Director, Deputy Chief Research and Development Officer, Department of Veterans Affairs

8:45 a.m.	Breakout Session	
9:30 a.m.	Presenter Preparation Time and Break	
9:45 a.m.	Plenary Session: Group Presentations and Discussion	
10:30 a.m.	Session III:	Connecting the Patient to the System
	Moderator:	*David Woods, Professor in Industrial and Systems Engineering, Ohio State University*
	10:30–11:45	Panel Presentations

Connecting Patients, Providers, and Payers
John Halamka, Senior Vice President and Chief Information Officer, CareGroup
Applying Financial Engineering to Health Services
John Mulvey, Professor of Operations Research and Financial Engineering, Princeton University

	11:45–12:00	Q&A
12:00 p.m.	Lunch	
1:00 p.m.	Breakout Session	
1:45 p.m.	Presenter Preparation Time and Break	
2:00 p.m.	Plenary Session: Group Presentations and Discussion	
2:45 p.m.	Closing Remarks	

Cochair Dale Compton

3:00 p.m.	Workshop Adjourns

Appendix F

Participants in Third Workshop

Workshop on Engineering and the Health Care System
Washington, DC
March 10–11, 2003

Mindy Aisen
Deputy Chief Research and Development Officer
Department of Veterans Affairs

Jim Benneyan
Assistant Professor
Mechanical, Industrial and Manufacturing Engineering
Northeastern University

Rebecca M. Bergman
Vice President, Science and Technology
Medtronic Inc.

John R. Birge
Dean, McCormick School of Engineering and Applied
    Science
Northwestern University

H. Kent Bowen
Bruce Rauner Professor in Business Administration
Harvard Business School

Patricia Flatley Brennan
Moehlman Bascom Professor
School of Nursing and College of Engineering
University of Wisconsin

Michael J. Breslow
Executive Vice President
Research and Development
VISICU Inc.

Thomas F. Budinger
Head, Department of Nuclear Medicine and Functional
    Imaging
E.O. Lawrence Berkeley National Laboratory

Carolyn M. Clancy
Director
Agency for Healthcare Research and Quality

W. Dale Compton
Lillian M. Gilbreth Distinguished Professor of Industrial
    Engineering
School of Industrial Engineering
Purdue University

Janet Corrigan
Director, Board on Health Care Services
Institute of Medicine
The National Academies

Denis Cortese
President and CEO
Mayo Clinic

Donna J. Dean
Deputy Director
National Institute of Biomedical Imaging and
    Bioengineering
National Institutes of Health

Robert S. Dittus
Director, Center for Health Services Research
Vanderbilt University Medical Center

Molla S. Donaldson
Senior Scientist for Quality of Care Research and Policy
Outcomes Research Branch
National Cancer Institute

David M. Eddy
Senior Advisor for Health Policy and Management
Kaiser Permanente

Gary Fanjiang
Fellow, National Academy of Engineering Program Office
The National Academies

G. Scott Gazelle
Director
MGH Institute for Technology Assessment

Linda Green
Armand G. Erpf Professor
Columbia School of Business

Paul F. Griner
Professor of Medicine, Emeritus
University of Rochester School of Medicine

Jerome H. Grossman (by phone)
Senior Fellow
Center for Business and Government
John F. Kennedy School of Government
Harvard University

John D. Halamka
Chief Information Officer
CareGroup Health System and Harvard Medical School

Carol Haraden
Vice President
Institute for Healthcare Improvement

Andrew Kusiak
Professor, Intelligent Systems Laboratory
University of Iowa

Eva K. Lee
Assistant Professor and Director for Operations Research
    in Medicine
School of Industrial and Systems Engineering
Georgia Institute of Technology

Eugene Litvak
Director, Program for Management of Variability in Health
    Care Delivery
Health Policy Institute
Boston University

Richard J. Migliori
CEO
United Resource Networks

John M. Mulvey
Professor, Operations Research and Financial Engineering
Princeton University

Woodrow Myers
Executive Vice President and Chief Medical Officer
WellPoint Health Networks

Richard P. O'Neill
Economic Group Manager
Office of Markets, Tariffs, and Rates
U.S. Department of Energy

James Phimister
J. Herbert Hollomon Fellow
National Academy of Engineering Program Office
The National Academies

Catherine Plaisant
Associate Director
Human-Computer Interaction Laboratory
University of Maryland

Peter J. Pronovost
Associate Professor and Medical Director
Center for Innovations in Quality Patient Care
Johns Hopkins University School of Medicine

Ronald L. Rardin
Program Director for Operations Research and Service
    Enterprise Engineering
National Science Foundation

Proctor P. Reid
Associate Director
National Academy of Engineering Program Office
The National Academies

Alvin E. Roth
George Gund Professor of Economics and Business
    Administration
Department of Economics
Harvard University

Donald M. Steinwachs
Professor and Chair
Department of Health Policy and Management
Bloomberg School of Public Health
Johns Hopkins University

Jan Twomey
Program Director, Manufacturing Enterprise Systems
    Program
National Science Foundation

Reha M. Uzsoy
Director, Laboratory for Extended Enterprises at Purdue
Purdue University

Kim J. Vicente
Jerome C. Hunsaker Distinguished Visiting Professor of
    Aerospace Information Engineering
Department of Aeronautics and Astronautics
Massachusetts Institute of Technology

Timothy J. Ward
Principal
Health Services Engineering Inc.

Kensall D. Wise
J. Reid and Polly Anderson Professor of Manufacturing
    Technology
University of Michigan

David D. Woods
Professor in Industrial and Systems Engineering
Institute for Ergonomics
Ohio State University

Yan Xiao
Professor
University of Maryland School of Medicine

Appendix G

Biographical information

Committee Co-chairs

W. DALE COMPTON is the Lillian M. Gilbreth Distinguished Professor of Industrial Engineering Emeritus at Purdue University. His research interests include materials science, automotive engineering, combustion engineering, materials engineering, manufacturing engineering, and management of technology. From 1986 to 1988, as the first National Academy of Engineering (NAE) Senior Fellow, Dr. Compton directed activities related to industrial issues and engineering education. He came to NAE from the Ford Motor Company, where he was vice president of research. Before that, he was professor of physics and director of the Coordinated Sciences Laboratory at the University of Illinois. Dr. Compton has served as a consultant to numerous government and industrial organizations and is a fellow of the American Physical Society, American Association for the Advancement of Science, Society of Automotive Engineers, and Engineering Society of Detroit. He has received the M. Eugene Merchant Manufacturing Medal from ASME and SME, the University of Illinois College of Engineering Alumni Award for Distinguished Service, and the Science Trailblazers Award from the Detroit Science Center and the Michigan Sesquicentennial Commission. Dr. Compton was elected a member of the NAE in 1981 and is currently NAE home secretary.

JEROME H. GROSSMAN, senior fellow and director of the Harvard/Kennedy School Health Care Delivery Project, is working to develop innovations and reforms in the medical care delivery system. Dr. Grossman is Chairman Emeritus of New England Medical Center, where he served as chairman and CEO from 1979 to 1995, where he founded the Health Institute, a research and development organization that works on problems in the health care system. He is also professor of medicine at Tufts University School of Medicine and an Honorary Physician at the Massachusetts General Hospital, where he worked full-time from 1966 to 1979. Dr. Grossman was a member of the founding team of several health care companies, including Meditech, a medical software company, and Tufts Associated Health Plan, Chartwell Home Therapies, and Transition Systems Inc., a medical-care information-management company.

Named to the Institute of Medicine (IOM) of the National Academy of Sciences in 1984, Dr. Grossman has chaired four committees and been a member of the Committee for Quality of Health Care in America. He was also chair of the National Academy of Engineering (NAE) Committee on the Impact of Academic Research on Industrial Performance. In 1999, he was appointed to the National Academies Council on Government-University-Industry Research Roundtable. Dr. Grossman was scholar-in-residence at the IOM in 1996. Dr. Grossman is a director/trustee of a number of organizations, including The Mayo Clinic Foundation, Penn Medicine (University of Pennsylvania Medical School and Health System), Stryker Corporation, Eureka Medical Inc., and Committee for Economic Development.

Committee Members

REBECCA M. BERGMAN, who joined Medtronic 17 years ago, has been a leader in the advancement of biologically oriented sciences. Currently vice president, science and technology, she is responsible for Medtronic's Materials and Biosciences Center, Technical Knowledge Center, innovation programs, and other corporate technology initiatives. Prior to becoming vice president, Becky held scientific and R&D management positions of increasing responsibility in the corporation. She has received several of Medtronic's highest honors, including membership in the Bakken Society, an honorary society for Medtronic's most distinguished scientific and technical contributors, and the Wallin

Leadership Award. In 2000, Becky played a key role in the development of Medtronic's "Vision 2010," a 10-year strategic plan for the corporation.

Mrs. Bergman holds a B.S. degree in chemical engineering from Princeton University and she has completed graduate studies in chemical engineering and materials science at the University of Minnesota, where she has been an adjunct professor and taught courses in biomedical engineering. Becky is a Fellow of the American Institute for Medical and Biological Engineering.

JOHN R. BIRGE is professor of operations management and Neubauer Family Faculty Fellow, Graduate School of Business, University of Chicago. Until June 2004, Dr. Birge was dean of the Robert R. McCormick School of Engineering and Applied Science at Northwestern University. His research is focused on the mathematical modeling of systems with uncertainty, stochastic programming, and large-scale optimization as they apply to power systems, finance, transportation, public policy, and manufacturing. He has taught courses on capital budgeting, financial engineering, and operations research. Dr. Birge is a member of the Institute for Operations Research and the Management Sciences, the Mathematical Programming Society, the Mathematical Association of America, the American Mathematical Society, the Society for Industrial and Applied Mathematics, the Institute of Industrial Engineers, and the Production and Operations Management Society. He has received the Institute of Industrial Engineers Medallion Award, an Office of Naval Research Young Investigator Award, and a National Science Foundation Research Initiation Grant. Dr. Birge was the E. Leonard Arnoff Memorial Lecturer on the Practice of Management Science and Ilyong Ham Distinguished Lecturer at Pennsylvania State University.

DENIS CORTESE is president and chief executive officer of Mayo Clinic and a specialist in pulmonary medicine . Prior to this appointment, he was chair of the Board of Governors at Mayo Clinic in Jacksonville, chair of the Board of Directors at St. Luke's Hospital in Jacksonville, Florida, and medical director of the Mayo Health Plan in Jacksonville. Dr. Cortese is a member of the Mayo Foundation Board of Trustees and a former member of the Mayo Clinic Rochester Board of Governors. Dr. Cortese served as a lieutenant commander in the U.S. Navy Medical Corps. He is well known for his work in the use of photodynamic therapy in lung cancer and is a director and former president of the International Photodynamic Association.

ROBERT S. DITTUS is the Harvie Branscomb Distinguished Professor, Albert and Bernard Werthan Professor of Medicine, Chief of the Division of General Internal Medicine and Public Health, Director of the Center for Health Services Research, Director of the Institute for Community Health, and Director of the Center for Improving Patient

Safety at Vanderbilt University; director of the Geriatric Research, Education and Clinical Center, and director of the Quality Scholars Program at the Veterans Administration Tennessee Valley Healthcare System. His career has focused on methodologies for improving clinical decision making, the use of simulation modeling to improve clinical and operational decision making, and the use of systems engineering and management-science techniques in clinical medicine and public health to improve the quality, safety, and efficiency of health care delivery.

G. SCOTT GAZELLE received his B.A. from Dartmouth College and his M.D. from Case Western Reserve University School of Medicine. After completing a residency in radiology at University Hospitals of Cleveland, where he was also chief resident, he completed a fellowship in abdominal imaging and interventional radiology at the Massachusetts General Hospital (MGH); he subsequently joined the faculty at MGH in the Division of Abdominal Imaging and Interventional Radiology. In 1996, he received an M.P.H. from the Harvard School of Public Health, where he majored in health care management. In 1999, he received a Ph.D. in health policy from Harvard University, where he concentrated in decision science. Currently, associate professor in radiology at Harvard Medical School and associate professor in the Department of Health Policy and Management at the Harvard School of Public Health, Dr. Gazelle is also director of the MGH Institute for Technology Assessment, the Dana-Farber/Harvard Cancer Center Program in Cancer Outcomes Research Training, the Technology Assessment and Outcomes Analysis Program of the Partners HealthCare System Center for Integration of Medicine and Innovative Technology, and the MGH Clinical Research Support Office. In addition, he is also senior scientist at the Partners Institute for Health Policy, and director of clinical research in the Department of Radiology at MGH. He is past president of the Association of University Radiologists, Radiology Research Alliance, and New England Roentgen Ray Society, and is current chair of the American College of Radiology Commission on Research and Technology Assessment and chair of the RSNA Research Development Committee and a member of the Medicare Coverage Advisory Committee. His research is focused on evaluating the benefits, costs, and appropriate uses of new medical technologies. Dr. Gazelle is the author of more than 150 scientific articles and two textbooks. He has also presented numerous papers, lectures, and workshops nationally and internationally.

CAROL HARADEN, vice president at the Institute for Healthcare Improvement (IHI), is a quality of care outcomes researcher, educator, and change leader. At IHI she is responsible for patient safety and idealized design development in medication use, intensive care units, and the flow of patients through the health care system. Dr. Haraden has been a dean in higher education, a clinician, a consultant, and a researcher. Prior to joining IHI, she was vice president for quality services at Fletcher Allen Health Care in Burlington, Vermont, where she was responsible for quality improvement, clinical and operational measurement, service excellence, risk management, safety, and organizational development. Dr. Haraden has written several grants and has served as the measurement consultant for a Robert Woods Johnson grant. Carol is a frequent speaker on program evaluation, measurement, and quality improvement and is the author of a chapter in the American Hospital Association publication, *Work Redesign*. She holds an adjunct appointment at the University of Vermont.

RICHARD MIGLIORI, is chief executive officer of United Resource Networks, a specialized care services company within UnitedHealth Group. United Resource Networks provides specialized solutions for complex medical conditions, such as transplantation, cancer, infertility and congenital heart disease. Their "products" include: quantifying specialized medical expertise, providing clinical consultation, and establishing comprehensive, value-driven contracts to help increase patient survival rates while simultaneously lowering costs for corporate America. Dr. Migliori spearheaded the design, organization, and management of national health care delivery networks and led the development of UnitedHealthcare's Care Coordination Model. Dr. Migliori was previously CEO of HealthSystem Minnesota, one of the largest multispecialty, integrated-care systems in the United States.

WOODROW MYERS is the former executive vice president and chief medical officer of WellPoint, where he managed WellPoint's Health Care Services Division, which includes overseeing medical policy, clinical affairs, and health services operations. He was also responsible for strategic initiatives to enhance the health care experience for WellPoint members and to simplify administration and improve communications with physicians and other health care professionals. Prior to joining WellPoint, Dr. Myers was director of healthcare management at Ford Motor Company. His responsibilities at Ford included addressing quality, cost, and access issues related to health benefits, occupational health, workers compensation, and disability programs. Prior to joining Ford, he was corporate medical director for Anthem Blue Cross Blue Shield, commissioner of health for the state of Indiana, and commissioner of health for New York City. Dr. Myers was an assistant professor of medicine at the University of California San Francisco and a Robert Wood Johnson Foundation Clinical Scholar and a fellow in critical care medicine at the Stanford University Medical Center. Dr. Myers received an M.D. from Harvard Medical School and an M.B.A. from Stanford University Graduate School of Business. He has received numerous medical and community service awards and has published extensively on medical issues important to public health.

WILLIAM P. PIERSKALLA is the former dean and current Distinguished Professor Emeritus of decisions, operations, and technology management at The Anderson Graduate School of Management at the University of California, Los Angeles. His current research interests include the management aspects of health care delivery, operations research, operations management, and global competition. He is a former president of the International Federation of Operational Research Societies, serves on the editorial staffs of five publications, and a recent past vice president for publications for the Institute for Operations Research and Management Sciences. Dr. Pierskalla has been president of the Operations Research Society of America and is a past editor of *Operations Research*. At the University of Pennsylvania, he has also been deputy dean for academic affairs, director of the Huntsman Center for Global Competition and Leadership, chair of the Health Care Systems Department in the Wharton School, and executive director of the Leonard Davis Institute of Health Economics. He has lectured internationally and written more than 50 articles on mathematical programming, transportation, inventory and production control, maintainability, and health care delivery. As a consultant to the American Red Cross, Dr. Pierskalla was involved in analyzing the blood supply management, including delivery, testing, and inventory.

STEPHEN M. SHORTELL is dean of the School of Public Health, Blue Cross of California Distinguished Professor of Health Policy and Management, and professor of organization behavior in the School of Public Health and Haas School of Business of the University of California, Berkeley. From 1982 to 1998, he was professor of sociology and A.C. Buehler Distinguished Professor of Health Services Management and a professor of organization behavior in the J.L. Kellogg Graduate School of Management at Northwestern University. His current research and interests are the strategy, structure, and performance of health care systems; organizational performance; organizational and managerial correlates of continuous quality improvement and health care outcomes; empirical analysis of physician-organizational relationships; and the evaluation of community health demonstration programs. Dr. Shortell is a member of the Institute of Medicine and has received an honorary American Hospital Association Lifetime Member Award, a Gold Medal Award from the American College of Healthcare Executives, a Distinguished Investigator Award from the Association for Health Services Research, the Baxter Health Services Research Prize, and the George R. Terry "Book of the Year" Award from the Academy of Management.

KENSALL D. WISE is the William Gould Dow Distinguished University Professor of Electrical Engineering and Computer Science and professor of biomedical engineering at the University of Michigan. His work has focused primarily on the development of integrated sensors for applications of microelectronics in new areas, including health care and environmental monitoring. He has worked on supporting technologies, such as micromachining, impurity-based etch-stops, wafer bonding, and wafer-level hermetic packaging, as well as on the devices themselves. Dr. Wise has long experience in a number of biomedical devices and has helped pioneer technologies for merging sensing microstructures with integrated circuits. An area of increasing interest in microsystems that combine sensors, microactuators, and signal processing electronics. Dr. Wise is a member of the National Academy of Engineering.

DAVID D. WOODS is professor of industrial and systems engineering at Ohio State University and a pioneer in cognitive systems engineering for human-computer decision making and in resilience engineering for safety management. Dr. Woods is past president and a fellow of the Human Factors and Ergonomic Society and a fellow of the American Psychological Society and the American Psychological Association. He received the Ely Award for best paper in the journal Human Factors (1994) and a Laurels Award from Aviation Week and Space Technology (1995) for research on the human factors of highly automated cockpits. As a board member of the National Patient Safety Foundation (1996-2002) and associate director of the Midwest Center for Inquiry on Patient Safety of the Veterans Health Administration (1999-2003), he has worked extensively on the interaction of engineering and health care. He is coauthor of *Behind Human Error* (1994), *A Tale of Two Stories: Contrasting Views of Patient Safety* (1998), and *Resilience Engineering* (2005). Dr. Woods has also investigated accidents in nuclear power, aviation, space, and anesthesiology and was an advisor to the Columbia Accident Investigation Board.

GEORGE BROWN COLLEGE
CASA LOMA LIBRARY LEARNING COMMONS